A PRACTICAL GUIDE
TO TRANSCRANIAL
MAGNETIC STIMULATION
NEUROPHYSIOLOGY AND
TREATMENT STUDIES

A PRACTICAL GUIDE TO TRANSCRANIAL MAGNETIC STIMULATION NEUROPHYSIOLOGY AND TREATMENT STUDIES

Robert Chen
Professor of Medicine (Neurology)
University of Toronto
Senior Scientist
Krembil Research Institute
University Health Network

Daniel M. Blumberger
Director and Chair
Temerty Centre for Therapeutic Brain Intervention
Centre for Addiction and Mental Health
Professor
Department of Psychiatry
University of Toronto

Paul B. Fitzgerald
Professor of Psychiatry and Director
Epworth Centre for Innovation in Mental Health
Epworth Healthcare and Monash University

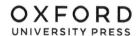

OXFORD
UNIVERSITY PRESS

OXFORD
UNIVERSITY PRESS

Oxford University Press is a department of the University of Oxford. It furthers
the University's objective of excellence in research, scholarship, and education
by publishing worldwide. Oxford is a registered trade mark of Oxford University
Press in the UK and certain other countries.

Published in the United States of America by Oxford University Press
198 Madison Avenue, New York, NY 10016, United States of America.

Library of Congress Cataloging-in-Publication Data
Names: Chen, Robert, 1964- editor. | Blumberger, Daniel M. (Daniel Michael), editor. |
Fitzgerald, Paul B., editor.
Title: A practical guide to Transcranial Magnetic Stimulation neurophysiology and treatment studies /
[edited by] Robert Chen, Daniel M. Blumberger, Paul B. Fitzgerald.
Description: New York, NY : Oxford University Press, [2022] |
Includes bibliographical references and index.
Identifiers: LCCN 2022000687 | ISBN 9780199335848 (paperback) |
ISBN 9780199335862 (epub) | ISBN 9780190495428 (online)
Subjects: MESH: Transcranial Magnetic Stimulation | Central Nervous System—physiology |
Central Nervous System Diseases—therapy |
Mental Disorders—therapy | Neuroimaging
Classification: LCC QP360 | NLM WL 141.5.T7 | DDC 612.8—dc23/eng/20220210
LC record available at https://lccn.loc.gov/2022000687

DOI: 10.1093/med/9780199335848.001.0001

1 3 5 7 9 8 6 4 2
Printed by Marquis, Canada

Contents

SECTION II RTMS AS TREATMENT OF NEUROLOGICAL AND PSYCHIATRIC DISORDERS

Preface

Transcranial magnetic stimulation (TMS) is a widely used noninvasive brain stimulation technique in basic and clinical neuroscience. Following the original description of TMS by Barker and colleagues in 1985, early TMS studies mostly involved the motor system, and TMS has become a valuable method to provide unique insights into motor physiology and pathophysiology. Subsequent studies have expanded the use of TMS to probe cognitive and sensory functions of the human brain, and further important insights were provided by combining TMS with other methods, including neuroimaging and electroencephalography. The development of TMS paradigms to induce brain plasticity paved the way for its use as a treatment for neurological and psychiatric disorders. Repetitive TMS (rTMS) is now an evidenced-based treatment for a number of neuropsychiatric disorders.

The authors of this text, a neurologist and two psychiatrists, are experienced in using TMS for both neurophysiological investigations and as treatment. While there are excellent review articles and textbooks on TMS, we aimed to fill a gap by providing a comprehensive practical guide that covers using TMS for investigations of normal neurophysiological processes as well as TMS to examine the pathophysiology of brain disorders and the use of rTMS as a treatment. Although the emphasis is on providing practical information, theoretical aspects are also covered to provide background information. Since TMS has been tested as a treatment in many neurological and psychiatric disorders, we selected disorders that are more commonly treated using rTMS and that reflect our interest and expertise. While we expect that the book will be useful to investigators new to the field of TMS, experienced users will also find useful practical information for both clinical and research settings.

Acknowledgments

The authors thank Mr. Craig Panner of Oxford University Press for his encouragement throughout the period of writing of this book, Dr. Christoph Zrenner, Dr. Jean-Philippe Miron and Dr. Sanjeev Kumar for their valuable comments and feedback. We are particularly grateful to Professor John Rothwell for his helpful review of a draft version this book.

SECTION

I

TMS NEUROPHYSIOLOGY

The History of TMS and Basic Principles of TMS and rTMS

1.1 INTRODUCTION

Transcranial magnetic stimulation (TMS) involves the use of a magnetic field to induce an electrical current in the brain to try to stimulate the brain or modify brain activity. The concept of using a magnetic field or some type of externally applied electricity to influence the brain or body is one which has a relatively long history, although most historical forms of magnetic and electrical stimulation do not closely resemble modern forms of brain stimulation. One of the first descriptions of the use of electrical stimulation in medicine dates from 46 AD, when Scribonius Largus, physician of the Roman emperor Tiberius, discussed the use of an aquatic animal like an electrical eel for medical applications. During and following the Renaissance, there was a substantial escalation in interest in the use of electricity for medical purposes. In the 1600s, the English physician William Gilbert described medical uses of "electricity," a term that he first used as an abstraction from the Greek word "electron," describing amber. A professor of medicine in Germany, Johann Gottlob Krüger, described the potential use of electricity for the treatment of paralysis in the 1743 and subsequently Christian Gottlieb Kratzenstein conducted experiments on electrification of the human body.

In the later part of the 1700s, Luigi Galvani at the University of Bologna in Italy described the capacity of electrical stimulation to produce twitching of muscles from the leg of a frog. Alessandro Volta went on to demonstrate that this effect, which was described as "galvanic," did not require contact with the animal (and also contributed to the development of the battery).[1] As these medical and scientific applications of electricity were being explored, the concepts of magnetism were progressively being developed, initially by Paracelsus in the 1500s and then by Anton Mesmer in the seventeenth century. Mesmer's concepts and his clinical approach were eventually discredited and contributed to the development of hypnosis more than to the physical sciences associated with magnetic stimulation. From the 1800s through to the early part of the twentieth century, therapeutic approaches using magnets and electrical therapies were popular, often justified in the belief that magnetic stimulation could provide some form of nutrient to the body.

1.2 THE DEVELOPMENT OF THE SCIENCES UNDERPINNING TMS

In the 1800s, Michael Faraday first described the basic principles of the relationship between magnetic fields and electricity that underpin modern TMS (e.g., as later described in his Lectures on the Forces of Matter, given at The Royal Institution of Great Britain, in December 1859).[2] This principle, as he described it, states that a current can be induced in a secondary circuit when its relationship to a primary circuit is altered in several specific ways, including that the primary current is turned on or off or the primary current is moved relative to the secondary current. Faraday described that this effect was mediated through the magnetic flux created by the changing circuit and that alterations in the magnetic flux would induce an electrical field.[2] The line integral of this electric field is referred to as the *electromotive force*, and this force is responsible for the induced current flow. The magnitude of this effect can be quantified and mathematically described. Importantly, the magnitude of the force is proportional to the rate of change in the magnetic flux.

Later that century, Nikola Tesla in the United States conducted a series of experiments investigating the physiological effects of high-frequency currents.[2] He used a number of flat, cone-, and helix-shaped coils that were to produce physiological effects. These *Tesla coils*, or *Oudin resonators*, consisted of primary and secondary large coils used to produce an ionization of the air between the coils. A patient would sit between the coils and experience a sensation described by Tesla as akin to the "bombardment of miniature hail stones."

Building on these developments, the Frenchman D'Arsonval was the first person to develop ideas that could be considered somewhat equivalent to modern TMS technology. He developed a large magnetic coil producing a 110-volt current at 42 Hz and applied this to human subjects. This produced a variety of sensations and physiological responses including dilation of blood vessels, vertigo, syncope, and phosphenes. *Phosphenes*, or visual flashes of light, are produced with modern TMS stimulation of the occipital visual cortex, and it is possible that this was the source of the experiences produced in D'Arsonval's experiments, although from knowledge of the capacity of technology of the day it seems more likely that they were the result of direct retinal stimulation.

Several years later (1902), a separate series of studies by Beer with similar results were reported in English,[3] and a device designed for use in the treatment of depression and other neuroses was actually patented by Pollacsek and Beer in Vienna. Follow-on experiments were reported by Thompson, who produced a large 32-turn coil in which a subject's head was placed and which produced some sight and taste sensations. Magnusson and Stevens produced two elliptical coils that were used to produce visual sensations including flickering and a luminous horizontal bar.[4] However, interest in this area seemed to die off in the first half of the twentieth century, particularly as a variety of other tools become available to study the central nervous system and to be used in the potential treatment of psychiatric disorders. A variety of electrical therapies were used in different parts of the world but with little persistent systematic investigation.

The next attempt to directly stimulate brain activity came about using direct electrical stimulation through the scalp in awake human subjects. This was attempted in the 1950s, but was only used to a limited degree due to the discomfort associated with this procedure. Low-intensity forms of electrical stimulation were used throughout the 1950s and 1960s, including in a variety of proposed therapeutic applications, but there was little theoretical understanding about the effects of these forms of stimulation on brain tissue. In 1980, it was found that a brief, high-voltage electrical pulse applied to the scalp was able to noninvasively stimulate the motor cortex reliably in normal human subjects.[5] However, the procedure was painful and was not widely used.

1.3 MODERN TMS

The modern field of TMS really began in Sheffield, England, in 1985. In the 1970s, Anthony Barker investigated the use of short, pulsed magnetic fields in the stimulation of peripheral nerves. In the 1980s, with colleagues, he developed a device capable of generating a sufficiently powerful magnetic field to stimulate cortical activity through the human scalp.[6] This device could produce single TMS pulses capable of inducing depolarization of cortical neurons. This type of stimulator was initially attractive to neurophysiologists and neurologists who were now able to study nerve conduction from the pyramidal neurons in the cortex all the way to the periphery. Over the course of 10 years, a variety of innovative protocols were developed to utilize TMS pulses in the investigation of cortical neurophysiology: many of these are still used today and will be described in subsequent chapters in this book. A substantive breakthrough in the use of TMS was the development of stimulators capable of providing repetitive pulses at frequencies of 1 Hz and greater. Studies soon demonstrated that repetitive stimulation could potentially modulate the excitability of the cortex, with the possibility of both increasing and decreasing cortical activity. This soon led to interest in the potential therapeutic use of these devices.

The first therapeutic applications tested with TMS stimulators were for the modulation of mood in depressive disorders. Studies in healthy control subjects suggested that mood could be altered in a positive direction, and initial clinical trials in depressed subjects provided promising results in the mid-1990s.[7] Over the past 30 years, an extensive series of clinical trials has explored the therapeutic use of TMS in a variety of disorders while the science underpinning its use in the protocols for its investigative use are progressively expanded.

1.4 BASIC PRINCIPLES

The use of TMS is fundamentally dependent on the basic law of magnetic induction as described earlier and first outlined by Michael Faraday. Faraday demonstrated that a current was induced in a secondary circuit when it was brought in close proximity to a primary circuit in which a time-varying current was flowing. The change in the initial electrical current produces a changing magnetic field inducing a secondary current in a nearby conducting material.

During TMS, a considerable electrical charge is stored in capacitors in the TMS device. This current is discharged rapidly so that the current passing through the TMS coil is switched on rapidly. The process of charge and discharge of the capacitors is regulated by a thyristor switch. The rapidly time-variable electrical field produces a substantial magnetic field capable of inducing an electrical field in the superficial layers of the cortex. If the induced electrical field is of sufficient strength, depolarization of pyramidal neurones can occur, either directly or indirectly through activation of connecting dendrites and interneurons.

It is notable that this process occurs efficiently because there is no effective resistance to the passage of the magnetic field across the scalp and skull. Therefore TMS acts as a way of inducing an electrical current in the brain, but without requiring direct electrical stimulation to the scalp. However, the distance between the stimulating coil and the brain tissue is not insignificant, and there is a rapid decrease in the strength of the magnetic field with distance.

There are two commonly utilized types of TMS pulses which are determined by the stimulator circuitry. A *biphasic pulse* is sinusoidal and is generally of shorter duration than a *monophasic pulse*, which involves a rapid rise from zero followed by a slow decay back to baseline. Typically, monophasic pulses have been most commonly used in investigational studies and biphasic pulses in stimulators capable of providing TMS at high frequencies, usually in therapeutic protocols. Monophasic and biphasic pulses may have different effects on neuronal activity and cannot be automatically used interchangeably. Newer stimulators with variable pulse configurations have recently been developed, although the optimal application of these is not yet clear.[8]

There are a range of coils typically used for TMS.[9] TMS experiments were initially done with circular coils, where the windings of the coil are concentrated in a band on the outside of a circle, often between 7 and 10 cm in diameter. This coil type cannot be focused accurately as the peak area of stimulation is under the rim of the outside of the coil.[10] The coil type most commonly used in both investigational and therapeutic circumstances is described as a *figure-of-eight–shaped coil* (Figure 1.1). This type of coil has two round coils placed side by side. This produces a more strongly focused field, and the central point of stimulation sits under the join between the two circular coils. Figure-of-eight coils in which the diameter of each round coil is around 7 cm are the most commonly utilized. These produce an area of cortical activation of approximately 2–3 cm^2 and to a depth of approximately 2 cm. In most studies, figure-of-eight coils are held over the cortex flat and at about 45 degrees from the midline position, perpendicular to the central sulcus. This induces a current moving from the posterior to anterior direction, perpendicular to descending pyramidal neurons and parallel to interneurons, which modulate pyramidal cell firing.[11] Figure-of-eight coils may be produced with an air core (i.e., space between the windings of the coil) or with an iron core. Iron-core coils are advantageous in that they tend to require less power to produce strong magnetic fields and they generate less heat.[12]

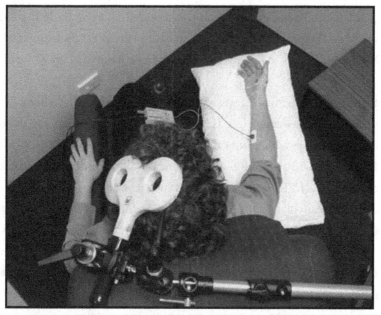

FIGURE 1.1 *A figure-of-8 Magstim coil held over the head in a custom-built stand. Electromyography (EMG) electrodes are placed to record muscle activity induced by stimulation of the motor cortex.*

By contrast, more traditional circular or figure-of-eight copper coils generate significant heat that increases as more pulses are delivered.[13] This heat generation can be managed by the use of an active cooling system, using air or a fluid to dissipate the heat generated.

There are also an increasing number of novel coil configurations. The wings of a figure-of-eight coil can be angulated in a manner that produces a deeper region of field penetration (e.g., double-cone coils). A more radical development is the family of *H coils*, which entail multiple coil windings developed to generate a greater depth of penetration, with stimulation of areas possible up to 6 cm below the cortical surface.[14] Another system has been described where multiple coils are used to generate stimulation of deeper brain regions. It is likely that the range of stimulation equipment available will continue to grow over the coming years.

1.5 REPETITIVE TMS

Initially TMS machines were developed that were able to produce a single pulse to evoke transient cortical activity. Within a relatively short period of time, however, technical developments occurred that allowed the repetitive application of TMS pulses, usually at frequencies somewhere between 1 and 20 Hz (Figure 1.2). The repetitive application of TMS (repetitive TMS; rTMS) opened the possibility of using external brain stimulation to modulate the activity of the brain. Most rTMS devices, especially initially, were able to achieve higher frequencies of stimulation by utilizing a bipolar stimulus pulse, as opposed to a unipolar stimulus, which is shorter and requires less energy to produce neuronal excitability. Thus, capacitors can charge and discharge rapidly, thereby achieving high stimulation rates. It is this ability to achieve such high stimulation rates that has made rTMS a valuable tool in the investigation and treatment of many neuropsychiatric disorders.

Repetitive TMS can either activate or inhibit cortical activity depending on stimulation frequency.[15] Low-frequency (~1 Hz) stimulation for a period of approximately 15 minutes or more induces a transient inhibition, or a decrease in activity, of the cortex.[16] The mechanisms behind such inhibition are unclear although there are similarities to long-term depression (LTD), a phenomena in which repeated low-frequency stimulation reduces activity in individual synapses in cellular experiments.[17] In contrast, stimulation at frequencies above 1 Hz has been shown to induce increased cortical activation,[18] analogous to the process of long-term potentiation (LTP).[17] This may be due to a transient increase in the efficacy of excitatory synapses. Potentiation of plasticity may also represent a mechanism through which rTMS produces brain changes. Plasticity in the cortex involves an adaptive rewiring of neurons in response to environmental change. Synaptic plasticity has long been conceptualized as a cellular substrate of learning and memory. As

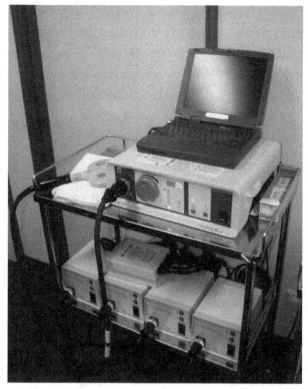

FIGURE 1.2 *Magstim SuperRapid with four separate capacitors ("booster modules" from 2002).*

theorized by Hebb, synaptic plasticity is represented by changes in synaptic strength in response to coincident activation of coactive cells, which manifests as LTP or LTD.[19] LTP depends, in part, on activation of a double-gated N-methyl-D-aspartic acid (NMDA) receptor that serves as a "molecular" coincidence detector. These calcium-permeable glutamatergic receptors are able to provide a long-term augmentation of postsynaptic signal once activated by an input sufficient to depolarize postsynaptic membrane and relieve tonic magnesium (Mg^{2+}) inhibition.[20] rTMS can cause neurons in the cortex to generate repeated and consistent firing of coactive cells, thereby producing plasticity in the cortex.

Although these are interesting ideas, unfortunately we still lack an understanding of whether they fundamentally underpin the effects of TMS when applied to cortical circuits, especially when this is done in the treatment of an illness such as depression. Therapeutic effects of rTMS could theoretically be related to local changes in cortical excitability, changes in the capacity of the target brain site (e.g., the dorsolateral prefrontal cortex) to regulate other disease-specific brain regions, changes in the strength of connections between relevant brain regions driven by repeated stimulation, or changes in the activity of distal brain regions altered through trans-synaptic activation. In fact, how these mechanisms play a role may be disease- and stimulation-specific: as such the mechanism of rTMS effects may well not be the same across different conditions.

Regardless of these unanswered questions, rTMS has definitively been established as a valuable tool for investigating the role of cortical areas in brain function as well as a safe, clinically effective, and useful therapeutic tool. Its use is only likely to continue to expand as therapeutic applications of rTMS progress and novel experimental methods, particular combining TMS with methods to assess brain activity, continue to be developed and applied.

REFERENCES

1. Becker RO, Marino AA. *The Origins of Electrobiology*. In Becker RO, Marino AA, eds. *Electromagnetism & Life*. Albany, NY: State University of New York Press; 1982:7–12.
2. Cheney M. *Tesla: Man Out of Time*. Breckenridge, CO: Twenty-First Century Books; 1983.
3. Beer B. Ueber das Auftraten einer objective Lichtempfindung in magnetischen Felde. *Klin Wochenschr*. 1902;15:108–109.
4. Thompson SP. A physiological effect of an alternating magnetic field. *Proc R Soc London Series B- Containing Papers of a Biological Character*. 1910;82:396–398.
5. Merton PA, Morton HB. Stimulation of the cerebral cortex in the intact human subject. *Nature*. 1980;285:227.
6. Barker AT, Jalinous R, Freeston IL. Non-invasive magnetic stimulation of human motor cortex. *Lancet*. 1985;1:1106–1107.
7. George MS, Wassermann EM, Post RM. Transcranial magnetic stimulation: A neuropsychiatric tool for the 21st century. *J Neuropsychiatry Clin Neurosci*. 1996;8:373–382.
8. Goetz SM, Luber B, Lisanby SH, Murphy DL, Kozyrkov IC, Grill WM, et al. Enhancement of neuromodulation with novel pulse shapes generated by controllable pulse parameter transcranial magnetic stimulation. *Brain Stimul*. 2016;9:39–47.
9. Barker AT. An introduction to the basic principles of magnetic nerve stimulation. *J Clin Neurophysiol*. 1991;8:26–37.
10. Jalinous R. Technical and practical aspects of magnetic nerve stimulation. *J Clin Neurophysiol*. 1991;8:10–25.
11. Amassian VE, Deletis V. Relationships between animal and human corticospinal responses. *Electroencephalogr Clin Neurophysiol Suppl*. 1999;51:79–92.
12. Epstein CM, Davey KR. Iron-core coils for transcranial magnetic stimulation. *J Clin Neurophysiol*. 2002;19:376–381.
13. Weyh T, Wendicke K, Mentschel C, Zantow H, Siebner HR. Marked differences in the thermal characteristics of figure-of-eight shaped coils used for repetitive transcranial magnetic stimulation. *Clin Neurophysiol*. 2005;116:1477–1486.
14. Deng ZD, Peterchev AV, Lisanby SH. Coil design considerations for deep-brain transcranial magnetic stimulation (dTMS). *Conf Proc IEEE Eng Med Biol Soc*. 2008;2008:5675–5679.
15. Fitzgerald PB, Fountain S, Daskalakis ZJ. A comprehensive review of the effects of rTMS on motor cortical excitability and inhibition. *Clin Neurophysiol*. 2006;117:2584–2596.
16. Chen R, Classen J, Gerloff C, Celnik P, Wassermann EM, Hallett M, et al. Depression of motor cortex excitability by low-frequency transcranial magnetic stimulation. *Neurology*. 1997;48:1398–1403.
17. Bear MF, Malenka RC. Synaptic plasticity: LTP and LTD. *Curr Opin Neurobiol*. 1994;4:389–399.
18. Siebner HR, Peller M, Willoch F, Minoshima S, Boecker H, Auer C, et al. Lasting cortical activation after repetitive TMS of the motor cortex: a glucose metabolic study. *Neurology*. 2000; 54: 956–963.
19. Hebb DO. *The Organization of Behavior: A Neuropsychological Theory*. New York: Wiley; 1949.
20. Rison RA, Stanton PK. Long-term potentiation and N-methyl-D-aspartate receptors: Foundations of memory and neurologic disease? *Neurosci Biobehav Rev*. 1995;19:533–552.

TMS and Neuronavigation Equipment

2.1 BASIC COMPONENTS OF TMS

2.1.1 TMS Equipment

Numerous commercially available transcranial magnetic stimulation (TMS) devices currently exist, all derived from the basic design first reported by Barker et al. in 1985.[1] In general, TMS circuits are comprised of a high-voltage power source that charges the capacitor. The capacitor then quickly discharges through an electronic switch, into the coil, to ultimately generate a briefly time-varying magnetic field pulse. Specifically, TMS devices are constructed of several components that form an oscillator (or RLC circuit): the internal resistors (R), present in the components and cables; the coil inductor (L); and the energy storage capacitor (C), which generates pulses. In addition to the resistor, coil, and capacitor, the main stimulator unit includes a voltage source, which produces the magnetic field, and a solid state switch, which is able to navigate large currents over very short periods of time. The return path for the energy within the coil flows through the diode and resistor, returning some energy to the capacitor while the rest dissipates, generating heat. The resonant frequency of the RLC circuit and ultimately the pulse shape is controlled by pulse-shaping circuitry within the main stimulator unit. Monophasic and biphasic pulse shapes are most commonly used (reviewed in Chapter 1).

The type of coil selected determines the depth, focality, and pattern of the induced electrical field as well as the targeted brain region or circuit. Coils are composed of windings of conductive wire filled with either a ferromagnetic material, or they are left empty and are surrounded by an insulator.[2,3] Important physical characteristics of the coil include its size and shape (i.e., circular, figure-of-eight, double cone, H-coils, etc.), the core material, the dimensions of the core and loops within the coil, and the number of winding turns.[4] In general, circular coils are less focal than figure-of-eight coils, and larger coils are associated with a slower decay with depth.[5] A brief review of the different types of available coils can be found in Chapter 1.

2.1.2 TMS-EMG and TMS-EEG Equipment

2.1.2.1 TMS-EMG

When a sufficiently strong TMS pulse is delivered over the motor cortex, this results in a muscle twitch in those muscle groups controlled by the stimulated area of cortex. This muscle response can be recorded from the target region in the form of motor evoked potentials (MEPs) using surface electrodes. While there are several configurations for electrode placement, one of the most common is the bipolar belly-tendon arrangement. Furthermore, a ground electrode is placed over an electrically inactive area, between the coil and recording electrodes (e.g., on the forearm) in order to reduce signal noise. The electromyography (EMG) signal is amplified so that it can be displayed on the computer screen for the identification of the motor "hot spot" and measurement of the motor threshold. The EMG signal is then filtered and digitized using an analog-to-digital converter, which converts the signals into the digital domain necessary for input into a computer.[6] Investigators may also wish to include auditory equipment as a measure of acoustic feedback to ensure muscle relaxation (Figure 2.1).

2.1.2.2 TMS-EEG

Current electroencephalogram (EEG) systems are constructed of several components including (1) electrodes, ranging from 8 to more than 250; (2) an amplifier that is responsible for converting, electronically stabilizing, and amplifying weak neuronal signals; and (3) an analog-to-digital converter. Because the TMS pulse causes high-amplitude transient electric artifacts, EEG systems must be specially designed to avoid amplifier saturation. Nevertheless, monitoring EEG responses closely following the TMS pulse poses several challenges, especially in the case of online analysis and visualization. Therefore, TMS-compatible EEG equipment including electrodes and amplifiers is a crucial component of combined TMS and EEG.

Electrodes. There are a number of requirements necessary specific to EEG electrodes to ensure accurate and safe data acquisition during stimulation. As discussed in Chapter 7 on combined TMS-EEG, eddy currents generated by the TMS time-varying magnetic field in conductive material can lead to artifacts associated with movement and heating of the electrodes.[7] As such, TMS-compatible electrodes should have a small diameter

(A)

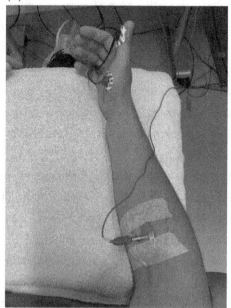

(B)

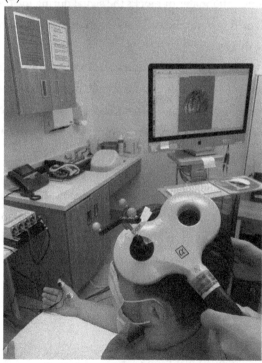

FIGURE 2.1 *Transcranial magnetic stimulation (TMS)-electromyogram (EMG) setup. (A) A common configuration for EMG electrode placement, known as the bipolar belly-tendon arrangement, in which the active electrode is attached to the skin overlying the belly of the target muscle (in this case, the abductor pollicis brevis) and the reference electrode is attached to the skin overlying the muscle tendon. A ground electrode is placed over an electrically inactive area, between the coil and recording electrodes (e.g., on the forearm). (B) The TMS-EMG setup including the electrodes over the hand muscle to capture motor evoked potentials (MEPs), the TMS coil placed over the primary motor cortex (M1) region, and the neuronavigation computer screen (reviewed in Section 2.2.2).*

to minimize the potential of overheating or movement and must be coated with a material that is most suitable for interactions with the skin.[8] For example, most commercially available electrodes are made of a plastic pellet electrode coated in silver epoxy (silver–silver chloride, Ag/AgCl electrodes), a minimally conductive material.[9,10] Cutting a slit out of ring electrodes has also been shown to be effective in reducing heating and conductivity.[11] Despite advances in electrodes design, numerous additional online and offline steps still need to be taken to ensure a low level of electrode impedance and high quality of data acquisition (reviewed in Chapter 7).

Amplifiers. One of the most significant early challenges in combing TMS and EEG was associated with the saturation of EEG amplifiers due to the large TMS-induced voltages. While the TMS pulse is brief, it could take the amplifiers hundreds of milliseconds to recover; thus key early neuronal responses were impacted. In response to this methodological limitation, several novel solutions were developed. In 1997, Ilmoniemi et al. decoupled the electrodes and amplifier during the TMS pulse (−50 μs to 2.5 ms post TMS) to avoid saturation.[12] This method was modified into what is known as a *sample-and-hold approach*, which attenuates or blocks the signal during the duration of the pulse. This can be accomplished in a number of ways including simply switching the amplifier off during TMS pulse delivery.[11,13]

An alternative approach to amplifier saturation that does not require decoupling of electrodes and amplifiers uses amplifiers with a wide operational range (e.g., >100 mV) to capture the entirety of the TMS pulse. In addition to this, an increased sampling rate (e.g., >5 kHz) and enhanced sensitivity of analog-to-digital conversion (e.g., <0.05μV/bit) allows for the recording of signals directly following the TMS pulse.[14] Another solution utilizes a preamplifier with a limited slew rate or rate of voltage change.[9,15] While it does not eliminate the presence of the TMS artifact from the ongoing signal, the continuous recording allows for the artifact to be removed via subtraction from a control or baseline signal.[10,15] Of course, each of these approaches is associated with different limitations and should be selected by investigators based on the study design and research question of interest.

2.1.3 How Similar Are TMS Devices?

The number of commercially available TMS devices has grown since the initial approval by the US Food and Drug Administration (FDA) of the NeuroStar rTMS device from Neuronetics. With this comes important questions regarding the clinical efficacy and overall similarity among these devices. Several additional rTMS devices have received FDA approval in recent years, given their substantial equivalency to the NeuroStar system. These devices are not, however, identical, with slight differences both in physical characteristics and stimulation parameters. In addition, the devices and coils have different capacities to sustain the magnetic field at higher intensities, in particular when using patterned forms of stimulation such as theta burst stimulation. It is worth consulting device manufacturers concerning the capabilities and intensities where roll-off occurs when choosing a device for an intended clinical or research purpose.

Few studies have investigated the comparative efficacy of available TMS devices. In an open-label retrospective study, Oliveira-Maia et al. found no difference in clinical responses among the 113 patients who received treatment with the Magstim device compared to 41 patients who received treatment with NeuroStar.[16] However, in a more recent open-label study in 247 patients, greater remission rates were observed in those treated using the MagVenture device compared to the NeuroStar device. Importantly, this finding remained significant after controlling for potential confounding variables including age, sex, severity, and comorbidity.[17] While compelling, this limited research does not provide definitive support for the superiority of one device over another; rather, it suggests that more research on this topic is needed.[18] In recent years a newer device called *controlled TMS* has come on the market, though it is not yet approved by the FDA. This device allows one to control the pulse width and directionality for more refined experiments.[19]

2.2 NEURONAVIGATION

2.2.1 Non-Navigation Methods

2.2.1.1 *The 5 cm Method*
The dorsolateral prefrontal cortex (DLPFC) represents an important site of stimulation for the treatment of depression and other psychiatric disorders. Given that the DLPFC is a cortical area that is functionally identified rather than a distinct anatomic region with an easily quantifiable stimulation response, accurately targeting of nonmotor regions is challenging. Initial rTMS studies for the treatment of depression targeted the DLPFC using the "5 cm anterior rule." This method involves measuring 5 cm anteriorly along the cortical surface from the motor "hot spot." The success of the 5 cm method in targeting the DLPFC has only been evaluated in one published study. In this study, Herwig et al. found that, using the 5 cm method, in only 7 of 22 study participants was the DLPFC (defined as Brodmann area 9) accurately located, compared to the neuronavigated and structural magnetic resonance imaging (MRI) location of the DLPFC. In the remaining 15 participants, the coil positioning was located over more posterior regions, mostly the premotor cortex.[20] In fact, it has been suggested that this study may have overestimated the success of the 5 cm method in localizing DLPFC. While this method is a relatively simple and fast estimation of the DLPFC, it does not account for individual neuroanatomy. Therefore,

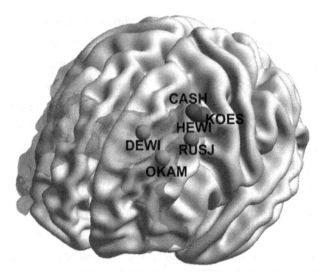

FIGURE 2.2 *An illustration of the variability across studies in the localization of the F3 site. Each point represents a study that aimed to identify the cortical site corresponding to the F3 electroencephalogram (EEG) electrode position. This image highlights the variability in identifying the cortical location for stimulation and overall limitation with this approach. The green region depicts Brodmann area 9 and the purple region depicts area 46.*
FROM FITZGERALD, *BRAIN STIMUL.* 2021;14(3):730–736.

the 5 cm method may be a suboptimal approach to targeting the DLPFC and may account for the modest therapeutic effects published in early rTMS treatment studies. More recently experts have advocated for more anterior and lateral approaches if this method of approximation is employed.

2.2.1.2 The 10-20 System and Beam F3

Perhaps the simplest and least expensive advance in coil targeting, particularly for the treatment of depression, has been the use of the F3 electrode as a target region for the DLPFC (Figure 2.3). This approach is based on the International 10-20 coordinate system, which uses four anatomical landmarks (i.e., nasion, inion, left and right preauricular point) as a standardized method for EEG electrode placement. Unlike the 5 cm method, this method takes into consideration individual variability in head size. Previous studies have demonstrated that the F3 electrode closely approximates the area represented by the Talairach coordinates that most closely approximate the hypofrontal activation of the DLPFC in depression.[22]

Conventional methods for properly identifying F3 involve using an electrode cap for placement. However, this process is subject to potential error based on the numerous measurements involved in proper cap placement and F3 location marking.[21] The "beam F3" method[23] represents an efficient, easy to use alternative approach for identifying the

(A)   (B)   (C)

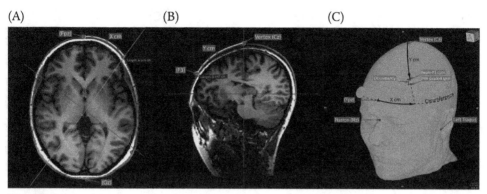

FIGURE 2.3 *Comparison of scalp sites for Beam F3 versus magnetic resonance imaging (MRI)-guided methods. Using the cardinal scalp measurements, the Beam F3 algorithm returned values for circumferential arc X and radial arc Y, thereby indicating a scalp location for F3 to be used in stimulating left dorsolateral prefrontal cortex (DLPFC) (A) and the image volume then resliced through the vertical plane from the vertex through point X. The Beam F3-generated measurement for arc Y was then traced along the scalp in this plane (B) to locate the Beam F3 point. The distance between the Beam F3 scalp site and the scalp site at minimum distance from the MRI-guided coordinate was then measured (C) to quantify the discrepancy. Finally, the image volume was again resliced in the vertical plane from the vertex through the MRI-guided scalp site rather than the Beam F3 site in order to measure empirical MRI-guided values for parameters X and Y for comparison to the Beam F3-generated values.*

FROM MIR-MOGHTADAEI ET AL., *BRAIN STIMUL.* 2015;8(5):965–973.

F3 electrode, one that does not require the use of an EEG cap. The beam F3 method uses stand-alone computer software/website (http://www.clinicalresearcher.org/software.htm), along with three measurements calculated by the administrator, to localize F3. In brief, the administrator inputs the distance from the nasion to the inion, followed by the left to right preauricular distance; the vertex is marked as the halfway point between these two measurements. Finally, the head circumference, measured at the eyebrow level and over the inion is entered into the computer. The program then generates two values, one representing a measurement from the midline along the circumference (i.e., X) and the second measurement from the vertex through point-X (i.e., Y); this point is the estimated location of F3 (Figures 2.3 and 2.4).

The distinct advantage of beam F3 over conventional 10-20 system measurement is that it simplifies the process with fewer measurements and, as a corollary, reduced potential for human error. In a small sample, a recent study found that the beam F3 and EEG cap methods resulted in a similar localization of the DLPFC; however, beam F3 was associated with a slightly more anterior placement, especially among those with smaller head sizes (Figure 2.5).[25] Compared to a more advanced fMRI-guided neuronavigational method, the beam F3 method has been shown to provide a fairly comparable approximation of the DLPFC when using a correction factor that is now built into the online software.[24]

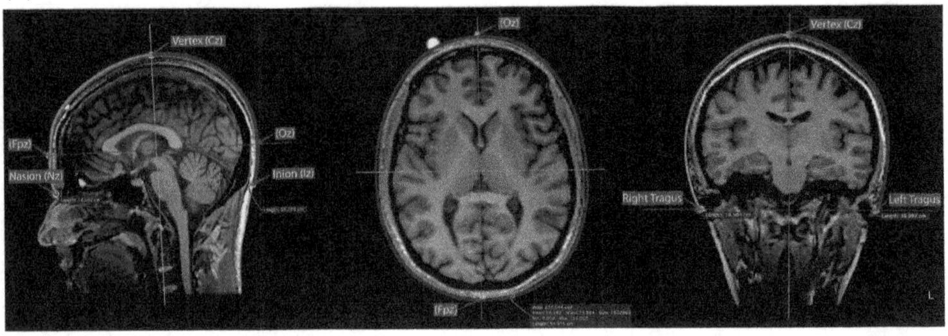

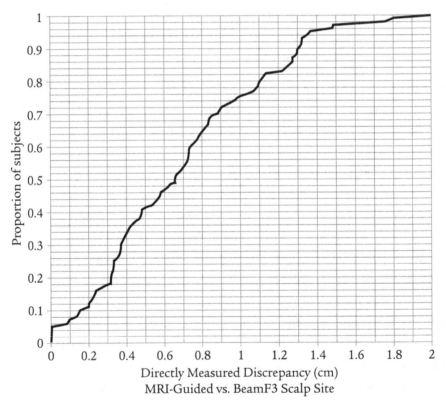

FIGURE 2.4 *Scalp measurements for Beam F3 localization of the left dorsolateral prefrontal cortex (DLPFC). (A) The length of the nasion to inion along the midline of the scalp surface, the position of the vertex (Cz) and FPz and Oz electrode locations. (B) The head circumference in the horizontal plane passing through FPz and Oz (i.e., 10% of the nasion-inion distance from each end). (C) The length of the left-to-right tragus along the scalp through the vertex.*

FROM MIR-MOGHTADAEI ET AL., *BRAIN STIMUL.* 2015;8(5):965–973.

FIGURE 2.5 *Cumulative distribution for the distance between Beam F3 and magnetic resonance imaging (MRI)-guided scalp sites. This graph displays the absolute values for the distance between the scalp location determined using Beam F3 versus the scalp location determined using the MRI-guided approach for left dorsolateral prefrontal cortex (DLPFC) stimulation.*

FROM MIR-MOGHTADAEI ET AL., *BRAIN STIMUL.* 2015;8(5):965–973.

2.2.2 Basic Approaches to Neuronavigation

Stereoscopic 3D-positioning system-guided neuronavigation introduces a number of advantages compared to traditional coil positioning approaches (Figure 2.6). In addition to improving the accuracy of locating nonmotor regions, neuronavigation improves reliability and reproducibility across testing sessions and TMS investigators.[26] Neuronavigation works by precisely monitoring the position and orientation of different "trackers" consisting of a reflective spheres arranged in a unique geometry. One tracker is affixed to the head and one to the coil so that the relative positioning of the trackers is precisely known. By extension, after calibration, each tracker, the relative position of the head, and the coil can be inferred: the coil tracker is registered to a 3D model of the coil based on the known coil geometry. Similarly, the head tracker is registered to a 3D model of the head. To guide the positioning of the coil, this 3D model is generated from individual structural MRI data by extracting the scalp surface and the cortex. It is also possible to co-register and overlay other imaging data such as fMRI, tractography, or

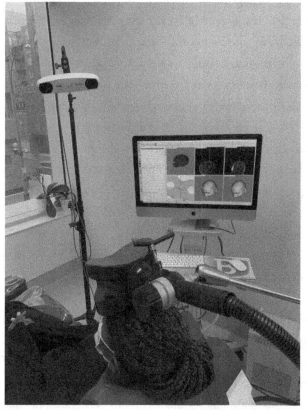

FIGURE 2.6 *Neuronavigational setup for repetitive transcranial magnetic stimulation (rTMS) treatment over the dorsomedial prefrontal cortex. The neuronavigation camera monitors the position and orientation of the coils through the use of trackers on the patient's head (obscured in this photo: refer to Chapter 7 for depiction) and coil. The coil tracker is registered to a 3D model of the coil based on the known coil geometry, while the head tracker is registered to a 3D model of the head.*

positron emission tomography (PET). If individual imaging data are not available, a 3D model based on a template brain can be resized to fit the individual head, thus enabling anatomical targeting using what is known as the "probabilistic approach."[26] In general, the 3D model of the head and the head tracker are linked or co-registered using the individual's cranial landmarks. This approach provides the operator with real-time feedback on coil positioning and orientation relative to the participant's neuroanatomy and head motion. In addition, the exact location of stimulation within the cortex can be recorded at each session along with coil orientation. A recent advanced method has been developed to be able to rapidly calculate the optimal coil orientation that maximizes the e-field for a given target region.[27] This approach will allow for the investigation of personalized e-field delivery in future treatment and neurophysiology studies.

2.2.3 Targeting Specific Cortical Regions

Various methods for targeting a specific stimulation site are possible. One method involves the reverse co-registration from a stereotaxic coordinate on the standard Montreal Neurological Institute (MNI-152) template brain on to each individual's anatomical MRI. The MNI coordinates for the left DLPFC (e.g., [x-38 y + 44 z + 26]) in treating depression were drawn from a recent study identifying this site as an optimal target based on clinical outcomes and resting-state functional connectivity.[28] However, other methods and approaches for targeting a specific stimulation site have emerged in research on depression and for probing other disorders or processes.

Regions other than the DLPFC (e.g., dorsomedial prefrontal cortex [DMPFC] and the orbitofrontal cortex [OFC]) are currently under investigation as rTMS targets in the treatment of depression and other psychiatric disorders. The DMPFC is typically targeted at the stereotaxic coordinate (X 0 Y + 30 Z + 30) with the coil vertex placed at the scalp point closest to the coordinate (X 0 Y + 60 Z + 60). This point is estimated to be approximately 25% of the distance from nasion to inion.[29] There are, however, additional refinements needed to target the DMPFC. First, due to its distance from the skull surface, an angled figure-of-eight coil is usually used to target this cortical region. Furthermore, the motor threshold for the lower extremity is used to determine the stimulus intensity needed to activate the DMPFC given that the DMPFC is located against the medial wall, similar to the lower extremity motor region. Finally, stimulation of the DMPFC is achieved by positioning the coil 90 degrees to the mid-sagittal line, orienting the coil e-fields in a direction that optimally stimulates midline structures. In contrast, the OFC is estimated over the AF8 electrode site (for the right OFC). As mentioned earlier, this site can be identified using an EEG cap or by first measuring 10% of the nasion-to-inion distance along the sagittal midline, followed by measuring 10% of the head circumference to the right. The coil is oriented with the handle held perpendicular to the axial plane of the head, thus causing the induced current to flow in an inferior to superior direction, stimulating the horizontal shelf of the OFC.[30]

2.2.4 Robotic TMS

After identifying the correct target location using neuronavigation, the coil can be manually held in place over the participant's head. Even in using the visual feedback functions available through neuronavigation software, certain factors, including participant head movements and administrator fatigue, make accurate and consistent coil positioning challenging. As such, TMS coil holders were developed to facilitate accurate and reliable coil positioning. While some TMS manufacturers provide adjustable coil holders, the coil must still be manually adjusted to account for any participant movement. Recent technological advances, however, have led to robotic-assisted TMS coil systems. When using a robotic system, the target coil position relative to the participant's head is converted to coordinates and input into the software that controls the arm. In continuously tracking the participant's head via an optical tracking system, the trajectory of the coil's path can be modified in real time to account for any movements.[31–33] Using a robotic coil positioning system also facilitates the reliable sequential targeting of multiple anatomical targets. Taken together, the integration of neuronavigation with a robotic-assisted TMS represents a feasible and reliable advancement in the accurate targeting of TMS stimulation.

REFERENCES

1. Barker AT, Jalinous R, Freeston IL. Non-invasive magnetic stimulation of human motor cortex. *Lancet.* 1985;1(8437):1106–1107.
2. Davey K, Epstein CM. Magnetic stimulation coil and circuit design. *IEEE Trans Biomed Eng.* 2000;47(11):1493–1499.
3. Epstein CM, Davey KR. Iron-core coils for transcranial magnetic stimulation. *J Clin Neurophysiol.* 2002;19(4):376–381.
4. Peterchev AV, Wagner TA, Miranda PC, Nitsche MA, Paulus W, Lisanby SH, et al. Fundamentals of transcranial electric and magnetic stimulation dose: Definition, selection, and reporting practices. *Brain Stimul.* 2012;5(4):435–453.
5. Deng ZD, Lisanby SH, Peterchev AV. Coil design considerations for deep transcranial magnetic stimulation. *Clin Neurophysiol.* 2014;125(6):1202–1212.
6. Groppa S, Oliviero A, Eisen A, Quartarone A, Cohen LG, Mall V, et al. A practical guide to diagnostic transcranial magnetic stimulation: Report of an IFCN committee. *Clin Neurophysiol.* 2012;123(5):858–882.
7. Pascual-Leone A, Dhuna A, Roth BJ, Cohen L, Hallett M. Risk of burns during rapid-rate magnetic stimulation in presence of electrodes. *Lancet.* 1990;336(8724):1195–1196.
8. Ilmoniemi RJ, Kicic D. Methodology for combined TMS and EEG. *Brain Topogr.* 2010;22(4):233–248.
9. Ives JR, Rotenberg A, Poma R, Thut G, Pascual-Leone A. Electroencephalographic recording during transcranial magnetic stimulation in humans and animals. *Clin Neurophysiol.* 2006;117(8):1870–1875.
10. Thut G, Ives JR, Kampmann F, Pastor MA, Pascual-Leone A. A new device and protocol for combining TMS and online recordings of EEG and evoked potentials. *J Neurosci Methods.* 2005;141(2):207–217.
11. Virtanen J, Ruohonen J, Naatanen R, Ilmoniemi RJ. Instrumentation for the measurement of electric brain responses to transcranial magnetic stimulation. *Med Biol Eng Comput.* 1999;37(3):322–326.

12. Ilmoniemi RJ, Virtanen J, Ruohonen J, Karhu J, Aronen HJ, Naatanen R, et al. Neuronal responses to magnetic stimulation reveal cortical reactivity and connectivity. *Neuroreport*. 1997;8(16):3537–3540.

13. Iramina K, Maeno T, Nohaka Y, Ueno S. Measurement of evoked electroencephalography induced by transcranial magnetic stimulation. *J Appl Physiol* 2003;93:6718–6720.

14. Bonato C, Miniussi C, Rossini PM. Transcranial magnetic stimulation and cortical evoked potentials: A TMS/EEG co-registration study. *Clin Neurophysiol*. 2006;117(8):1699–1707.

15. Thut G, Northoff G, Ives JR, Kamitani Y, Pfennig A, Kampmann F, et al. Effects of single-pulse tran- scranial magnetic stimulation (TMS) on functional brain activity: A combined event-related TMS and evoked potential study. *Clin Neurophysiol*. 2003;114(11):2071–2080.

16. Oliveira-Maia AJ, Garcia-Guarniz AL, Sinanis A, Pascual-Leone A, Press D. Comparative efficacy of repetitive transcranial magnetic stimulation for treatment of depression using 2 different stimulation devices: A retrospective open-label study. *J Clin Psychiatry*. 2016;77(6):e743–744.

17. Davila MC, Ely B, Manzardo AM. Repetitive transcranial magnetic stimulation (rTMS) using different TMS instruments for major depressive disorder at a suburban tertiary clinic. *Ment Illn*. 2019;11(1):7947.

18. Fitzgerald PB. An update on the clinical use of repetitive transcranial magnetic stimulation in the treat- ment of depression. *J Affect Dis*. 2020;276:90–103.

19. Goetz SM, Luber B, Lisanby SH, Murphy DL, Kozyrkov IC, Grill WM, et al. Enhancement of neuro- modulation with novel pulse shapes generated by controllable pulse parameter transcranial magnetic stimulation. *Brain Stimul*. 2016;9(1):39–47.

20. Herwig U, Padberg F, Unger J, Spitzer M, Schonfeldt-Lecuona C. Transcranial magnetic stimulation in therapy studies: Examination of the reliability of "standard" coil positioning by neuronavigation. *Biol Psychiatry*. 2001;50(1):58–61.

21. Fitzgerald PB. Targeting repetitive transcranial magnetic stimulation in depression: Do we really know what we are stimulating and how best to do it? *Brain Stimul*. 2021;14(3):730–736.

22. Fitzgerald PB, Maller JJ, Hoy KE, Thomson R, Daskalakis ZJ. Exploring the optimal site for the localiza- tion of dorsolateral prefrontal cortex in brain stimulation experiments. *Brain Stimul*. 2009;2(4):234–237.

23. Beam W, Borckardt JJ, Reeves ST, George MS. An efficient and accurate new method for locating the F3 position for prefrontal TMS applications. *Brain Stimul*. 2009;2(1):50–54.

24. Mir-Moghtadaei A, Caballero R, Fried P, Fox MD, Lee K, Giacobbe P, et al. Concordance between beamf3 and MRI-neuronavigated target sites for repetitive transcranial magnetic stimulation of the left dorsolateral prefrontal cortex. *Brain Stimul*. 2015;8(5):965–973.

25. Nikolin S, D'Souza O, Vulovic V, Alonzo A, Chand N, Dong V, et al. Comparison of site localization techniques for brain stimulation. *J ECT*. 2019;35(2):127–132.

26. Lefaucheur JP. Why image-guided navigation becomes essential in the practice of transcranial magnetic stimulation. *Neurophysiol Clin*. 2010;40(1):1–5.

27. Gomez LJ, Dannhauer M, Peterchev AV. Fast computational optimization of TMS coil placement for individualized electric field targeting. *NeuroImage*. 2021;228:117696.

28. Fox MD, Buckner RL, White MP, Greicius MD, Pascual-Leone A. Efficacy of transcranial magnetic stim- ulation targets for depression is related to intrinsic functional connectivity with the subgenual cingulate. *Biol Psychiatry*. 2012;72(7):595–603.

29. Downar J, Geraci J, Salomons TV, Dunlop K, Wheeler S, McAndrews MP, et al. Anhedonia and reward- circuit connectivity distinguish nonresponders from responders to dorsomedial prefrontal repetitive transcranial magnetic stimulation in major depression. *Biol Psychiatry*. 2014;76(3):176–185.

30. Feffer K, Fettes P, Giacobbe P, Daskalakis ZJ, Blumberger DM, Downar J. 1Hz rTMS of the right orbito- frontal cortex for major depression: Safety, tolerability and clinical outcomes. *Eur Neuropsychopharmacol*. 2018;28(1):109–117.

31. Pennimpede G, Spedaliere L, Formica D, Di Pino G, Zollo L, Pellegrino G, et al. Hot Spot Hound: A novel robot-assisted platform for enhancing TMS performance. *Annu Int Conf IEEE Eng Med Biol Soc*. 2013;2013:6301–6304.

32. Kantelhardt SR, Fadini T, Finke M, Kallenberg K, Siemerkus J, Bockermann V, et al. Robot-assisted image-guided transcranial magnetic stimulation for somatotopic mapping of the motor cortex: A clinical pilot study. *Acta Neurochirurgica*. 2010;152(2):333–343.

33. Matthaus L, Giese A, Wertheimer D, Schweikard A. Planning and analyzing robotized TMS using virtual reality. *Stud Health Technol Inform*. 2006;119:373–378.

Single-, Paired-, Triple-Pulse TMS for Motor Physiological Studies

S INGLE- AND PAIRED-PULSE TRANSCRANIAL MAGNETIC STIMULATION (TMS) techniques are useful in measuring cortical excitability and cortical connectivity. This chapter focuses on measurements at the motor cortex (M1).

3.1 SINGLE-PULSE TMS MEASUREMENTS

3.1.1 Determining the Location of the Optimal Position or Hotspot

The first step in studies of M1 excitability is to determine the location of the optimal position for obtaining motor-evoked potentials (MEP), also known as the *motor hot spot*. Surface electromyography (EMG) is recorded from the target muscles of interest. The TMS machine should initially be set at suprathreshold intensity. For a figure-of-eight coil, the coil should initially be moved in steps of 1–2 cm in the medial-lateral and anterior-posterior (AP) directions to estimate the position that produces the highest MEP amplitude. When optimal position is approximately located, the coil is moved in steps of approximately 0.5 cm to locate the optimal position. Since there is substantial pulse-to-pulse variability in MEP amplitudes, several (generally 3–5) pulses should be observed to estimate the MEP amplitude at one location. It may be preferable to determine the optimal position for one direction (e.g., medial-lateral) and then the optimal position for the perpendicular (e.g., AP) direction. Once the optimal position is determined, it should be marked on the scalp (e.g., using a marker pen) such that the markers are visible with the coil in place. In some experiments, it may be preferable to use a cap such as a swim cap. However, some study participants find tight caps uncomfortable especially for long experiments, and even tight caps may move during experiments. Frameless stereotaxic neuronavigation (discussed in Chapter 2) may be used, but two studies found no relevant differences in using navigated TMS in comparison to conventional TMS for determining the location for stimulating the hand area of M1.[1,2] However, it may be useful to ensure that the same spot is stimulated on different days in the same participant. An automated method using individual magnetic resonance imaging (MRI) and a robotized TMS system to determine the optimal position has also been developed.[3] Since the central sulcus is at 30–45 degrees to the mid-sagittal line, the coil is most commonly held at 30–45 degrees to the mid-sagittal line with the handle pointing backward to induce posterior-to-anterior (PA) current across the central sulcus, which produces the lowest motor threshold.

For a circular coil, the optimal position is less critical than that for a figure-of-eight coil. Initially, the coil can be centered over the vertex and then moved in steps of about 1 cm to locate the optimal position for the target muscle. It should be noted that with monophasic TMS machines, the side of the circular coil that induces anticlockwise current in the brain (viewed from above), with PA current in the right hemisphere and AP direction in the left hemisphere, results in lower motor threshold (MT) for the right hemisphere. Flipping the coil will produce current flow in the opposite direction, with lower MT for the left hemisphere.

3.1.2 Motor Threshold

MT is a useful measure of corticospinal excitability of the motor cortex (M1) and is generally defined as the lowest intensity that produces a recordable response in a target muscle. It is often expressed as a percentage of stimulator output, and therefore the values vary between different machines and coils, with lower MT indicating higher excitability. MT may be determined with the target muscle at rest or during muscle activation. For the resting MT (RMT), when conducting electrophysiological experiments and especially when the RMT is a measured variable, it is advisable to monitor the muscle activity visually on a computer screen and via speakers at high gain to ensure muscle relaxation. For the active MT (AMT), the target muscle is activated at a constant level, typically between 10% and 20% of maximum voluntary contraction to avoid muscle fatigue. It is preferable to monitor the level of background muscle contraction. There are two main methods to determine the MT.[4,5]

The *relative frequency method* is the most commonly used. For RMT, the criterion is typically the lowest stimulus intensity that evokes MEPs of 50 μV or greater in at least 5 out of 10 trials for hand muscles. For AMT, the amplitude criterion is usually 100 μV or 200 μV. With the coil at the optimal position, stimulus intensity is increased by steps of 5% of maximum stimulator output (MSO) from a low intensity (such as 30% MSO) until MEPs are consistently obtained. It is then decreased by steps of 2% MSO until MEP amplitudes fall below 50 μV, and then increased or decreased by steps of 1% until the MT is obtained.

The *adaptive method* is based on the threshold tracking technique. A freely available computer program can be used to run the maximum likelihood threshold tracking algorithm. An upper and a lower boundary for MT are first defined. The algorithm selects the TMS intensity and adjusts it based on whether an MEP is evoked or not. Lower numbers of TMS pulses are needed to determine the MT using this method compared to the relative frequency method.

Other methods to determine the MT include a *two-threshold method* with determination of a low threshold (highest intensity that evokes no response) and a high threshold (lowest intensity that evokes response at every trial).[6] Another method is the *supervised parametric estimation method* based on sigmoid curve fitting of the response probability as a function of stimulus intensity.[7]

Some studies have used visible muscle twitch to determine RMT.[8] It should be noted that the RMT determined with this approach is usually higher than that using surface EMG because EMG is more sensitive than visual determination of muscle twitch. Moreover, the degree of muscle relaxation cannot be monitored.

MT is lower for intrinsic hand muscles compared to proximal arm, trunk, and lower limb muscles.[5,9] This is likely related to the different sizes of cortical representation in the motor cortex and the strength of corticospinal projections, with the strongest projection to intrinsic hand muscles.

MT increases with age.[10] Pharmacological agents that block voltage-gated sodium channel such as phenytoin,[11] carbamazepine,[12] and lamotrigine[12] increase the motor threshold, whereas modulation of major neurotransmitters such as gamma aminobutyric acid (GABA), dopamine, and acetylcholine had inconsistent or no effects on MT.[13] These finding suggest that MT reflects axonal excitability. In practical terms, one needs to be aware that the medications that participants take may influence MT.

3.1.3 Measurements of MEP Size and Latency

MEP latency (Figure 3.1) is generally taken as the onset of the MEP. The most widely used measure of MEP size is the peak-to-peak amplitude. Since MEPs occur at known latencies after TMS, automated algorithms can be used to obtain MEP amplitudes unless the recordings are contaminated by significant artifacts. MEP area may also be used, especially in proximal and truncal muscles where the MEPs are polyphasic and the amplitudes are lower, but generally it offers little advantage over peak-to-peak amplitude. In

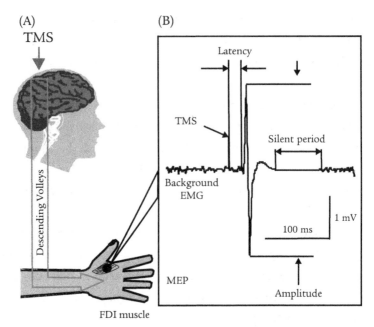

FIGURE 3.1 *Transcranial magnetic stimulation (TMS) and measurement of motor-evoked potential (MEP). (A) When TMS is applied to the primary motor cortex, it produces descending volleys in the spinal cord. This in turn activates the spinal motoneurons and a MEP can be recorded in the target muscle (e.g., first dorsal interosseous muscle) with surface electromyogram (EMG). (B) MEP measurements. When TMS is delivered during voluntary muscle contraction, a MEP is followed by a silent period with no background EMG activity. MEP latency is defined as the time from TMS delivery to the onset of MEP. MEP amplitude is usually measured as the peak-to-peak value. Silent period can be measured from the onset or end of MEP to the first recovery of background EMG activity.*
MODIFIED FROM NI AND CHEN, *TRANSLAT NEURODEGENERATION.* 2015;4:22 AND NI ET AL., *J NEUROPHYSIOL.* 2011;105:749–756, WITH PERMISSION.

some studies, it may be useful to express MEP as a percentage or ratio to the maximum *compound muscle action potential* (CMAP), which is the maximum M wave from peripheral nerve stimulation. This gives an estimate of the portion of spinal motor neurons activated by TMS and provides normalization for individual differences in CMAP, which may be affected by diseases (Figure 3.2).[14]

Effects of muscle activation on MEP amplitude. Muscle activation decreases MEP latency, increases MEP amplitude and duration, and the slope of the MEP recruitment curve.[15] This is related to increase in both cortical and spinal excitability.[16] It has been speculated that the increase in MEP duration may be related to the contribution of propriospinal inputs to the activation of alpha motorneurons.[17]

3.1.4 MEP Recruitment Curve

The *recruitment curve* refers to the increase in MEP amplitude with higher stimulus intensities; it is also known as the *input-output curve* or the *stimulus-response curve*. The curve is

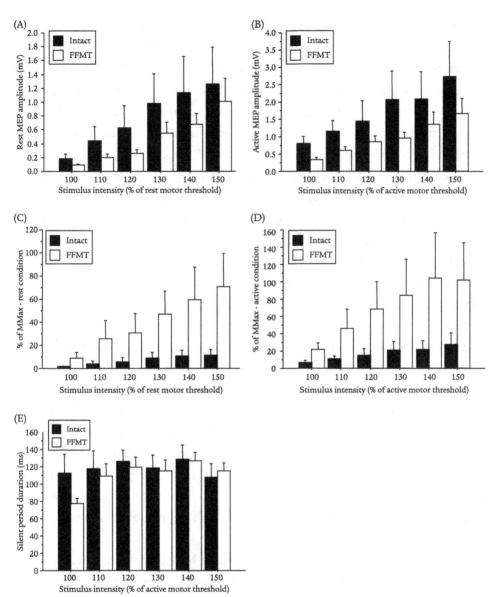

FIGURE 3.2 *Example of measurements of motor-evoked potential (MEP) recruitment curve and silent period duration in patients with free functioning muscle transfer (FFMT). (A,B) MEP recruitment curves based on MEP amplitudes for the rest (A) and active (B) conditions for the intact and the FFMT sides. (C,D) MEP recruitment curves based on %MMax (MEP amplitude divided by the maximum compound muscle action potential [MMax] from peripheral nerve stimulation) for the rest (C) and active (D) conditions at different TMS intensities. (E) The silent period durations at different transcranial magnetic stimulation (TMS) intensities. The FFMT muscles have lower MMax than muscles on the intact side. Therefore they showed higher MEP recruitment when amplitudes are expressed as a %MMax compared to muscles of the intact side. Each error bar represents one standard error.*

FROM CHEN ET AL., *CLIN NEUROPHYSIOL.* 2003;114:2434–2446, WITH PERMISSION.

sigmoid-shaped, with the initial flat part turning to the steep part of the curve at the MT. The steep part of the recruitment curve, from 100% MT to about 150% MT, is approximately linear in shape until the plateau is reached (Figure 3.2). The MEP recruitment curve can be modeled using a sigmoid function,[15] while the linear portion can be assessed with linear regression. Compared to lower intensities near the MT, higher TMS intensities excites higher threshold neurons and those further from the center of the motor representations. The slopes of linear portion of the MEP recruitment curves are steeper in intrinsic hand muscles compared to proximal hand muscles or lower limb muscles, and this likely reflects the strength of corticospinal projections.[9] The plateau of the recruitment curve represents the maximum MEP amplitude elicited by TMS. It is generally lower than the maximum CMAP, largely due to desynchronization of descending volleys from TMS leading to phase cancellation.[18]

The MEP recruitment curve is a useful way to assess corticospinal excitability. For example, it is altered after interventions that change cortical excitability and is often abnormal in diseases. It is more time-consuming than measurement of MEP at a single stimulus intensity but provides additional information. For example, if MEP amplitude at a single TMS intensity is increased after a plasticity intervention, MEP recruitment curve can determine if the changes are due to a "shift to the left" of the recruitment curve, a steeper slope of the curve, and whether the maximum MEP or the plateau of the recruitment curve is increased. These changes likely have different physiological bases. However, more participants are likely needed to demonstrate changes in recruitment curve compared to MEP amplitude at a single stimulus intensity. For example, MEP recruitment curve is a useful method to examine changes in cortical excitability in experimental setting such as transient ischemia,[19] in participants with amputation,[19] or in professional musicians.[20]

There is considerable pulse-to-pulse variation in MEP amplitude. Navigated TMS with control of coil tilt, location, and orientation may reduce some of the variability of MEP amplitude[21] although another study found no difference.[2]

3.1.5 Central Motor Conduction Time

The *central motor conduction time* (CMCT) refers to the conduction time in the brain and spinal cord along the corticospinal tract from the motor cortex to spinal motor neurons, or to bulbar motor neurons in cranial nerve innervated muscles (Figure 3.3). It is determined by subtracting the MEP latency from TMS by the peripheral conduction time. MEP latency is obtained with the target muscle under slight voluntary contraction (10–20% of maximum) because MEP latencies are shorter by about 2 ms in the

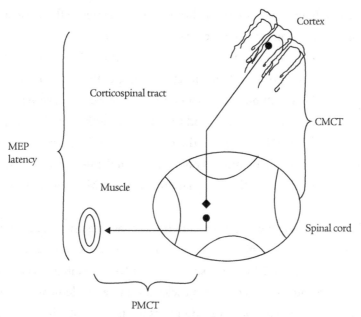

Cortex

Corticospinal tract

CMCT

MEP
latency

Muscle

Spinal cord

PMCT

FIGURE 3.3 *Schematic representation of the calculation of central motor conduction time (CMCT). The latencies of muscle response to cortical stimulation represent the sum of central and peripheral conduction times. CMCT is calculated by subtracting the peripheral conduction time (PMCT) from the motor evoked potential (MEP) latency elicited by motor cortical stimulation.*
FROM UDUPA AND CHEN R, *HANDBOOK OF CLINICAL NEUROLOGY.* 2013;116:375–386, WITH PERMISSION.

active compared to the rest condition. At rest, temporal summation of D and I waves at the spinal motor neuron is required to achieve firing threshold, whereas the earliest descending corticospinal volley can discharge spinal motor neurons in the active condition. TMS is usually set to produce maximum MEP amplitude, at about 140% RMT or 170% AMT.[4] The MEP with the largest amplitude and shortest latency from five consecutive stimuli, best done by superimposing the responses, is used for the calculation because this provides an estimate of the optimal central motor conduction for a particular patient.

Several methods can be used to obtain the peripheral motor conduction time from spinal motor neuron to the target muscle. The first is to use the F-wave latency. With peripheral nerve stimulation, the M wave occurs from direct activation of the muscle from nerve stimulation. The F-wave is due to antidromic activation of the motor axon which activates the spinal motor neuron, and the impulse conducts back orthodromically to the target muscle. Typically, the shortest F-wave latency of 10–20 trials is used; the formula is CMCT = $(F + M\text{-}1)/2$.[22,23] One millisecond is subtracted as an estimate of activation time of the spinal motor neuron. The advantage of the F-wave method is that it is relatively easy to perform but is only applicable to distal muscles. A practical point is that F-wave amplitudes are much smaller than M wave amplitudes, and they occur at much longer latencies (about 22–28 ms for median nerve stimulation at the wrist compared to 3–4 ms for the M wave) and may not be present in every trial.

Another approach to obtain the peripheral conduction time is to apply magnetic stimulation to the appropriate vertebral level. This excites the motor nerve roots at the spinal foramina.[24] This method is applicable to most muscles. However, it underestimates the peripheral conduction time and therefore overestimates CMCT, particularly for lower limb muscles. This is because the distance from the nerve root exiting from the spinal cord to the spinal foramina is not included in the peripheral conduction time calculations. Therefore, this method may falsely increase CMCT in patients with nerve root lesions.

A third method is to apply transcutaneous high-voltage electrical stimulation over the cervical spine. The cathode is placed over the spinous process of the target segment; the anode is placed 5–6 cm cranially on the spine for muscles innervated by cervical roots[25,26] and over the contralateral iliac crest for muscles innervated by lumbar and sacral roots. The advantage of this method is that it stimulates the nerve roots shortly after they exit from the spinal cord,[26] but it is not widely used because it is painful.

3.1.6 The Triple Stimulation Method

The maximum MEP amplitude from TMS is always below the maximum CMAP from peripheral nerve stimulation largely because of desynchronization and phase cancellation of the descending corticospinal impulses. The *triple stimulation test* (TST) is a collision technique used to synchronize the discharges of spinal motor neurons activated by TMS and avoid phase cancellations.[18,27]

The technique involves delivering TMS first, followed by two peripheral nerve stimuli with appropriate delays (Figure 3.4). The first peripheral stimulus is a supramaximal stimulus applied to a distal nerve, such as median nerve at the wrist. It collides with the impulses coming down the arm from activation of spinal motor neurons by TMS. The impulses that do not collide continue to travel up the arm. The second peripheral stimulus is a supramaximal stimulus in the proximal arm, such as Erb's point. The descending impulses collide with the remaining ascending impulses from the first peripheral nerve stimulation. After the collision, the only nerve fibers with descending impulses are the original fibers activated by TMS, but they are now synchronized. This is the TST test response. The TST control trial is performed with peripheral nerve stimuli alone. The response is the ratios of the second deflection of the TST test to the TST control trials. TST ratio is close to 100% in normal participants, indicating that TMS can activate virtually all descending corticospinal fibers.

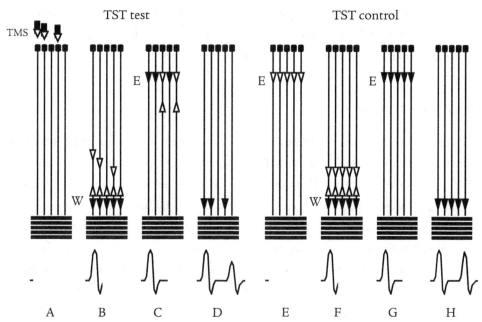

FIGURE 3.4 *Principle of triple stimulation technique (TST).The motor tract is simplified to five spinal motor neurons, and the horizontal lines represent the muscle fibers of the five motor units. Black arrows depict action potentials that evoke a response (i.e., a trace deflection) and open arrows those that collide. TST test is shown in (A–D). (A) A submaximal transcranial magnetic stimulation (TMS) excites three spinal motor neurons (1, 2, and 4) out of five (large open arrows). (B) TMS-induced action potentials descend in the axons of these three spinal motor neurons. The three action potentials in axons 1, 2, and 4 are desynchronized. After a delay, a supramaximal stimulus is applied to the peripheral nerve close to the target muscle (W, wrist). The orthodromic wave gives rise to a first negative deflection of the EMG trace. The antidromic action potentials collide with the descending action potentials on motor axons 1, 2, and 4. (C) The action potential on axons 3 and 5 continue to ascend. After a second delay, a supramaximal stimulus is applied to the proximal nerve, close to the spinal motor neuron (Erb's point, E). In axons 3 and 5, the descending action potentials collide with the ascending action potentials. (D) A synchronized response from the three motor neurons that were initially excited by TMS is recorded as the second deflection of the TST test trace. TST control is shown in (E–H). (E) A supramaximal stimulus is applied at Erb's point. (F) After a delay, a supramaximal stimulus applied at the wrist (W) is recorded as the first deflection of the TST control trace. (G) After another delay, a second supramaximal stimulus is applied at Erb's point. (H) A synchronized response from the five motor axons is recorded as the second deflection of the TST control trace. The test response is quantified as the ratio of second deflections of the TST test (D) to TST control (H).*

FROM CHEN ET AL., CLIN NEUROPHYSIOL. 2008;119:504–532, WITH PERMISSION.

TST allows precise quantification of corticospinal conduction because it avoids phase cancellation due to desynchronization of corticospinal volleys. It is considered more sensitive than standard TMS methods in detecting corticospinal conduction deficits. For example, TST can be used to demonstrate corticospinal tract involvement in amyotrophic lateral sclerosis, including those with lower motor neuron syndrome.[28] It has diagnostic utility in multiple sclerosis, with high test-retest reliability in long-term follow-up[29] and may correlate better with motor dysfunction compared to central conduction based on MEP.[30] However, TST is more technically challenging than standard TMS, and some participants may find the procedure uncomfortable.

3.1.7 TMS Mapping

TMS mapping is used to determine the location and extent of muscle representations in the motor cortex. Typically, the stimulation begins at the optimal position (hot spot). The coil is moved systematically in the medial, lateral, anterior, and posterior directions along a grid. Most commonly a 1 cm grid is used, although some studies have used a 0.5 cm grid. It may be drawn on a tight-fitting swim cap or on the scalp. After stimulation at the optimal position, the coil is moved 1 cm in one direction (e.g., lateral) and the same stimuli are applied. It is moved another centimeter in the same direction until no MEP from the target muscle can be obtained or the average MEP amplitude falls below a target amplitude, such as 10% or 25% of the average at the optimal position, indicating that the "edge" of the map has been reached. The coil is then moved 1 cm to another direction from the optimal position (e.g., medial) and the same process repeated for all directions to be tested. At the end of the mapping, inactive positions should lie along the circumference of the map, with the active positions inside.[31,32] An alternative method is to stimulate a grid (e.g., 7 × 7 cm) in a pseduorandom manner; the grid may need to be expanded to ensure that outermost stimulation sites evoked no response. A refinement of this technique is to create a subject-specific region of interest using approximately 50 pulses, then apply approximately 100 pulses pseudorandomly within the region of interest with neuronavigation; the map results are analyzed with digital reconstruction methods.[33,34] The number of pulses delivered at each position is a tradeoff between the time required for the study and the accuracy of mapping. One study showed that with 10 stimuli per site, the location of the center of gravity (COG) was within 1 mm; with 5 stimuli per site, COG deviation was within 2 mm of that calculated with 20 stimuli per site.[35] The stimulation intensity is typically set at about 110–120% RMT. The time between TMS pulses may be shortened to 1.5–2 s to reduce the time required for mapping.[33,36]

TMS mapping is used to determine the location of the COG and map size. The COG is calculated from the amplitude weighted average of the MEP amplitude at each stimulation site and is determined separately for the AP and medial-lateral directions. Its scalp location is often expressed in relation to the vertex (Cz). The TMS map area refers to the number of active positions on the stimulation grid and may be defined as the number of positions with MEP amplitudes that are two-third, one-half, or one-third of the maximum or with any response evoked. The map volume is the sum of average MEP amplitude recorded from all site. However, the measures of map area or volume should be interpreted with caution. Due to spread of the stimulating current, the finding that MEPs can be evoked at a stimulation site does not imply that there is cortical representation of the target muscle at that site. Moreover, changes in map size may be caused by changes in the size of cortical representation or changes in excitability.[19] For intrinsic hand muscles, TMS map area, volume and COG were found to be stable over time.[37,38]

The accuracy of TMS mapping has been improved with the use of TMS neuronavigation systems, which may be used with digital reconstruction methods.[33,34] A navigated TMS mapping and functional MRI (fMRI) study showed high between session reliability for the COG, but the spatial extent of muscle representation has low reliability for both navigated TMS and fMRI.[39] As expected, TMS mapping of the hand representation was feasible for all participants but was achieved only in some participants for foot (90%), face (70%), and tongue (40%) muscles.[39] Navigated TMS mapping that follows the shape of the central sulcus may improve the resolution of TMS maps,[40] and a technique that projects the stimulated sites to gyral anatomy may decrease inter-individual variability of cortical maps.[41]

Robot-assisted TMS is a promising method to further improve TMS mapping.[42,43] Map volume, COG location, and highest MEP amplitude (hot spot magnitude) had good to excellent reliability, while map area had moderate to poor reliability with robot TMS mapping.[44] The map area of smaller excitability regions with borders based on 25–75% of peak MEP amplitude correlated with motor function of the dominant hemisphere.[45]

Studies that involved co-registration of TMS sites and comparison to areas activated on functional imaging studies showed good concordance between COG measured by TMS and functional imaging studies, and the COG lies within the precentral gyrus.[35] However, a study suggested that the COG for first dorsal interosseous muscle is not over the hand knob of the M1 in some participants and may be displaced anteriorly.[46] One study found that the location of activation determined by fMRI differed from that determined by TMS by an average of 13.9 mm, with the difference being bigger in participants with higher threshold and lower MEP amplitude.[47] Thus, TMS and fMRI provide complementary information on cortical maps.[39]

3.1.8 Different Current Directions of TMS Activate Different Cortical Circuits: D and I Waves

A single electrical stimulus to the exposed motor cortex (M1) of cats and monkeys elicited multiple (up to 8) descending volleys in the corticospinal tract separated by 1–1.5 ms, indicating an approximate 600 Hz discharge rate.[48] The first wave (direct or D wave) is due to excitation of the corticospinal axon. The later waves (indirect or I waves) are due to synaptic activation of corticospinal neurons and are numbered sequentially, with the first wave termed I1, the second wave I2, etc. Recordings in awake patients with implanted ep-idural spinal electrodes confirmed that D and I waves occur in humans after electrical or magnetic brain stimulation (Figure 3.5). However, the population of cortical neurons ac-tivated by TMS depends on the direction of the induced current. Medially directed cur-rent (lateral-medial [LM] direction) activates corticospinal axons directly leading to the D wave and produces MEPs with the shortest latency. PA-directed current preferentially induces the I1 wave, whereas AP-directed current preferentially recruits the later I3 wave

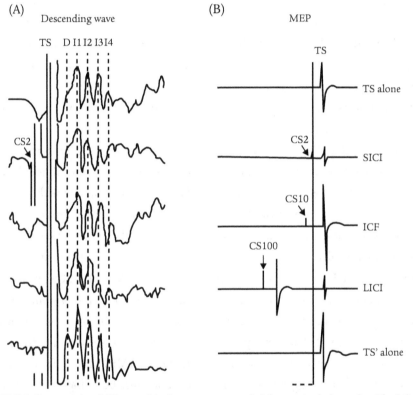

FIGURE 3.5 *Example of direct and indirect waves recorded from spinal electrodes. The left panel (A) shows descending corticospinal waves recorded from a cervical epidural electrode at the C7 level from −5 ms to 15 ms from the test stimulus (TS) onset. The right panel (B) shows motor-evoked poten-tial (MEP) recordings from −200 ms to 100 ms from TS. Dashed lines indicate the peaks of direct (D wave) and indirect waves (I1–I4 waves). TS alone generated MEP of ~1 mV and produces I1–I4 waves. Short interval intracortical inhibition (SICI) represents a trial in which TS was conditioned by a sub-threshold conditioning stimulus at 2 ms before TS (CS2). Intracortical facilitation (ICF) represents a trial in which TS was conditioned by a subthreshold CS10. Long interval intracortical inhibition (LICI) represents a trial in which TS was conditioned by a suprathreshold CS100. Note that late I waves (I3, I4) were suppressed but the I1 wave was not affected by SICI and LICI. ICF facilitated MEP but had little effect on I waves. TS' alone with higher intensity than TS produced larger MEP and descending waves. A D wave was also generated by TS'.*

MODIFIED FROM NI ET AL., *J PHYSIOL.* 2011;589:2955–2962, WITH PERMISSION.

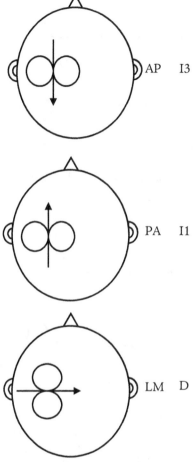

AP   I3

PA   I1

LM   D

FIGURE 3.6 *Effects of induced current directions on recruitment of direct and indirect waves. The arrows show the induced current directions from a figure-of-eight coil held at different orientations. Induced current in the posterior-anterior (PA) direction preferentially induces the first indirect (I1) wave. Induced current in the anterior-posterior (AP) direction preferentially induces the third indirect (I3) wave, while lateral-medial directed current preferentially induces the direct (D) wave.*

and leads to MEPs with the longest latency (Figures 3.6 and 3.7).[49–52] MT is lowest with the induced current in the PA direction. These findings are likely due to the different orientations of groups of cortical fibers, with the PA and AP directions activating different groups of cortical neurons and the LM current activating the axon of the corticospinal neuron (Figure 3.8). With TMS at higher intensities, the different I waves are recruited regardless of the current direction. However, there is also evidence that I waves at the same latency are evoked by different current directions, for example I3 waves evoked by PA and AP directions, are mediated by different circuits. In addition, late I waves were more inhibited by short-latency afferent inhibition (SAI) generated by the AP compared to the PA direction.[53]

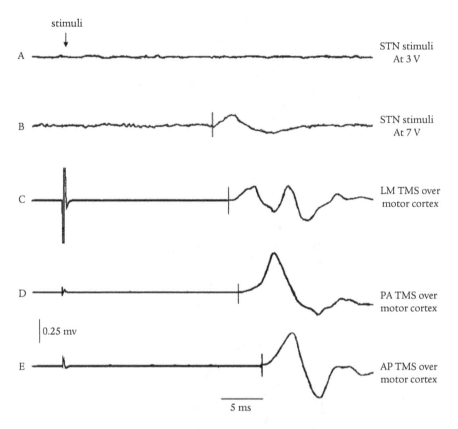

FIGURE 3.7 *Examples of motor-evoked potentials (MEPs) from the contralateral first interosseous muscle following subthalamic (STN) stimulation and transcranial magnetic stimulation (TMS) of the motor cortex (M1). Each trace represents the average of 20 trials. (A) STN stimulation at 3 V produced no MEP. (B) STN stimulation at 7 V produced MEP with a latency of 20 ms, due to activation of the internal capsule. (C) Lateral-medial (LM) direction TMS over M1 produced MEP with latency of 22 ms. (D) Posterior-anterior (PA) direction TMS produced MEP with latency of 23.5 ms. (E) Anterior-posterior (AP) direction TMS produced MEP with a latency of 26.5 ms.*
FROM KURIAKOSE ET AL., *CEREBRAL CORTEX* 2010;20:1926–1936, WITH PERMISSION.

There are considerable individual variations in the recruitment of late I waves by TMS. The difference in MEP latencies induced by AP- and LM-directed currents, which ranges from 0 to 6 ms, is a measure of late I wave recruitment by AP current direction *in a given participant.*[54] A large difference implies activation of late I waves, while a small difference implies predominant activation of early I waves by AP TMS.[54]

D and I waves induced by TMS can be recorded in patients with epidural spinal cord electrodes with the leads externalized. The most common setting is spinal cord stimulation for the treatment of pain,[55-57] and this is generally limited to patients with implanted spinal electrodes in the immediate (few days) postoperative setting (Figure 3.5). D and I waves can also be studied in human participants using a *peristimulus time histogram* (PSTH). This technique requires the participant to produce a slight voluntary contraction

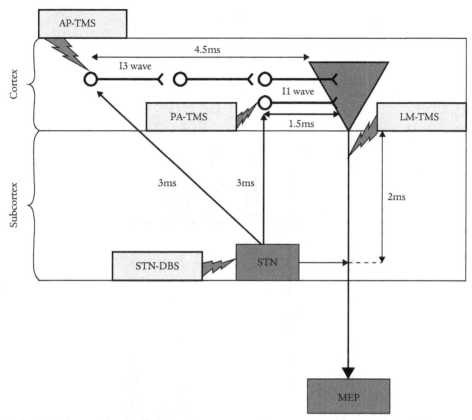

FIGURE 3.8 *Possible site of activation by transcranial magnetic stimulation (TMS) at different current directions. Lateral-medial (LM) directed TMS activates the axon of corticospinal neurons. Motor-evoked potential (MEP) latency following anterior-posterior (AP) TMS is 4.5 ms longer than LM TMS due to activation of I3 neuron. MEP latency following posterior-anterior (PA) TMS is 1.5 ms longer than LM TMS due to activation of I1 neuron. MEP latency following suprathreshold subthalamic nucleus (STN) stimulation is 2 ms shorter than LM TMS with activation of the internal capsule.*

to activate a single motor unit recorded with a needle EMG electrode. The probably of the unit firing at different times after TMS is plotted[51,53] to show peak increases in firing probability occurring at different times for different current directions (Figure 3.9).

3.1.9 Facial Muscles

Facial muscles are under both volitional and emotional control but recording facial MEPs presents specific challenges. Recording from the orbicularis oculi muscles is affected by the blink reflex. The first phase of the blink reflex (R1) is only ipsilateral to the stimulation and occurs at latencies (9–10 ms) similar to the expected MEP latencies, while the bilateral second phase of the blink reflex (R2) occurs at much longer latency and should not be confused with facial MEP (Figure 3.10).[58] Another potential confound is activation of the facial or the trigeminal nerve by magnetic stimulation, which has shorter

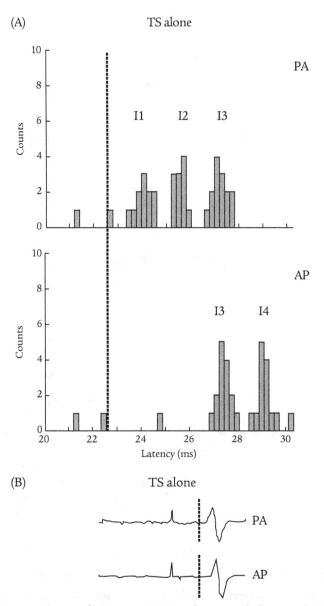

FIGURE 3.9 *Peristimulus time histogram (PSTH) and motor-evoked potential (MEP) recordings in one subject. Data from test stimulus (TS) alone with needle and surface electromyogram (EMG) recordings from the first dorsal interosseous muscle. (A) PSTH was constructed with the bin size set at 0.2 ms. The abscissa indicates the time after transcranial magnetic stimulation (TMS). The ordinate indicates the number of spikes in each bin. The dashed lines show the direct (D) wave latency. Data from posterior-anterior (PA) and anterior-posterior (AP) current directions were compared. (B) Simultaneously recorded surface EMG recording (average of 100 trials). The dashed lines represent the MEP latency for LM current direction. This latency is shorter than that produced by PA and AP current directions. Moreover, MEP latency for PA current direction was shorter than that for AP current direction.*

Modified from Ni et al., *J Neurophysiol.* 2011;105:749–756, with permission.

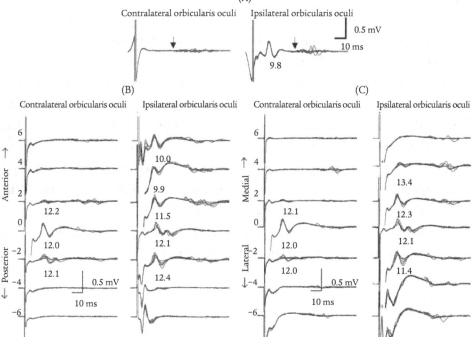

FIGURE 3.10 *Responses of the contralateral and ipsilateral orbicularis oculi (OOc) muscles at rest, with transcranial magnetic stimulation (TMS) at different scalp sites. For comparison (A) shows the blink reflex elicited with the center of the coil applied over the supraorbital notch (three superimposed trials). The number below the trace of the I-OOc denotes the onset of the early response of the blink reflex (R1). There is no R1 in the contralateral OOc. The arrows indicate the onset of the late response of the blink reflex (R2) at 35.6 ms in the ipsilateral and 35.9 ms in the contralateral OOc. Responses in the anterior-posterior axis are shown in (B), and with TMS at different scalp sites in the coronal plane in (C). Each trace represents five superimposed trials in one subject. Stimulus intensity was 70% of the maximal stimulator output in all sites. The numbers preceding the traces denote the distance (in cm) with respect to the optimal stimulation site, with anterior being positive and posterior negative in B and with medial being positive and lateral negative in C. Zero represents the optimal position for the contralateral OOc response. The numbers below the responses denote the onset latencies (in ms). TMS elicited a maximal response in the contralateral OOc muscle when the coil was placed in the optimal site. When the coil was displaced 2 cm in any direction, there was a pronounced reduction in amplitude, and further displacement resulted in no response. In (B), the ipsilateral OOc muscle showed responses of similar shape and amplitude between 2 cm posterior to the optimal site and 6 cm anterior to the optimal site. The onset latency decreased with progressively more anterior placement of the coil, eventually approaching the latency of the early response of the blink reflex. In (C), the ipsilateral OOc muscle showed a response with similar shape and amplitude with the coil placed 2 cm medial or lateral to optimal site. Stimulation at 4 and 6 cm lateral to the optimal site produced a large, short-latency response due to direct facial nerve stimulation.*

FROM PARADISO ET AL., J PHYSIOL. 2005;567(PT 1):323–336, WITH PERMISSION.

latencies (2–4 ms) than facial MEP.[59] Stimulation artifacts may also obscure some of the MEP responses due to the close proximity between the TMS coil and the recording electrodes. In addition to examining latencies, the effects of muscle activation can help to distinguish between MEPs from TMS and responses from nerve stimulation because TMS responses increase in amplitude and decrease in latency with muscle activation, whereas the responses to direct nerve stimulation shows little change with muscle activation. While contralateral responses can be recorded from lower facial muscles such as the orbicularis oris or the triangularis (depressor anguliioris) muscles, it is controversial whether there are reliable responses in ipsilateral lower facial muscles.[58,60,61] In the upper face, contralateral response can be recorded from the orbicularis oculi muscle, and the ipsilateral response may be confounded by the R1 blink reflex.[58] Response from the orbicularis oculi muscles can also be obtained by stimulation over the vertex, presumably from activation of the cingulated motor area, at latencies of 6–8 ms.[59]

3.1.10 Leg Muscles

Leg muscles have higher MTs than arm muscles in part due to their representation located in the medial area of the motor cortex near the midline, away from the scalp. PSTH studies showed that TMS activates monosynaptic projections to leg muscles.[62] In some normal participants, MEP could not be elicited by a figure-of-eight coil or even a circular coil.[9] Background muscle activation will increase the probability of evoking MEPs. If a figure-of-eight coil is used, the optimal coil orientation is with the handle pointing laterally away from the hemisphere to be stimulated (e.g., handle pointing the right if the left M1 is being stimulated) to induce current in the medial-lateral (away from the interhemispheric fissure) direction, with induced current in the left-to-right direction for stimulation of right M1 and the opposite direction for stimulation of the left M1.[4,63] However, a double-cone coil will reliably evoke response from normal participants. Both the figure-of-eight and double-cone coils elicit predominately the I1 wave near threshold intensities.[64] There is more discomfort to the participant compared to recording from hand muscles due to higher stimulation intensities used.

3.1.11 Ipsilateral Motor Evoked Potentials

Ipsilateral MEP (iMEP) can be recorded in upper limb muscles. iMEP requires background muscle activation and is of much lower amplitude and longer latencies, by 2–7 ms, compared to contralateral MEP.[65–67] Its detection generally requires rectification and averaging of multiple trials (Figure 3.11). iMEPs are likely mediated by ipsilateral oligosynaptic pathways, such as the reticulospinal or propriospinal pathway. The cortical circuits

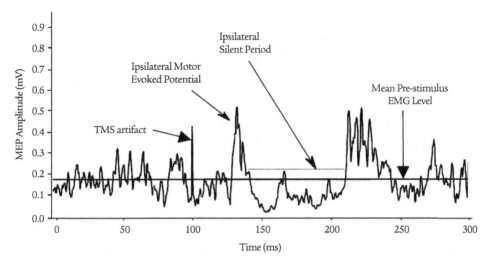

FIGURE 3.11 *Example of an ipsilateral motor-evoked potentials (iMEP) followed by an ipsilateral silent period (iSP). Recording from right first dorsal interosseous (FDI) muscle with the subject maintaining a 50% maximum voluntary contraction. Rectified and averaged electromyogram (EMG) from 10 trials. The right motor cortex was stimulated at 100 ms (stimulus artifact) at 75% of stimulator output with induced current in the anterior-medial direction. An iMEP (onset: 128.1 ms, peak amplitude: 0.532 mV, offset: 143.3 ms) occurred followed by iSP (onset: 143.3 ms, offset: 212.0 ms). The iSP was interrupted by an increase in the EMG signal at ~166 ms. Following the iSP, there was a period of rebound EMG.*

From Chen et al., *J Neurophysiol.* 2003;89:1256–1264, with permission.

involved in iMEP are different from contralateral MEP as they have different cortical map locations,[65,68] with the COG for iMEP being shifted anteriorly and medially compared to contralateral MEP. There is no directional preference for iMEP, whereas contralateral MEP has lowest threshold with induced current in the AP direction.[66] Another study reported that the hot spots for iMEP are mostly located in secondary motor areas, such as the supplementary motor area or the premotor cortex, with no consistent somatotopy for proximal versus distal muscles.[67] One study found that iMEP are more easily obtained in proximal muscle such as biceps than in distal muscles, but most participants showed inhibition rather than facilitation in the triceps muscle.[65] However, another study using 100% stimulator output and hot spot assessment in a grid with neuronavigation reported that iMEP was present in the first dorsal interosseous (FDI) in all normal participants tested and had higher amplitudes than iMEP in the biceps muscle.[67] In the trapezius and pectoralis muscles, iMEP could be recorded with small background contractions in most participants.[69] In the wrist extensors and biceps, it is increased with neck rotation toward the side of TMS and decreased by neck rotation away from the side of TMS.[65,70] In the biceps, it is increased with neck extension and decreased with neck flexion, decreased with activation of the contralateral biceps (homonymous activation), and increased with activation of the contralateral triceps muscle (heteronymous activation).[70] These findings suggest that the asymmetric tonic neck reflexes modulate iMEP, and this is consistent with the suggestion that iMEPs are mediated by the reticulospinal pathway. However, another study found no effect of head rotation on biceps iMEP amplitude, and head rotation to either side decreased FDI iMEP amplitude.[67] The ipsilateral to contralateral MEP amplitude ratio has been suggested as a measure of the relative importance of the reticulospinal versus corticospinal pathways for a given muscle.[71] In older adults, higher relative reticulospinal connectivity was associated with greater grip strength.[71]

3.1.12 Silent Period

When TMS is delivered during voluntary muscle contraction, there is a period of disruption of the background EMG activity after the MEP; this is referred to as the *silent period* (SP).[72] It is also known as the *contralateral SP* or the *cortical SP* (Figure 3.1). The first part of the SP (~50 ms) is at least partly related to spinal inhibition including motor neuronal refractoriness and Renshaw inhibition.[73] The second part of the SP is due to cortical inhibition, as shown by testing of spinal H reflexes,[73] transcranial electrical stimulation, and stimulation of the cervicomedullary junction[74] and by recording of descending corticospinal waves evoked by TMS during the SP.[56] The generation of SP is not from the same circuit as the MEP since the SP and MEP have different topographies[75] and SP can be evoked at lower stimulus intensities than MEP.[76,77] The SP increases with stimulus intensities but is not strongly related to MEP amplitude.[74,76] Increasing the level of background contraction slightly decreases SP duration.[78,79] Since administration of the GABA reuptake inhibitor tiagabine and both oral and intrathecal administration of $GABA_B$ receptor[80,81] agonist baclofen lengthens the SP, SP duration is considered a marker of cortical $GABA_B$ receptor-mediated inhibition. This is consistent with the duration of $GABA_B$-mediated inhibition in cell slice studies, an inhibition that lasts several hundred milliseconds.[82] Prolongation of the SP with ethanol,[83] lorazepam,[84] and zolpidem, an agonist of benzodiazepine receptor subtype BZ1,[85] suggest that $GABA_A$ receptors may also be involved. Pregabalin also lengthens the SP.[86] Moreover, short-interval intracortical inhibition (SICI) is decreased during SP, which may be due to $GABA_B$ receptor-mediated presynaptic inhibition of $GABA_A$ effects.[87]

The SP represents a simple, single-pulse TMS method to examine cortical inhibition and has been reported to be abnormal in many neurological and psychiatric disorders. At least 5 trials, and ideally 10 trials or more, should be performed, with the duration of the SP averaged across trials. Assessing the SP at multiple stimulus intensities with the stimulus-response curve fitted to a Boltzmann function may provide more accurate measure than a single stimulus intensity.[88] It is advisable to provide participant feedback to produce a constant level of background muscle contraction. Since the duration of the

SP can be 200–300 ms, the duration of the EMG recording should be sufficiently long to capture a period of at least 100 ms before TMS and 400 ms after TMS. There are different ways to measure the SP duration, and there is no consensus. The SP may be measured in single trials and then averaged, or measured using a rectified, averaged EMG trace from multiple trials. The beginning of the SP occurs at near the end of the MEP and is difficult to measure accurately. Therefore, most investigators used either the time of TMS delivery or the onset of the MEP to mark the beginning of the SP. The end of the SP can be marked by the return of any EMG activity (absolute SP) in single traces or the return of EMG activity to a predetermined level of the baseline, such as 25%, 50%, or 100%, which requires rectification and averaging of the EMG recording from multiple trials. Since the manual marking of the end of the SP can be subjective and time-consuming, several groups have published automated methods to measure the SP.[89-94]

Some participants have a period of EMG activity in the SP followed by another period of EMG silence before the return of sustained EMG activity. This has been termed the *late excitatory potential* or *breakthrough EMG*. It increases with the level of muscle contraction and decreases with stimulus intensity.[95] It may be due to spinal mechanisms as a result of sudden lengthening of muscles as force drops, which activates muscle spindles and excite spinal motor neurons.[96] The criteria for determining the end of the SP should specify whether the breakthrough EMG or return of sustained EMG is considered the end of the SP. Since breakthrough EMG may be of spinal origin, it has been recommended that breakthrough EMG be considered part of the SP.[97] Detailed recommendations for the measurement and reporting of SP have been provided.[97]

3.1.13 Ipsilateral Silent Period

The *ipsilateral SP* (iSP) refers to interruption of ongoing voluntary EMG activity with stimulation of the ipsilateral motor cortex. There is considerable evidence that iSP is mediated by interhemispheric inhibition due to transmission through the corpus callosum. It is absent or delayed in patients with congenital or acquired lesions of the corpus callosum,[98,99] and stimulation of the internal capsule through deep brain stimulation electrodes near the internal globus pallidus did not evoke iSP.[100] However, a study with deep brain stimulation near the subthalamic nucleus reported iSP,[101] and, in a patient with agenesis of the corpus callosum, iSP was present although the latency was prolonged and the degree of EMG suppression was decreased compared to reference values.[102] This findings suggest that non-callosal pathway could also be involved in generating iSP, although iSP is considered a useful measure of transcallosal inhibition. It is particularly useful for proximal arm and leg muscles, where it is difficult to use the twin-coil method to study interhemispheric inhibition.

To measure iSP, the participant needs to maintain a constant level of background contraction. Fifty percent of maximum contraction is suitable for distal hand muscles[66] but for proximal arm muscles such as the biceps or triceps, 10% contraction may be sufficient. The iSP is of smaller magnitude and shorter duration than the contralateral SP (Figure 3.11). Although iSP may be visible in single trials, unlike the contralateral SP, the EMG interruption is usually not complete and is best analyzed with rectification and averaging of multiple trials using automated methods.[66,103] The parameters for iSP include onset and offset latencies, duration (offset–onset latency), iSP area, and iSP depth,[103] which refers to the average depth of inhibition during the iSP. iSP area and depth are calculated in relation to the level of background EMG. The iSP of distal hand muscles is increased by voluntary activation of contralateral hand muscles, suggesting that voluntary activation increases the interhemispheric suppression of contralateral M1.[104] A detailed recommendation for the measurement of iSP has been provided.[97]

3.2 PAIRED-PULSE TMS STUDIES

Paired-pulse TMS, typically with a conditioning pulse followed by a test pulse, is a powerful method to examine cortical inhibition and facilitation. The effects of the conditioning-test pulse combination are compared to that of the test pulse alone to assess the inhibitory or facilitatory effect on the motor cortex. Some protocols involve conditioning stimulation of the motor cortex and some involve conditioning stimulation outside the motor cortex. The test pulse is applied to the motor cortex. The more commonly applied paired-pulse protocols are summarized in Table 3.1.

3.2.1 Short-Interval Intracortical Inhibition (SICI)

Short-interval intracortical inhibition (SICI) is a widely used paradigm originally described by Kujirai et al.[105] Sanger et al.[106] introduced the term SICI (Figure 3.5). It involves a subthreshold conditioning stimulus (CS) followed by a test stimulus (TS) administered 1–5 ms later. There is good evidence that the inhibition is cortical since the CS did not suppress the response to weak transcranial electrical stimulation,[105] and epidural spinal recordings showed that it suppressed late I waves evoked by the TS (Figure 3.5).[107,108] Detailed studies of the effects of interstimulus intervals on SICI showed that there are two phases of maximum inhibition at about 1 ms and 2.5 ms.[109,110] This is supported by the finding that transcranial direct current stimulation has opposite effects on these two phases of SICI.[111] The inhibition at 1 ms may be partially related to neuronal refractoriness,[109] but synaptic inhibition also contributes.[110] The role of synaptic inhibition in mediating SICI at 1 ms is supported by the finding that GABA level as assessed by magnetic resonance spectroscopy

Table 3.1. Summary of the properties of different forms of paired pulse cortical inhibition and facilitation

	SICI	LICI	SICF	ICF	SIHI	LIHI	CBI	SAI	LAI
				METHOD					
Conditioning stimulus/S1 for SICF)	Sub-threshold TMS	Supra-threshold TMS	Supra-threshold TMS	Sub-threshold TMS	Supra-threshold TMS	Supra-threshold TMS	Cerebellar stim	Median nerve stim.	Median nerve stim
Test stimulus/S2 for SICF	Supra-threshold TMS	Supra-threshold TMS	Sub-threshold TMS	Supra-threshold TMS	Supra-threshold TMS	Supra-threshold TMS	Supra-threshold TMS	Supra-threshold TMS	Supra-threshold TMS
Interstimulus interval (ms)	1-6	50-200	1.0-1.5, 2.3-3.0, 4.1-5.0	8-30	8-12	~40-50	5-7	~20	~200
Proposed neurotransmitter/ receptor	$GABA_A$?dopamine	$GABA_B$	?Glutamate ($\downarrow$ by $GABA_A$)	Glutamate	?	$GABA_B$	?	ACh $\uparrow$ by $GABA_A$	$GABA_A$

ACh = acetylcholine, CBI = cerebellar inhibition, ICF = intracortical facilitation, GABA = γ-aminobutyric acid, GABAA = $GABA_A$ receptor type A, $GABA_B$ = GABA receptor type B, LICI = long interval intracortical inhibition, LIHI = long interval interhemispheric inhibition LAI = long interval interhemispheric inhibition, SAI = short latency afferent inhibition, SICI = short interval intracortical inhibition, SICF = short interval intracortical facilitation, SIHI = short interval interhemispheric inhibition, $\downarrow$ = decreased, $\uparrow$ = increased, $\leftrightarrow$ = no change, ? = unknown correlated with SICI at 1 ms but not at 2.5 ms.[112] The inhibition at 2.5 ms is related to synaptic inhibition. SICI has been observed in facial, proximal arm, trunk, leg muscles,[9] diaphragm[113] and the anal sphincter.[114] It has been suggested that SICI may serve to prevent unwanted muscle activation. It is progressively decreased just before muscle activation,[115] while volitional inhibition[116] and suppression of movements during an urge[117] increases SICI. A study reported that participants with greater resting SICI had faster reaction time and more accurate inhibition of manual responses.[118] SICI is lower in the left hemisphere compared to the right hemisphere,[10,119] and it decreases with age.[120,121]

SICI may be studied with the target muscle at rest or during voluntary contraction. Voluntary muscle contraction reduces SICI,[122] which may partly be related to increased short-interval intracortical facilitation (SICF) with muscle contraction although at low CS intensities of about 0.7 AMT, SICI can be demonstrated independently of SICF at low levels of contraction.[123] Therefore, the background EMG level should be carefully controlled and measured during determination of SICI.

Typically, SICI is calculated as a ratio of the conditioned MEP (CS-TS) to that evoked by TS alone, with ratios below 1 (or 100%) meaning inhibition and ratios above 1 indicating facilitation. Some studies report the percentage of inhibition (1 – MEP ratio). A threshold tracking method in which the stimulator is adjusted to produce a predetermined MEP amplitude can also be used.[109,124] SICI is measured by the increase in stimulator output required to produce the same response in the presence of the CS. A study compared serial tracking of SICI with increasing interstimulus interval (ISIs) from 1 to 7 ms, with all the ISI tracked in parallel and conventional amplitude measurements. Serial tracking and conventional SICI were closely related.[120] However, variability between participants was lowest for conventional SICI and greatest for serial tracking SICI, and only conventional SICI decreased with age. Thus, conventional SICI may be more sensitive to loss of inhibition.

Effects of CS intensity on SICI. The relationship between CS intensity and SICI is characterized by a U-shaped curve.[9] At very low CS intensities, there is no inhibition, and inhibition increases with higher CS intensities, with maximum at about 0.6–0.8 RMT or 0.8–0.9 AMT.[9] The inhibition reduced with further increase in CS and turned into facilitation at higher CS intensities. This facilitation is like due to SICF,[125,126] since they are evoked at similar ISIs. Therefore, SICI represents the net effect of both inhibition and facilitation, and the balance between inhibition and facilitation depends on the interstimulus interval and the CS intensities used.

Effect of TS intensity and MEP amplitude. SICI increases with test MEP amplitude from about 0.2 mV to 1 mV.[106,110] An analysis of data from 35 studies also found that SICI increases with higher test MEP amplitude.[10] Therefore, in the studies comparing two groups or before and after an intervention, the test MEP amplitudes should be matched for proper comparison of SICI.

Topography of SICI. SICI can be obtained in both upper and lower facial muscles and is reduced with muscle activation.[58,61] It is also observed in proximal arm and leg muscles.[9]

Effect of current direction. SICI is conventionally studied with induced current in the PA direction. SICI can also be studied with AP current which requires higher stimulus intensities. The extent of SICI is greater with AP compared to PA directions at interstimulus interval of 3 ms but not at 2 ms.[127,128] Different cortical circuits are likely involved with SICI in different current directions.

To comprehensively study SICI, it is recommended to study a range of interstimulus interval and CS intensities to distinguish between changes in inhibition and facilitation. The ISIs for both the peaks and troughs of SICF should be included[129] to distinguish between the effects of SICI and SICF. For example, if differences between a patient group and controls are seen at the right side of the U-shaped CS intensity recruitment curve and most prominently at ISIs for SICF peaks (e.g., approximate ISIs of 1.5 or 2.9 ms), the difference is likely due to SICF. If differences between patients and controls are seen at the troughs where there is no SICF (e.g., ~2 ms) and on the left side of the U-shaped CS intensity recruitment curve, the differences are likely due to SICI. However, in some instances, detailed studies of SICI and SICF may not be possible due to time constraints. If SICI can only be investigated at a single CS intensity and ISI, a CS intensity of about 90% AMT and an ISI of 2 ms is recommended to avoid the influence of SICF. In studies that look for changes of SICI with interventions, the pre-intervention SICI can be adjusted to produce about 50% inhibition by adjusting the CS intensities so that the SICI level is sensitive to change. The CS intensity should be on the left side of the CS intensity recruitment curve to avoid the influence of SICF.

Pharmacology of SICI. SICI is increased with drugs that enhance $GABA_A$ receptor transmission, such as alcohol[83] and benzodiazepines. Dopamine agonists, glutamatergic antagonists, and norepinephrine antagonists also increased SICI. It is decreased with norepinephrine agonists, while dopamine antagonists have variable effects. It is unaffected by voltage-gated sodium channel blockers.[11,12]

3.2.2 Intracortical Facilitation

Similar to SICI, ICF is elicited by a subthreshold CS followed by a suprathreshold TS but at longer ISIs of 8–30 ms (Figure 3.5).[105] ISIs of 10 and 15 ms are commonly used. The facilitation is likely in part mediated by cortical mechanisms since the condition stimulus did not change spinal H reflexes in the active abductor digiti minimi muscle.[130] However, there may be spinal contribution as the H reflex from the flexor carpi radialis and soleus muscles recorded at rest were increased[131] and epidural recording did not show an increase in I waves (Figure 3.5).[132] ICF is due to mechanisms different from SICI and requires slightly higher CS intensities than SICI.[130] Glutamate likely mediates ICF as ICF is deceased by glutamate receptor antagonist dextromethorphan.[133] Chronic administration of the serotonin reuptake inhibitor paroxetine increased ICF.[134] An analysis of data from 35 studies found that ICF decreases with higher test MEP amplitude.[10]

SICI and ICF have robust effects in most normal participants and are often studied together. However, there is still considerable subject-to-subject variability for both measures.[105–107]

3.2.3 Long-Interval Intracortical Inhibition (LICI)

Long-interval intracortical inhibition (LICI) is elicited by suprathreshold CS and TS at ISIs from 50 ms to about 200 ms[135,136] (Figure 3.5).[106] It is due to cortical inhibition based on absence of change in spinal excitability[73] and reduction of descending corticospinal waves.[56,137] However, a study that used cervicomedullary stimulation as TS showed that spinal inhibition contributes to LICI during muscle fatigue.[138] Pharmacological studies suggest that LICI is mediated $GABA_B$ receptors as it is increased by the $GABA_B$ receptor agonist baclofen.[139] LICI is related to the SP as both are elicited by suprathreshold CS, the TS for LICI is delivered during the SP, and both are mediated by $GABA_B$ receptor-mediated inhibition. SP may measure the duration while LICI measures the depth of $GABA_B$ receptor-mediated inhibition. However, LICI and SP can be affected differently in diseases.[140] Thus, LICI and SP are mediated by overlapping but not identical mechanisms. A study reported that participants with greater resting LICI had faster reaction time and more accurate inhibition of manual responses.[118]

As expected, LICI increases with higher CS intensities but decreases with higher test MEP amplitudes,[106,141] suggesting that higher threshold cortical neurons are less sensitive to LICI. While SICI is decreased with voluntary muscle activation, LICI can be observed during voluntary muscle contraction[136,142] but decreases slightly with higher levels of contraction.[143] A study found that LICI is strongest with weak to moderate muscle contraction compared to rest or maximum voluntary contraction.[144]

3.2.4 Late Cortical Disinhibition

Immediately following LICI, there is a period of increased cortical excitability known as late cortical disinhibition (LCD).[145,146] Increasing the CS intensity increases the latency of LCD as it increases the duration of LICI and SP. During LCD, SICI is decreased[145] and SICF[146] is increased. It may be more prominent during muscle activation.[147] LCD is potentially a presynaptic $GABA_B$ receptor-mediated inhibition.[145–147] LCD was increased when participants were trained to increase MEP amplitudes.[148]

3.2.5 Short-Interval Intracortical Facilitation

Short-interval intracortical facilitation (SICF), also known as *facilitatory I-wave interaction*, is elicited by paired suprathreshold pulses[149] or a suprathreshold first stimulus (S1) followed by a subthreshold second stimulus (S2).[150,151] It is now generally known as SICF (Figure 3.12).[23,152] The facilitation critically depends on the ISI between the two pulses, with facilitation observed at ISI of 1.1–1.5 ms (peak 1), 2.3–3 ms (peak 2), and 4.1–5.0 ms (peak 3), with no facilitation at the troughs between the peaks. Peak 3 has lower amplitude and slightly shorter duration than peaks 1 and 2, while the interval between peaks 2 and 3 is slightly longer than that between peaks 1 and 2.[153] The mechanism of SICF is thought to be caused by first pulse subliminally depolarizing but not discharging some cortical neurons. This makes the neurons more excitable, and they are discharged by the second pulse.[154] The facilitation begins at S1 intensities of about 0.7 RMT and increases with higher S2 intensities; it can also be elicited in active muscles.[150] SICF, at least for peak 1, is of cortical origin since no facilitation was seen when magnetic S2 was replaced by transcranial electric stimulation[150,151] and descending I waves (I2 and I3) were increased by SICF.[155] Electrical cervicomedullary stimulation at threshold or above also lead to peaks 2 and 3, suggesting a spinal component could be involved in generating these peaks.[153]

While most studies were performed in hand muscles, SICF is also present in proximal arm and leg muscles[151] with similar peak latencies. It is likely related to the monosynaptic corticomotoneuronal system as muscles with weaker corticospinal projection, such as the biceps, have less SICF than hand muscles and the tibialis anterior muscle.[151] Pharmacology studies showed that SICF is decreased by drugs that increase $GABA_A$ receptor function such as lorazepam, vigabatrin, phenobarbital, and ethanol but is unaffected by the $GABA_B$ receptor agonist baclofen. Thus, $GABA_A$ receptor function appears to play a role in controlling SICF peaks. In contrast, the N-methyl-D-aspartate (NMDA) receptor antagonist memantine and sodium channel blockers carbamazepine and lamotrigine did not influence SICF.[156]

3.2.6 Effects of Genetic Variation on Cortical Circuits

Brain derived neurotrophic factor (BDNF) plays important role in synaptic plasticity and is widely expressed in the mammalian brain. Met allele of BDNF single nucleotide polymorphism (SNP) at codon 66 (Val66Met) is associated with decreased activity-dependent secretion of BDNF in animal studies. A study found that BDNF met carriers have lower SICI, LICI, and SICF compared to val/val homozygotes.[157] Moreover, participants with higher SICI also had higher SICF, suggesting that an excitatory/inhibitory (E/I) balance is maintain in the brain. The E/I ratio was higher in participants with the

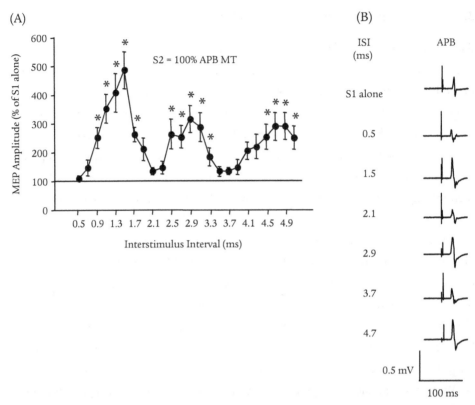

FIGURE 3.12 *Short-interval intracortical facilitation (SICF). (A) SICF recorded from the abductor pollicis brevis (APB) muscle. The intensity of the second stimulus (S2) was at 100% resting motor threshold (MT). The motor-evoked potential (MEP) amplitudes, expressed as percentages of the MEP amplitude evoked by the first stimulus (S1) alone, are plotted against interstimulus intervals (ISIs). Averaged data from 11 subjects. Error bars represent standard error. Asterisks indicate significant difference from control values (t-tests with Bonferroni correction). (B) Representative single trials from one subject. The first stimulus (S1) was adjusted to produce MEPs of 0.3–0.6 mV, and the second stimulus (S2) was at 100% of the motor threshold for the APB muscle being studied. Different ISIs were used. There are three distinct periods of MEP facilitation, separated by troughs in which the MEPs are similar to control (S1 alone) values.*

ADAPTED FROM CHEN AND GARG, *J NEUROPHYSIOL.* 2000;83:1426–1434, WITH PERMISSION.

val/val genotype than in met carriers. Further investigations are needed to confirm these findings due to the limited sample size of the study.[157]

3.3 CONDITIONING STIMULATION FROM THE CEREBELLUM OR PERIPHERAL NERVES

3.3.1 Cerebellar Inhibition

Cerebellar inhibition (CBI) is elicited by CS of the cerebellum followed by TS of the contralateral motor cortex. It was first described using cerebellar electrical stimulation[158] followed by introduction of cerebellar magnetic stimulation[159] (which is less painful that electrical stimulation) as the CS. Inhibition of the contralateral motor cortex occurs at 5–7 ms after the cerebellar stimulation.[159,160] It is thought that the cerebellar stimulation activates Purkinje cells in the cerebellum, which inhibits the cerebellar nuclei (dentate, fastigial, interpositus). These cerebellar output nuclei have excitatory projection to the contralateral thalamus, which in turn has excitatory projection to the motor cortex. Therefore, the net effect of cerebellar stimulation is inhibitory to the contralateral M1 (Figure 3.13). If the induced current direction in the motor cortex is in the AP direction instead of the usual PA direction, the maximum inhibition is at 7 ms instead of 5 ms. CBI for these two current directions in the motor cortex is likely mediated by different circuits since they are affected differently by paired associative stimulation and a motor learning tasks.[161] CBI decreases with activation of the target muscle and decreases with higher test MEP amplitude.[160,162] CBI may decrease with age.[163]

To study CBI, a double-cone coil, which has deeper penetration than a flat figure-of-eight coil, is used.[164,165] A figure-of-eight coil may activate neck muscles and peripheral nerves, leading to M1 inhibition starting at 7–8 ms.[164] The threshold for activating the corticospinal pathway with the double-cone coil placed at the midline (inion) is first determined. It is recommended that rectified, averaged MEP of multiple trials during

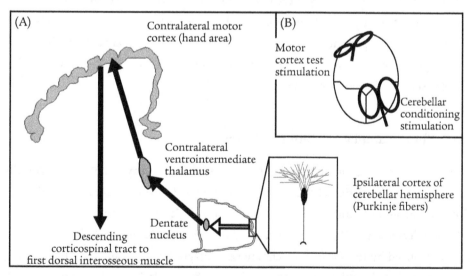

FIGURE 3.13 *Pathway involved in cerebellar inhibition (CBI). (A) Suggested pathway linking the cerebellum to the contralateral motor cortex via the contralateral ventrointermediate nucleus of the thalamus. The closed arrows indicate excitatory connections and the open arrow indicates inhibitory connection. Inhibitory Purkinje fibers are activated by transcranial magnetic stimulation (TMS) of the cerebellar hemispheres with a double-cone coil. (B) Posterior view of a double-cone coil over the right cerebellar hemisphere and a figure-of-eight coil over the left motor cortex.*
From Pinto and Chen, *Exp Brain Res.* 2001;140:505–510, with permission.

voluntary contraction be used for threshold determination[160,162] as using single trials on-line may overestimate the pyramidal tract threshold.[166] The double coil centered at about 3 cm lateral to the inion on a line joining inion and the external auditory meatus with the induced brain current in the upward direction was found to produce optimal inhibition.[159,164] The intensity should be at least 5–10% less than the active threshold for pyramidal tract activation. One study suggested that even at these intensities subtle activation of the corticospinal tract may still be produced, which could potentially lead to MEP inhibition through antidromic activation of the corticospinal pathway; thus, CS intensities of 15–20% below the active threshold should be used.[166] As high-intensity stimulation with the double-cone coil is uncomfortable, some investigators used 70% stimulator output if the brainstem motor threshold was higher than 75%.[161] Since there is debate whether the thresholds for corticospinal tract activation are lower at the lateral or midline positions, and with either up or down induced brain current, it has been suggested that these positions should be checked.[167]

The evidence that the CBI involves that cerebellar pathway includes the finding that the inhibition was absent in patients with cerebellar ataxia or lesion of the cerebellothalamocortical pathway, but was present in patients with lesions of the afferent pathways to the cerebellum.[159,168,169] Moreover, intermittent theta burst stimulation of cerebellum increases[170] while continuous theta burst stimulation decreases[171] functional connectivity between the cerebellum and cortical areas as tested by resting state fMRI, providing further evidence that magnetic stimulation over the posterior fossa activates the cerebellum.

A study with 83 participants reported that CBI has a measurement error of about 15% when repeated on the same or different days, demonstrating fair to good reliability.[172] CBI is decreased in older compared to younger adults.[163]

3.3.2 Short-Latency Afferent Inhibition

Short-latency afferent inhibition (SAI) is elicited by sensory stimulation, typically median nerve stimulation at the wrist, followed by M1 TMS at an ISI of 20–22 ms.[53] Epidural recordings confirmed that the inhibition is cortical since late I waves from TMS are decreased.[173] Pharmacological studies suggested that acetylcholine is involved as it is reduced by the muscarinic cholinergic antagonist scopolamine,[174] but $GABA_A$ receptor-mediated inhibition is also involved as SAI is decreased by lorazepam[175,176] while the $GABA_B$ receptor agonist baclofen had no effect.[176] The pathway mediating SAI is not fully understood, but the short latency implies that a relatively direct pathway is involved. It takes about 20 ms for the afferent impulse to reach the primary somatosensory cortex (S1), which accounts for the N20 component of somatosensory evoked potentials. SAI could be due to a projection from S1 to M1 or from the sensory thalamus directly to M1.

Inhibition can also be obtained by stimulation of digital nerves in the hand, with the latency being 2–3 ms longer due to conduction time from the fingers to the wrist.[173] With index finger (digit 2) stimulation, SAI is more pronounced in distal compared to proximal arm muscles, whereas stimulation of the big toe did not produce inhibition in arm or leg muscles.[177] A study using selective TMS of the FDI and abductor digiti minimi (ADM) muscles and stimulation of the index and little finger found that homotopic stimulation (e.g., digit 2 and FDI) resulted in SAI at an ISI of 23 ms whereas heterotopic stimulation (e.g., digit 5 and FDI) showed short latency facilitation at the same latency.[178] SAI was absent in the lower face, tested with stimulation of the mandibular branch of the facial nerve at ISIs of 5–30 ms[61] but was present at ISIs of 15–30 ms with stimulation of the trigeminal nerve.[179] The authors suggested that, in the facial motor cortex, SAI is evoked by low-threshold cutaneous afferents.[179]

The stimulus intensity for median nerve stimulation at the wrist is typically that required to produce a visible twitch,[53,173] although multiples of the sensory threshold can also be used.[53] The cathode is proximal to optimally direct the stimulation centrally. The ISI between median nerve stimulation can be fixed at between 20 and 22 ms, or varied according to the N20 latency of median nerve somatosensory evoked potentials to account for between-participant variations in conduction time from the median nerve to the somatosensory cortex.[173,180] The inhibition begins about 1 ms after the N20 peak and last until 7–8 ms after the N20 peak. The latency of N20 peak plus 2–4 ms produces maximum inhibition.[173] With TMS inducing PA current in a typical experimental setup that preferentially induces the I1 wave, the degree of SAI increases with the intensity of median nerve stimulation and decreases with higher test MEP amplitude.[53] However, with the TS inducing current in the AP direction, which preferentially induces the I3 wave, there was less SAI compared to the PA current although late I waves induced by the PA direction are preferentially decreased by SAI. These findings suggest that the I3 waves elicited by PA and AP directions are mediated by different neuronal populations.[53] The hypothesis that SAI evoked by PA versus AP currents is mediated by different circuits also is supported by the findings of TMS pulse durations,[181] and visual attention[182] affected PA and AP SAI differently. At least 10 trials of TS alone and 10 trials of CS-TS in combination should be tested. Changes in SAI have been reported with training with changes in performance but findings have been variable.[183]

In the lower limb, tibial nerve stimulation at the ankle led to MEP inhibition of the tibialis posterior muscle at approximately 35 ms and facilitation at approximately 50 ms, but the inhibition appeared to be of spinal origin while the facilitation is likely cortical.[184]

Another study confirmed that big toe stimulation did not produce SAI and produced MEP facilitation in leg muscles at approximately 55 ms.[185]

3.3.3 Long-Latency Afferent Inhibition

Long-latency afferent inhibition (LAI) represent inhibition of the motor cortex at about 200 ms after median nerve stimulation.[186] Similar inhibition can also be obtained by digit stimulation. Spinal F-wave amplitude was unchanged, supporting the hypothesis that LAI is due to cortical inhibition.[187] LAI was found in lower facial muscle at an ISI of 200 ms following stimulation of the mandibular branch of the facial nerve[61] but not with stimulation of trigeminal afferents,[179] suggesting that LAI could be due to muscle twitch activated by facial nerve stimulation. It likely involves $GABA_A$ but not $GABA_B$ receptor-mediated inhibition as it is decreased by lorazepam and is unaffected by baclofen.[176] The pathway mediating LAI is not known, but the long latency suggests that areas activated by somatosensory input in functional imaging studies, such as the secondary somatosensory area and the basal ganglia, could be involved. Since LAI can be tested with the same experimental setting as SAI, with the difference being the ISI between median nerve stimulation and TMS, it is often tested with SAI in the same experimental run. The factors that influence SAI and LAI have been reviewed in detail.[188]

3.4 STIMULATION OF OTHER CORTICAL AREAS: INTRAHEMISPHERIC (IPSILATERAL) CORTICAL CONNECTIONS TO THE MOTOR CORTEX

The functional connection from different cortical areas to the M1 can be studied using a dual-pulse or twin-coil TMS method, with CS applied to a cortical area and TS applied to the M1. The main findings of published intrahemispheric connection studies are summarized in Table 3.2.

3.4.1 Dorsal Premotor Cortex to M1

A challenge with studying the dorsal premotor cortex (PMd)-to-M1 connection is the close proximity between the two cortical sites. The regular figure-of-eight coil (mid-diameter 7 cm) is too big, and custom-made smaller coils are required. Civardi et al. used two 4 cm coils with the conditioning coil placed 3–5 cm anterior to the hot spot for the FDI muscle to study the left PMd-to-M1 connection. M1 inhibition was observed with CS at 0.9 AMT and facilitation with CS at 1.2 AMT at an ISI of 6 ms. Voluntary

TABLE 3.2. Findings of intrahemispheric cortco-cortical interactions studied with dual site TMS

Cortical area	Conditioning Stimulus coil				Test Stimulus coil			ISI (ms)	Condition	Interaction	Reference
	Location	Size (cm)	Induced current direction	Intensity	Size (cm)	Induced current direction	Intensity				
L-PMd	3-5 cm ant to M1	4	AP	0.9 AMT	4	PA	FDI, rest 1.2 RMT, active 0.2-0.5 mV	6	Rest, ↓ with activation	↓	Civardi 2001
				1.2 AMT			FDI, 1.2 RMT,		Rest	↑	
L-PMd	3 cm ant to M1	5.5e	AP	1.1 RMT	5.5e	PA	FDI, 1 mV	6	Rest	↑	Koch 2007
L-PMd	3 cm ant to M1	5.5	AP	0.8 AMT, 0.9 RMT	9e	PA	FDI	4,6	Rest	↔	Baumer 2009
	5 cm ant to M1 & 6 cm lat to vertex			0.8 AMT, 0.9 RMT				2-10		↔	
	as close as technically possible			0.8, 0.9 AMT; 0.9, 1.1 RMT				2-10		↓0.9 AMT, 8 ms; 1.1 RMT, 2, 4 ms	
L-PMd	4.5 cm dorsolateral and 3 cm anterior to M1	2.5e	AP	0.9 AMT	7e	PA	FDI, 0.5-1.5 mV	4, 6	Rest	↓	Weissbach 2015
				0.8 AMT or 1.1 RMT				4,6,8		↔	
L-PMd	2.5 cm anterior and 1 cm medial to M1	4	AP	0.9 AMT	5	PA	FDI, 1 mV	4,6	Rest	↓ young, ↔ older	Ni 2015
				1.1 AMT				4		↑ young, ↓ older	

(continued)

TABLE 3.2. CONTINUED

	Conditioning Stimulus coil				Test Stimulus coil						
Cortical area	Location	Size (cm)	Induced current direction	Intensity	Size (cm)	Induced current direction	Intensity	ISI (ms)	Condition	Interaction	Reference
L-PMd	Anterior-medial to M1, 3-4 cm between coils	5.6x10.4	PA (2nd phase biphasic)	0.7,0.9 RMT	5.6x10.4	PA (2nd phase biphasic)	FDI, 0.5 mV	1.2, 2.4, 2.8, 4.4	Rest	↑	Groppa 2011, Groppa 2012
L-PMd	2.5 cm ant and 1 cm medial to M1	4	AP	0.9 AMT	5	PA	FDI, 1.5 mV	4,6,8	Rest Grasping	↔ ↑	Vesia 2018
L-PMv (BA44)	NV	7e	MP	0.8 RMT	7e	PA	FDI, 1.2RMT	6,8	Rest Power grip Precision grip	↑ ↔ ↑	Davare 2008
L PMv, BA6 or 44	3 cm anterior and 2.5 cm lateral to M1	5.5	PM	0.8 AMT 0.9 AMT 0.9 RMT 1.1 RMT	9e	PA	FDI	4,6,8 2-10 2,4,6 2,4,10	Rest	↑ ↔ → →	Baumer 2009
L-DLPFC (BA46)	NV	5e	PM	1.05 RMT	7e	PA	FDI, APB, 1 mV	6, 8, 12	Free choice task Specified choice task	↑SOA 100 ms ↑SOA 75 ms	Hasan 2013
L-DLPFC (BA9)									Free or specified choice	↔	
L& R DLPFC	NV, BA46	4	AP	0.8, 1.2 RMT	5	PA	FDI, 1 mV	4-20	Rest, 20% MVC	↔	Brown 2019

Region	Coil location	Distance	Orientation	Intensity	Pulses	Coil	Muscle	ISI	Condition	Effect	Reference
L & R DLPFC	5 cm ant to M1	4	AM	1.1 RMT	4	PA	FDI, 1 mV	2-30	Rest	↓ 2, 10, 15 20 L hemisphere, ↔ R hemisphere	Wang 2020
Pre-SMA	"as close as possible" to 4 cm anterior to Cz	?	P	1.2 RMT	?	PA	FDI, 1-1.5 mV	6	action selection -conflict	↑	Mars 2009
									non-conflict	↔	
LSMA	4 cm ant to TA M1	7	L	1 AMT for TA	7	PA	FDI, 0.5 mV	2-12	Rest	↔, increasing SICF at 6 ms	Shirota 2012
SMA	4 cm ant to vertex	2.5	Lateral	1.4 AMT	7	PA	FDI, 1 mV	6	Rest	↑	Arai 2012
RPPC, cIPS	P4	7e	PA	0.9 RMT	5e	PA	FDI, 1 mV	4,15	Rest	↑	Koch 2007
				0.7,1,1.1,1.3 RMT				4,15		↔	
L PPC	P3		AP	0.9 RMT				4,15		↔	
	P3		PA	0.9 RMT				4,6		↑	
				1.1 RMT				4,6		↔	
aIPS, mIPS,	NV	5e		0.9 RMT	C,10e			4		↔	
R and L aIPL	NV	7e	PA	0.9 RMT	7e	PA	FDI, 1 mV	2,4	Rest	↓	Karabaanov 2013
L cIPL and pIPL								8		↑	
R cIPL and pIPL								2-8		↔	

TABLE 3.2. CONTINUED

Cortical area	Conditioning Stimulus coil				Test Stimulus coil			ISI (ms)	Condition	Interaction	Reference
	Location	Size (cm)	Induced current direction	Intensity	Size (cm)	Induced current direction	Intensity				
L Medial superior parietal BA5	NV	5i	PA	0.9 RMT	5i	PA	FDI, 1 mV	4-50	Rest	↔	Ziluk 2010
								6	D1 and D2	→	
								40	vibration	↑	
L aIPS	NV	5i	PA	0.9 RMT	5i	PA	FDI, 1.2 RMT	4	Rest	→	Vesia 2013
									Grasp planning	↑	
L SPOC								4-10	Rest	↔	
								4	Transport planning	↑	
L SPOC	NV	4i	PA	0.9 RMT	5i	PA	ADM 0.5 mV	6	Grasp planning, ADM, 6ms	↑	Vesia 2017
							FDI, 1.25 mV;	4,6,8	Rest	↔	
									Action planning	↑	
L S1	NV	2.5	AP	1.4,1.6 AMT	2.5	PA	FDI, 1.25 mV	1	Rest	→	Brown 2019

In all studies, the test stimulus coil was over the motor cortex ipsilateral to the location of the conditioning stimulus coil. Abbreviations. aIPL: anterior inferior parietal lobule, AM: anterior-medial, AP: anterior-posterior, APB: abductor pollicis brevis, BA: Brodmann area, BI: branding iron style, C: circular, cIPS: caudal inferior parietal sulcus, D1: digit 1 (thumb), D2: digit 2 (index finger), DLPFC: dorsolateral prefrontal cortex, e: outer diameter; i: inner diameter, L: left, MP: medial-posterior, MVC: maximum voluntary contraction, O: outer diameter, PA: posterior-anterior, PM: posterior-medial, PMd: dorsal premotor cortex, PMv: ventral premotor cortex, S1: primary somatosensory cortex, SICF: short-interval intracortial facilitation, SMA: supplementary motor area. SPOC: superior parietal-occipital cortex, TA: tibialis anterior contraction slightly reduced the inhibition, and the inhibition was observed only with the conditioning-induced current direction in the AP but not in the PA direction.[189] Koch et al.[190] confirmed that CS at 1.1 RMT placed 3 cm anterior to the motor hot spot facilitated the response to M1. However, another study that placed the coil at 3 cm (8% of distance between nasion and inion) or 5 cm anterior to the M1 hot spot found no inhibition or facilitation, whereas when the coils were placed "as close as technically possible," inhibition was observed at an ISI of 8 ms with 0.9 AMT.[191] In another study, the left PMd was stimulated at 4.5 cm dorsolateral and 3 cm anterior to M1 with a small 2.5 cm coil, and inhibition was observed at 4 and 6 ms at a CS intensity of 90% AMT in normal participants, while a CS at 80% AMT or 110% RMT had no effect on left M1 excitability.[192] Another study applied a CS at 2.5 cm anterior and 1 cm medial to the M1 hot spot, using a 4 cm coil for PMd stimulation and a 5 cm coil for M1 stimulation. Inhibition was observed with a CS at 90% AMT at ISI of 4 and 6 ms, and facilitation with a CS at 110% AMT at ISI of 4 ms in young adults but not in older individuals.[193] However, it has been suggested that the CS in some of these studies might have been applied rostral to the PMd in the left dorsolateral prefrontal cortex.[191,194] Due to the close proximity of the PMd to M1, some studies used custom-designed small coils (56 mm) with the maximum point of stimulation shifted toward the edge of the coil, with an effective distance of 3–4 cm between the two coils.[194,195] With TS to the left M1 *before* CS to left PMd, M1 facilitation was observed at a ISI of 1.2 ms (CS intensity 0.7 or 0.9 RMT),[195] 2.4–2.8 ms, and at about 4.4 ms.[194] The facilitation at 1.2 ms decreased with muscle activation. This is similar to SICF and is consistent with the suggestion that the I wave may be generated from the PMd-to-M1 connection. Diffusion tensor imaging showed that the fractional anisotropy from PMd to M1 correlated with the increase in PMd facilitation during an action selection task.[195] A study used a 40 mm coil to stimulate PMd at 2.5 cm anterior and 1 cm medial to the M1 optimal position for the hand muscles and 50 mm coil to stimulate M1. No interaction was found at rest, but there was M1 facilitation in specific hand muscles during the preparation for an upcoming grasping action.[196]

3.4.2 Ventral Premotor Cortex to M1

The left ventral premotor cortex (PMv) can be targeted by applying a custom 55 mm CS coil at 3 cm anterior and 2.5 cm lateral to the FDI hotspot, inducing current in the medial-posterior direction. The TS coil of M1 needs to be lifted and the intensities adjusted to accommodate the coils. Neuronavigation showed the CS targeted was Brodmann's area (BA) area 6 or 44.[191] Targeting BA44 (caudal portion of the pars opercularis of the inferior frontal gyrus) using neuronavigation can also be used.[197] At CS intensities of 0.8 AMT, M1 excitability was facilitated, but higher CS of 0.8 or 0.9 RMT led to M1 inhibition.[191,197] The inhibition changed to facilitation during a precision grip.[197] Thus, whether the effects are inhibitory or facilitatory critically depends on the CS intensity.[191]

3.4.3 Dorsolateral Prefrontal Cortex to M1

A study used neuronavigation with individual MRI to target BA46 for both right and left dorsolateral prefrontal cortex (DLPFC) with a 40 mm coil and the ipsilateral M1 with a 50 mm coil. No effects of right or left DLPFC stimulation at intensities of 80% and 120% RMT on M1 was found at an ISI of 4–20 ms with target muscle at rest or during slight (20% maximum) tonic voluntary contractions.[198] Another study tested the DLPFC-M1 connection at rest but used an intensity of 110% RMT and located the DLPFC without neuronavigation (5 cm anterior to FDI hot spot). M1 inhibition was observed after left DLPFC stimulation at an ISI of 2 and 10–20 ms, but no change was observed in the right hemisphere.[199]

A study used neuronavigation with individual MRI to locate the left DLPFC (BA46) with a custom 5 cm coil at an intensity of 105% RMT, oriented to induce current in the posterior-medial direction. A regular 7 cm coil was used for M1 stimulation. With an ISI of 6, 8, 12 ms tested, the facilitatory effects were maximum at 12 and were modulated by a free choice or specified choice selection task involving the hand. Targeting a more medial area of the DLPFC, BA9, showed no modulation with the task.[200] In this study, a complete rest condition was not tested.

The effects of DLPFC on M1 assessed with dual-site TMS may be more prominent in the left than the right hemisphere, are sensitive to the stimulus intensities used, and are modulated by task performance.

3.4.4 Pre-Supplementary Motor Area or SMA-to-M1

A study used two "branding iron" type 70 mm TMS coils over the left pre-supplementary motor area (SMA) defined as 3 cm anterior to the optimal site for the right tibialis anterior muscle and over the hand area of left M1. No effect on M1 was found with SMA stimulation at ISI of 2–12 ms but SMA stimulation increased SICF at ISI of 6 ms.[201] Another study used a small 25 mm coil located 4 cm anterior to the vertex for SMA stimulation. M1 facilitation was observed but only with laterally directed SMA current at ISI of 6 ms and an intensity of 140% AMT.[202] In a study that examined action under conflict, the conditioning coil was placed "as close as possible" to a position 4 cm anterior to the Cz position, which was over the pre-SMA, with the handle of the coil pointing anteriorly (inducing posterior-directed current). At an ISI of 6 ms, M1 facilitation was observed during action selection under conflict and not in nonconflict trials.[203] A study using two

50 mm coils with SMA stimulation at 4 cm anterior to Cz with posterior-directed induced current at 140% AMT showed facilitation at an ISI of 6 ms in younger but not in older participants. The facilitation correlated with bimanual performance.[204]

3.4.5 Posterior Parietal Cortex-to-M1 Interaction

Several studies have been performed in the posterior parietal cortex (PPC), with some variations in the protocol used and in the results obtained. The first study used a large 70 mm figure-of-eight coil to stimulate the right PPC at P4, close to the right caudal intraparietal sulcus (cIPS) and oriented to induce posterior to anterior current, and a small 50 mm coil to stimulate the right M1.[205] Facilitation was observed at an ISI of 4 and 15 ms at a CS intensity of 90% RMT but not at lower (70% RMT) or higher (110% and 130% RMT) CS intensities. The finding was also specific to the induced posterior-to-anterior current because reversing the CS current direction abolished the facilitation. Other approaches included using a small 50 mm coil to deliver the CS and a circular coil for the TS[205] or two custom 70 mm (external diameter) "branding iron" style coils with neuronavigation. With CS intensity at 90% RMT, stimulation of anterior inferior parietal lobule (IPL) cause ipsilateral M1 inhibition at 2 and 4 ms for both right and left hemispheres.[206] However, stimulation of central and posterior IPL caused M1 facilitation in the left hemisphere but no facilitation was found in the right hemisphere,[206] which showed different results from a previous study.[205] Moreover, the precise location of the hot spot for inhibition and facilitation from IPL stimulation showed considerable inter-individual variation.[206] The interaction between the left superior parietal occipital cortex (SPOC, identified using neuronavigation) and left M1 has also been examined with a 50 mm coil at M1 and a 40 mm coil at SPOC. The SPOC-M1 connection to different hand muscles was selectively increased during the preparation of different types of grasping.[207]

3.4.6 Medial Superior Parietal Lobule (Area 5) to M1

Two 50 mm inner diameter custom coils with neuronavigation were used to stimulate area 5 and left M1. The CS for area 5 was set at 90% RMT and current oriented to produce posterior-to-anterior current. At rest, no significant change in M1 excitability was found from ISIs of 4 to 50 ms. During vibration of the thumb and index finger, M1 was inhibited at 6 ms and facilitated at 40 ms compared to rest.[208] Another study confirmed that there was no significant effect of superior parietal lobule stimulation on M1 excitability at rest at ISIs of 4 to 10 ms, but the greater degree of inhibitory interaction correlated with a stronger illusion induced by a rubber hand illusion paradigm.[209]

3.4.7 Interactions Between Posterior Parietal Cortex, Ventral Premotor Cortex, and M1

This interaction can be tested using three TMS coils. Neuronavigation was used to place the left PMv coil over the pars opercularis of the inferior frontal gyrus and the PPC coil over the central portion of the left IPL. When PPC stimulation at 80% RMT, which had no effect on M1 excitability, preceded PMv stimulation by 6–15 ms, the inhibitory effect of PMv stimulation at ISIs of 4 and 6 ms was abolished.[210] This effect is likely mediated by connection between PPC and PMv. This triple stimulation technique can be used to study the interactions between different cortical regions.

3.4.8 Interaction Between Somatosensory Cortex and M1

A study used two small (25 mm) coils to test the interactions between left somatosensory cortex (S1) and M1.[211] S1 stimulation inhibited M1 excitability at an ISI of 1 ms and intensities of 140% and 160% AMT. Since the S1-M1 inhibition did not correlate with SICI, voluntary muscle contraction abolished SICI but not S1-M1 inhibition, and SAI increased in the presence of S1-M1 inhibition but increased in the presence of SICI, the results could not be explained by SICI in M1 and supports the notion of a short-latency inhibition of S1 on M1.

Intrahemispheric cortico-cortical connections are often studied with small TMS coils rather than standard size figure-of-eight coils due to the close proximity of the cortical areas being studied. One needs to be cautious in interpreting the coil sizes reported in different studies (Table 3.2). Manufacturers often refer to coil sizes as mid-diameters while many investigators report external or inner diameters. There is no standard way of measuring coil sizes. For example, the standard figure-of-eight coil may be reported as a 7 cm or 9 cm coil.

3.5 INTERHEMISPHERIC CORTICAL CONNECTIONS

3.5.1 Interhemispheric Inhibition Between Motor Cortices

Interhemispheric inhibition (IHI) was originally described for inhibition of the primary motor cortex (M1) from stimulation of the contralateral M1.[212] Studies of IHI are conducted with two coils, with CS applied to one motor cortex and TS applied to the opposite motor cortex (Table 3.1). IHI consists of two phases with maximum inhibition at ISI of 8–10 ms for short-latency IHI (SIHI) and at 40–50 ms for long-latency IHI (LIHI) (Figure 3.14).[66,213] A study that examined ISIs at 0.1 ms increments reported

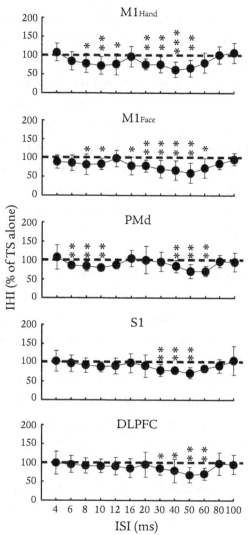

FIGURE 3.14 *The time courses of interhemispheric inhibition (IHI). Time courses of IHI (n = 12) from five different cortical areas (M1$_{Hand}$, M1$_{Face}$, PMd, S1, and dorsolateral prefrontal cortex [DLPFC]) to the left motor cortex. The abscissa indicates the ISI. The ordinate indicates the amplitude of conditioned motor-evoked potential (MEP) expressed as a percentage of the MEP amplitude from TS alone. The dashed lines indicate the MEP amplitude generated by test stimulus (TS) alone (100%). Values less than 100% represent inhibition and values greater than 100% represent facilitation. There are two phases of IHI with maximum inhibition at ISIs of ~10 and ~50 ms for M1$_{Hand}$, M1$_{Face}$, and PMd. For S1 and DFPFC, the early phase of IHI is absent and only the late phase is evident. *P<0.05, **P<0.01, ***P<0.001, compared with TS alone.*

ISI, interstimulus interval; M1, primary motor cortex; PMd, dorsal premotor cortex; S1, primary somatosensory cortex.

FROM NI ET AL., CEREBRAL CORTEX. 2009;19:1654–1665, WITH PERMISSION.

that the maximum SIHI occurred at 9.6 ms on average.[214] As expected, IHI increases with higher CS intensities but is not significantly influenced by the current direction of the CS.[66,213] However, when trial-to-trial variations of the MEP amplitude evoked by the CS were examined, trials with higher CS MEP amplitudes were paradoxically associated with lower SIHI and LIHI.[215] While the mechanisms underlying this observation are not known, one explanation is that spontaneous fluctuations in cortical excitability, which may be related to phases of the mu rhythm, could be synchronized between right and left M1. IHI decreases with higher test MEP amplitude.[212,216] Target muscle contractions contralateral to either the conditioning or test stimuli reduced SIHI and LIHI.[217] Since there is no long-range inhibitory projection across the corpus callosum, IHI is likely mediated by excitatory connections across the corpus callosum that project to inhibitory circuits in the contralateral hemisphere.

IHI is due to cortical inhibition because a test response elicited by anodal electrical stimulation was not suppressed,[212] and there is suppression of descending I waves.[218] However, subcortical mechanisms may contribute because MEPs from pyramidal tract stimulation at the level of the pyramidal decussation were also suppressed by the CS.[219] The hypothesis that SIHI is mediated by the corpus callosum is supported by the finding that it correlates with fractional anisotropy of callosal motor fibers measured by MRI.[220] Some studies found that SIHI is stronger from the dominant to the nondominant hemisphere[221,222] although other studies found no difference.[223] Pharmacological studies showed the LIHI is increased by the GABA$_B$ receptor agonist baclofen, whereas the benzodiazepine midazolam has no effect on SIHI or LIHI.[224] Therefore, LIHI is likely related to GABA$_B$ receptor-mediated inhibition. While both IHI and iSP are related to transcallosal inhibition, they are not mediated by the same circuits and represent complementary measures of ipsilateral inhibition, although LIHI may be related to iSP.

3.5.2 IHI from Other Cortical Areas to the Contralateral Motor Cortex

The main findings of published studies of other areas are summarized in Table 3.3. In addition to stimulation of the contralateral M1, IHI can also be elicited by conditioning stimulation of other cortical areas in the contralateral hemisphere including the face areas of M1, dorsal premotor cortex (PMd), DLPFC, and S1. At these locations, LIHI could be elicited at lower CS intensities than SIHI (Figure 3.14).[213]

Stimulation of right or left PMd at CS intensities of 0.9 RMT produced SIHI (ISI 8 and 10 ms) of the contralateral M1, while the CS over the M1 did not result IHI.[225] However, another study found that SIHI from PMd and M1 both began at a CS intensity of 1.6 AMT.[213] A study reported that right PMd stimulation at 80% AMT and ISI of

TABLE 3.3. Findings of interhemispheric cortco-cortical interactions studied with dual site TMS

Cortical area	Conditioning Stimulus coil				Test Stimulus coil					Interaction	Reference
	Location	Size (cm)	Orientation	Intensity	Size (cm)	Orientation	Intensity	ISI (ms)	Condition		
R PMd	2.5 cm ant, 1 cm medial to M1	5.5e	A,P,M,L	0.9, 1.1 RMT	9e	PA	FDI, 1 mV	8,10	Rest,	↓	Mochizuki 2004
L PMd	cm medial to M1		M	RMT					contraction	↓	
R DLPFC	5 cm ant to M1									↔	
L PMd	3 cm (8% nasion-inion) ant to M1	5.5e	M	1.1RMT	7e	PA	FDI, 1 mV	8	Rest	↓	Koch 2006
R M1	FDI hotspot	F8	M	AMT+ 5%SO	F8	AP	FDI, 0.2-0.4 mV	4-5	Active	↑	Hanajima 2001
R M1	FDI hotspot	5e	PA	FDI 0.5 mV	5e	PA	FDI 0.5 mV	2-6	Rest	↑ (max at 4.5 ms)	Ni 2020
L PMd	3 cm (8% nasion-inion) ant to M1	7e	PA	0.8AMT	7e	AP	FDI, 1 mV	6,8	Rest	↑	Baumer 2006
						PA		8		↑	
							FDI, 0.4-0.5 mV	6,8	Active, 10% MVC	↔	
L M1	FDI hotspot			0.6AMT			FDI, 1 mV	6	Rest	↑	
L M1				0.8AMT		AP		6,8		↑	
L M1							FDI, 0.4-0.5 mV	8	Active, 10% MVC	↑	

(continued)

TABLE 3.3. CONTINUED

Cortical area	Conditioning Stimulus coil				Test Stimulus coil						
	Location	Size (cm)	Orientation	Intensity	Size (cm)	Orientation	Intensity	ISI (ms)	Condition	Interaction	Reference
RM1 hand	FDI hotspot	8e	M	FDI, 1mV	9.5e	PA	FDI, 1 mV	8-12, 20-50	Rest	→	Ni 2009
RM1 face	Masseter hotspot							8-10, 16-60		→	
RDLPFC	5cm ant to M1,NV							30-60		→	
RPMd	2.5cm ant, 1cm medial to M1,NV							6-10, 40-60		→	
RS1	NV							30-50		→	
RcIPS	P4	5e	PA	0.9RMT	7e	PA	FDI, 1 mV	6-8,12	Rest	↑	Koch 2009
				0.7, 1.1 RMT				2-20		↔	
				0.9RMT		AP		13.5		↔	
aIPS	NV					PA		10-12		→	
LcIPS	P3							4-20		↔	
LcIPS	P3			1.1RMT				6,12		↑	

In all studies, the test stimulus coil was over the motor cortex, contralateral to the location of the conditioning stimulus coil. Abbreviations. aIPL: anterior inferior parietal lobule, APB: abductor pollicis brevis, BA: Brodmann area, BI: branding iron style, C: circular, cIPS: caudal inferior parietal sulcus, D1: digit 1 (thumb), D2: digit 2 (index finger), DLPFC: dorsolateral prefrontal cortex, e: outer diameter; F8: figure-of-eight, size not stated; L: left, M: medial, MP: medial-posterior, NV: neuronavigation, PA: posterior-anterior, PM: posterior-medial, PMd: dorsal premotor cortex, PMv: ventral premotor cortex, S1: primary somatosensory cortex, SO: stimulator output

8 ms facilitates but at 110% RMT inhibits left M1 excitability while at rest.[226] With right PMd stimulation at 110% RMT, another study did not find SIHI in left M1, but LIHI was observed at ISI of 40 ms at rest.[227] The right PMd-M1 interactions are modulated during movement preparation.[226,227]

Stimulation of aIPS at 0.9 RMT at ISI of 10–12 ms (SIHI) was found to produce contralateral M1 inhibition.[228]

3.5.3 Interhemispheric Facilitation

A small interhemispheric facilitation (IHF) between the motor cortices has been reported at an ISI of 4–5 ms.[229] This facilitation appears to require specific conditions including small test MEP (~0.3 mV in the FDI muscle) in preactivated muscle evoked by induced current in the AP direction to produce the I3 wave and the conditioning pulse-induced current in the medial direction. Another study showed that IHF can be produced by low-intensity CS (60–80% AMT) whereas higher intensities lead to IHI at an ISI of 6–8 ms with the target muscle at rest or during slight voluntary contraction.[230] A study reported resting IHF using PA-induced current for both conditioning and test stimuli set to produce 0.5 mV MEP in the contralateral FDI muscle at an ISI of 2–6 ms, with maximum IHF at 4.5 ms.[214] In addition to right M1 to left M1 IHF, right PMd to left M1 IHF could be observed.[226,230]

IHF was also observed with stimulation of the right cIPS (P4 position) at 0.9 RMT at an ISI of 6 or 12 ms but not at 10 ms, and with the TS inducing PA-directed current but not AP-directed current. Similar IHF was reported for the left cIPS, but at a higher conditioning intensity of 1.1 RMT.[226] Thus, the precise conditions under which IHF can be observed depend on the CS intensity, ISI, and the current direction of the TS.

A triple-coil study further tested the interactions between the right cIPS/angular gyrus (RAG) and the left angular gyrus (LAG) and left M1.[231] RAG stimulation at 70% RMT and ISI of 15 ms increased left M1 excitability but inhibited the first SICF peak in left M1 and inhibited the response to RAG stimulation followed by M1 stimulation. Moreover, combined RAG and LAG stimulation increased left M1 LICI. These findings suggest that RAG affects left M1 cortical circuits and may involve heterotopic connections.

In summary, double-coil TMS can be used to investigate the functional connectivity of different cortical areas to the M1. With the exception of IHI between the motor cortices, the degrees of inhibition and facilitation for cortico-cortical connections are generally smaller and are often more difficult to reproduce than intracortical circuits such as SICI, ICF, and SICF. The findings often critically depend on the CS intensities and the current directions of both the conditioning and test pulses. The inhibition or facilitation are often modulated in the behavioral context.

3.6 INTERACTION BETWEEN CORTICAL CIRCUITS

The cortical circuits described interact with each other. Their interactions can be studied with a triple stimulation technique that compares the effects of each circuit alone to that of the two circuits applied simultaneously.[152,232] The aim is to examine whether the effects of two circuits applied together is less than (suggests inhibitory interaction) or more than (suggests facilitatory interaction) the expected additive effects.

Sanger et al.[85,106] studied the interactions between SICI and LICI. They found that inhibitory effects of LICI and SICI applied together were less than the expected additive effects of the two inhibitory circuits, suggesting there are inhibitory interactions between SICI and LICI (Figure 3.15).

These studies have to be carefully designed to account for the finding that SICI and LICI are influenced by MEP amplitude. For example, if the first inhibitory circuit lowers the MEP amplitude, the change in inhibitory effect of the second circuit in the presence of the first circuit may be due to changes in MEP amplitude instead of true inhibitory

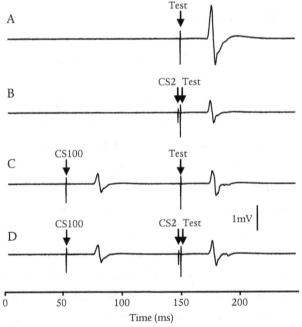

FIGURE 3.15 *The effect of long-interval intracortical inhibition (LICI) on short-interval intracortical inhibition (SICI). Averaged electromyogram (EMG) tracings from a representative study participant are shown. (A) Response to the test pulse alone (58% of maximum stimulator output). (B) Addition of a CS2 pulse (conditioning stimulus, 2 ms before test pulse, 0.8 motor threshold (MT), 30% of maximum stimulator output) inhibited the test motor-evoked potential (MEP), demonstrating SICI. (C) Addition of a CS100 pulse at low intensity of 1.1MT (48% of maximum stimulator output) did not inhibit the response to the test pulse. (D) addition of both CS100 (1.1MT) and CS2 pulses (0.8MT) reduced the inhibitory effect of CS2 and led to higher test MEP amplitude compared to those shown in B.* FROM SANGER ET AL., *J PHYSIOL.* 2001;530:307–317, WITH PERMISSION.

TABLE 3.4. Stimulus conditions used in a triple-pulse TMS paradigm testing for Circuit 1 in the presence of Circuit 2

Condition	Stimuli used					Tested circuit
	CS2	CS1	CS1'	TS	TS'	
A				+		TS alone
B		+		+		Circuit 1 alone
C	+			+		Circuit 2 alone
D					+	TS alone with adjusted TS intensity
E	+				+	Circuit 2 alone with adjusted TS intensity
F		+			+	Circuit 1 alone with adjusted TS intensity
G	+	+			+	Circuit 1 in the presence of Circuit 2

+ = presence of stimulus; CS1 = conditioning stimulus 1 (for Circuit1); CS2 = conditioning stimulus 2 (for Circuit2); TS = test stimulus; TS' = test stimulus with adjusted intensity.

Note that MEP amplitudes in condition A and E are matched, i.e. TS' is adjusted such that CS2 plus TS' yield an MEP of similar amplitude as TS alone. From Ni et al, *Brain Stimulation* 2011; 4: 281-293

interaction. Therefore, control conditions that applied higher TS intensities so that the MEP amplitudes in the presence of the first circuit are the same as "standard" MEP amplitudes (e.g., 1 mV in the FDI muscle) are necessary to examine the second circuit in the presence of the first. A sample experimental design is shown in Table 3.4. The design allowed comparisons between Circuit 1 in the presence of Circuit 2 (G/E) to Circuit 1 alone, matched for MEP amplitude (A/B) and TS intensity (F/D). In order to apply this design in a single experimental run, a system that allows TMS with at least three different stimulus intensities to be delivered in the same coil at short intervals is needed.

A number of interactions between different cortical circuits have been studied. Table 3.5 shows the published findings. A more detailed review of the triple stimulation method to study cortical interactions is available.[232]

3.7 ASSESSMENT OF CORTICAL VERSUS SPINAL EXCITABILITY

MEP amplitudes measured by TMS reflect both cortical and spinal excitability. If an intervention changes MEP amplitude, further studies are needed to determine if it occurs at the cortical or spinal level, or both. These involve stimulation at or below the level of the axon of the corticospinal neurons. If changes are observed with MEP from TMS but not with stimulation at the corticospinal axons or with subcortical stimulation, then the changes are largely mediated at the cortical level. The different methods that can be used are listed here.

TABLE 3.5. Summary of known interaction among cortical circuits

Target circuit	Conditioning circuit								
	SICI	ICF	LICI	iSP	SIHI	LIHI	SAI	LAI	CBI
SICF							↑		
CBI			↓						
LAI									
SAI	↓								
LIHI	↓	↔	↓		↔				
SIHI	↓	↔	↓			↔			
iSP	↓								
LICI					↓	↓	↓	↓	
ICF			↔	↑	↔	↔		↔	↑
SICI			↓	↓	↓	↔	↓	↔	↓

↑: conditioning circuit facilitates the target circuit, ↔: conditioning and target circuits do not affect each other- their effects are additive, ↓: conditioning circuit inhibits the target circuit

CBI: cerebellar inhibition, ICF: intracortical facilitation, iSP: ipsilateral silent period, LAI: long-latency afferent inhibition, LICI: long-interval intracortical inhibition, LIHI: long-latency interhemispheric inhibition, SAI: short-latency afferent inhibition, SICI: short-interval intracortical facilitation, SIHI: short-interval interhemispheric inhibition, SP: silent period

Based on.[1-3]

1. Ni Z, Muller-Dahlhaus F, Chen R, Ziemann U. Triple-pulse TMS to study interactions between neural circuits in human cortex. Brain Stimul. 2011;4(4):281–293.
2. Udupa K, Ni Z, Gunraj C, Chen R. Effects of short-latency afferent inhibition on short-interval intracortical inhibition. JNeurophysiol. 2014;111(6):1350–1361.
3. Cash RF, Isayama R, Gunraj CA, Ni Z, Chen R. The influence of sensory afferent input on local motor cortical excitatory circuitry in humans. Journal of Physiology (London). 2015;593(7):1667–1684.

1. *Different TMS current directions.* Medially directed current in the motor cortex preferentially evokes the D wave, which is likely due to activation at the axon of corticospinal neurons. Posteriorly or anteriorly directed currents have longer latencies, preferentially activate I waves, and are likely due to activation of cortical neurons through interneurons. If changes are seen with MEP from posteriorly or anteriorly directed current but not with medially directed current, it is likely due to changes in cortical excitability. Relatively low-intensity stimulations should be used because higher intensities will lead to activation of both D and I waves regardless of current direction. The advantage of this method is that it is easy to perform and relatively painless. However, the MEP latencies of each individual needs

to be verified as there are individual variations in the ability to recruit D and I waves with different current directions.[54]

2. *Anodal transcranial electrical stimulation (TES).* This method uses a high-voltage (up to 750 V), brief electrical current (~100 μs) applied to the scalp.[233] TES activates neurons at the axon, preferentially producing D waves.[234] The anode is placed over the motor cortex. For upper limb muscles, this is typically defined as the TMS hot spot and the cathode is placed on the vertex. For stimulation of leg representation, the anode can be placed at Cz and the cathode at Fz.[235] The advantage of this method is that it may provide clearer separation between D and I waves than using TMS in different current directions, although high-intensity TES also produces I waves. The disadvantage is that the stimulation is painful due to activation of scalp structures.

3. *TES at the level of pyramidal decussation (cervicomedullary stimulation).* The electrodes are placed over the mastoid processes bilaterally, about 5 cm lateral to the inion.[236,237] The stimulation intensities are increased in a stepwise manner until stable response is obtained. The advantage of this method is that the responses are not contaminated by cortical response. However, it is even more painful than TES over the motor cortex. The population of corticospinal fibers activated may be different from that of TMS of the motor cortex, although one study suggested that similar population of fibers are activated.[238] However, cervicomedullary stimulation produces a single volley in contrast to multiple volleys from cortical stimulation,[239] which may have different effects on spinal motor neurons.

4. *TMS at the level of pyramidal decussation.* This method also stimulates the pyramidal tract at the level of the foramen magnum. A double-cone coil placed at over or just below the inion induces upward current in the brain, with the participant's head tilted forward at 30–45 degrees.[237,240] Magnetic stimulation is usually given during voluntary contraction to lower the response threshold. This method is less painful than electrical stimulation at the same location.

5. *Spinal electrical stimulation.* High-voltage electrical stimulation is used to activate the descending tracts in the spinal cord projecting to leg muscles.[237,241] The response amplitudes are often small, and voluntary muscle activation will increase the response. To stimulate the fibers projecting to leg muscles, the cathode can be placed at C7 and the anode placed 10 cm below,[235] or the cathode can be placed in the upper thoracic spine between T1 and T6, and the anode 5–10 cm above it.[241,242] This procedure is painful.

6. *H-reflex.* H-reflex is a monosynaptic reflex from activation of Ia afferents that synapse to the spinal motor neuron in the spinal cord. It can be used to estimate spinal excitability. In some muscles such as the gastrocnemius muscle, the H-reflex is

relatively easy to obtain. In the arm, it can be obtained from the flexor carpi radialis muscle in most participants. However, it is difficult to obtain in many other limb muscles at rest although it can be recorded from more muscles with background contraction and averaging.

7. *F-wave*. F-waves are obtained from supramaximal stimulation of peripheral nerves. The impulses travel antidromically to the cell body of the spinal motor neuron, then turn back and travel orthodromically to the target muscle. It is mainly recorded in distal muscles but can be obtained in more muscles than the H-reflex. However, F-wave is not elicited in every trial. Typically, 20 trials are performed, and F-wave persistence and amplitudes are used to estimate spinal excitability. Moreover, the spinal motor neuron pool activated by F-waves is different from that activated by TMS and voluntary muscle contraction.

8. *Recording of descending corticospinal waves*. This can only be done in patients who had spinal epidural electrodes implanted, typically for treatment of chronic pain. Changes in descending I waves provide good evidence for changes in cortical excitability. However, changes in cortical excitability do not exclude changes in spinal excitability.

3.8 NUMBER OF TMS PULSES REQUIRED AND OPTIMAL INTERTRIAL INTERVALS TO ASSESS CORTICOSPINAL EXCITABILITY

MEP amplitudes from TMS vary considerably from trial to trial, in part related to different phases of EEG. Therefore, multiple trials are needed to assess corticospinal excitability. A guideline from the International Federation of Clinical Neurophysiology recommended 8–10 trials per condition for paired TMS studies.[5] A meta-analysis that examined four studies concluded that five stimuli provide excellent within-session MEP amplitude reliability, and 10 stimuli are required to achieve consistent between-session reliability in MEP amplitude.[243] However, another study suggested that 30 stimuli are needed to obtain MEP amplitudes with a 100% probability of achieving a 95% confidence interval, based on the results of using 40 stimuli as the gold standard.[244] In a study that used neuronavigated TMS, the minimum number of trials to obtain reliable measurement according to internal consistency analysis was 18 for MEP amplitude, 20 for SICI, and 23 for ICF.[245]

Many studies used intertrial intervals of 5–6 s. A study tested intertrial intervals from 1 to 10 s in three blocks of 10 trials each. There were significant effects of intertrial interval but the effects were not consistent from participant to participant, and there was also sig-nificant effect of block number.[246] Another study tested intertrial intervals from 5 to 20 s and reported that MEP amplitudes were higher and less variable for intertrial interval of 15 and 20 s compared to 5 s, although all the intertrial intervals tested had good within- and between-session reliability.[247] With intertrial intervals of 5 s, measurement of the MEP re-cruitment curve with decreasing stimulus intensity led to higher MEP amplitude than with increasing stimulus intensity. This effect was not observed with intertrial intervals of 20 s.[248]

While there is debate regarding the optimal number of trials for single and paired TMS measures, a large number of trials (in the range of 20–30) as well as longer intertrial intervals (in the order of 15–20 s) could potentially provide a better estimate of MEP amplitude than a lower number of trials and shorter intertrial intervals. However, in de-signing studies, one has to consider that using a large number of trials and long intertrial intervals will lead to longer experimental duration and may lead to participant fatigue and reduce the number of parameters that can be assessed. In practice, about 15 trials for each condition are likely sufficient as the gain in reliability decreases with increasing number of trials.

3.9 CLINICAL DIAGNOSTIC UTILITY OF TMS

TMS has established clinical diagnostic utility in several neurological disorders.[4,23]

3.9.1 Multiple Sclerosis

CMCT and TST studies can provide evidence of subclinical lesions for the diagnosis of multiple sclerosis. CMCT and MEP latency may be related to disease severity and fa-tigue.[249] Composite TMS indices based on CMCT as well as measures of corticospinal excitability, such as motor thresholds, SICI, iSP, and IHI, correlate with disability and has potential for disease monitoring.[250,251]

3.9.2 Amyotrophic Lateral Sclerosis

CMCT and TST studies can be used to demonstrate upper motor neuron dysfunction to support the diagnosis for amyotrophic lateral sclerosis (ALS). SICI determined by a threshold tracking method is also useful in the early diagnosis of ALS,[252] although SICI abnormalities are not specific to ALS. Reduced SICI may also be a marker of poor prog-nosis in ALS.[253] Patients who have no motor response (inexcitable motor cortex) may have a more malignant disease course.[254]

3.9.3 Myelopathy

CMCT measurements can be used together with other diagnostic modalities in the diagnosis and follow-up of patients with cervical myelopathy.[23,255,256] In a group of 231 patients, CMCT demonstrated 98% sensitivity and specificity for the diagnosis of compressive cervical myelopathy using MRI as the gold standard.[257] It may also be useful for determining the level of compression by recording from muscles above and below the level of compression.[26] CMCT to the tibialis anterior muscle improved after surgery for cervical spondylotic myelopathy.[258]

3.9.4 Other Disorders

TMS has potential clinical utility in cerebellar disorders, facial nerve disorders, dementia, movement disorders, stroke, migraine, and chronic pain.[23]

3.9.5 Use of Navigated TMS in Presurgical Mapping

Precise mapping of the somatotopic representation in M1 and the language areas is important to allow maximum resection of brain tumors while preserving motor and language functions. TMS is a useful noninvasive tool to map the location of the motor cortex and the language areas preoperatively.[259] Neuronavigated TMS is approved by the US Food and Drug Administration (FDA) for presurgical mapping of motor and language functions. In a study of 155 patients, navigated TMS reliably predicted the response to intraoperative TES to locate the motor cortical area,[260] and results are more accurate than with fMRI.[261] Navigated TMS was also reliable for mapping of the M1 in patients with recurrent glioma.[262] SICF may improve the efficacy of navigated TMS for mapping of the lower extremities compared to single-pulse TMS.[263]

For language mapping, rTMS is delivered during a language task such as a picture naming task. Several studies showed that the results of language mapping with navigated TMS correlated well with the results of invasive direct cortical stimulation.[264,265] In a study of 216 patients with brain tumors, the lesion-to-tract distances derived from navigated TMS–based diffusion tensor imaging fiber tracking was found to predict the occurrence of postoperative motor or language deficits.[266]

3.10 CONCLUSION

Single-, paired-, and triple-pulse TMS techniques are powerful methods to study motor cortical excitability, inhibition, facilitation, cortical representations, and interactions between cortical areas. Details of the technique, including stimulus intensities, current direction, precise coil locations, and interstimulus intervals, critically influence the results. These techniques have wide applicability in the field of motor and cognitive neuroscience and have clinical applications.

REFERENCES

1. Julkunen P, Säisänen L, Danner N, et al. Comparison of navigated and non-navigated transcranial magnetic stimulation for motor cortex mapping, motor threshold and motor evoked potentials. *Neuroimage.* Feb 1 2009;44(3):790–795. doi:10.1016/j.neuroimage.2008.09.040
2. Jung NH, Delvendahl I, Kuhnke NG, Hauschke D, Stolle S, Mall V. Navigated transcranial magnetic stimulation does not decrease the variability of motor-evoked potentials. *Brain Stimul.* Apr 2010;3(2):87–94. doi:10.1016/j.brs.2009.10.003
3. Harquel S, Diard J, Raffin E, et al. Automatized set-up procedure for transcranial magnetic stimulation protocols. *Neuroimage.* Jun 2017;153:307–318. doi:10.1016/j.neuroimage.2017.04.001
4. Groppa S, Oliviero A, Eisen A, et al. A practical guide to diagnostic transcranial magnetic stimulation: Report of an IFCN committee. *Clin Neurophysiol.* May 2012;123(5):858–882. doi:10.1016/j.clinph.2012.01.010
5. Rossini PM, Burke D, Chen R, et al. Non-invasive electrical and magnetic stimulation of the brain, spinal cord, roots and peripheral nerves: Basic principles and procedures for routine clinical and research application. An updated report from an I.F.C.N. Committee. *Clin Neurophysiol.* Jun 2015;126(6):1071–1107. doi:10.1016/j.clinph.2015.02.001
6. Mills KR, Nithi KA. Corticomotor threshold to magnetic stimulation: Normal values and repeatability. *Muscle Nerve.* May 1997;20(5):570–576. doi:10.1002/(sici)1097-4598(199705)20:5<570::aid-mus5>3.0.co;2-6
7. Tranulis C, Guéguen B, Pham-Scottez A, et al. Motor threshold in transcranial magnetic stimulation: Comparison of three estimation methods. *Clin Neurophysiol.* Jan-Feb 2006;36(1):1–7. doi:10.1016/j.neucli.2006.01.005
8. Pridmore S, Fernandes Filho JA, Nahas Z, Liberatos C, George MS. Motor threshold in transcranial magnetic stimulation: A comparison of a neurophysiological method and a visualization of movement method. *J ECT.* Mar 1998;14(1):25–27.
9. Chen R, Tam A, Bütefisch C, et al. Intracortical inhibition and facilitation in different representations of the human motor cortex. *J Neurophysiol.* Dec 1998;80(6):2870–2881. doi:10.1152/jn.1998.80.6.2870
10. Corp DT, Bereznicki HGK, Clark GM, et al. Large-scale analysis of interindividual variability in single and paired-pulse TMS data. *Clin Neurophysiol.* Jul 6 2021;doi:10.1016/j.clinph.2021.06.014
11. Chen R, Samii A, Caños M, Wassermann EM, Hallett M. Effects of phenytoin on cortical excitability in humans. *Neurology.* Sep 1997;49(3):881–883. doi:10.1212/wnl.49.3.881
12. Ziemann U, Lönnecker S, Steinhoff BJ, Paulus W. Effects of antiepileptic drugs on motor cortex excitability in humans: A transcranial magnetic stimulation study. *Ann Neurol.* Sep 1996;40(3):367–378. doi:10.1002/ana.410400306
13. Ziemann U, Reis J, Schwenkreis P, et al. TMS and drugs revisited 2014. *Clin Neurophysiol.* Oct 2015;126(10):1847–1868. doi:10.1016/j.clinph.2014.08.028
14. Chen R, Anastakis DJ, Haywood CT, Mikulis DJ, Manktelow RT. Plasticity of the human motor system following muscle reconstruction: A magnetic stimulation and functional magnetic resonance imaging study. *Clin Neurophysiol.* 2003;114(12):2434–2446.
15. Devanne H, Lavoie BA, Capaday C. Input-output properties and gain changes in the human corticospinal pathway. *Exp Brain Res.* Apr 1997;114(2):329–338. doi:10.1007/pl00005641
16. Di Lazzaro V, Restuccia D, Oliviero A, et al. Effects of voluntary contraction on descending volleys evoked by transcranial stimulation in conscious humans. *J Physiol.* Apr 15 1998;508 (Pt 2)(Pt 2):625–633. doi:10.1111/j.1469-7793.1998.625bq.x
17. Brum M, Cabib C, Valls-Solé J. Clinical value of the assessment of changes in MEP duration with voluntary contraction. *Front Neurosci.* 2015;9:505. doi:10.3389/fnins.2015.00505

18. Magistris MR, Rösler KM, Truffert A, Myers JP. Transcranial stimulation excites virtually all motor neurons supplying the target muscle: A demonstration and a method improving the study of motor evoked potentials. *Brain*. Mar 1998;121 (Pt 3):437–450. doi:10.1093/brain/121.3.437

19. Ridding MC, Rothwell JC. Stimulus/response curves as a method of measuring motor cortical excitability in man. *Electroencephalogr Clin Neurophysiol*. Oct 1997;105(5):340–344. doi:10.1016/s0924-980x(97)00041-6

20. Rosenkranz K, Williamon A, Rothwell JC. Motorcortical excitability and synaptic plasticity is enhanced in professional musicians. *J Neurosci*. May 9 2007;27(19):5200–5206. doi:10.1523/jneurosci.0836-07.2007

21. Schmidt S, Bathe-Peters R, Fleischmann R, Rönnefarth M, Scholz M, Brandt SA. Nonphysiological factors in navigated TMS studies: Confounding covariates and valid intracortical estimates. *Hum Brain Mapp*. Jan 2015;36(1):40–49. doi:10.1002/hbm.22611

22. Mills KR. *Magnetic Stimulation of the Human Nervous System*. Oxford University Press; 1999.

23. Chen R, Cros D, Curra A, et al. The clinical diagnostic utility of transcranial magnetic stimulation: Report of an IFCN committee. *Clin Neurophysiol*. 2008;119(3):504–532.

24. Chokroverty S, Picone MA, Chokroverty M. Percutaneous magnetic coil stimulation of human cervical vertebral column: Site of stimulation and clinical application. *Electroencephalogr Clin Neurophysiol*. Oct 1991;81(5):359–365. doi:10.1016/0168-5597(91)90025-s

25. Claus D. Central motor conduction: Method and normal results. *Muscle Nerve*. Dec 1990;13(12):1125–1132. doi:10.1002/mus.880131207

26. Chan KM, Nasathurai S, Chavin JM, Brown WF. The usefulness of central motor conduction studies in the localization of cord involvement in cervical spondylytic myelopathy. *Muscle Nerve*. Sep 1998;21(9):1220–1223. doi:10.1002/(sici)1097-4598(199809)21:9<1220::aid-mus18>3.0.co;2-v

27. Rosler KM, Petrow E, Mathis J, Aranyi Z, Hess CW, Magistris MR. Effect of discharge desynchronization on the size of motor evoked potentials: An analysis. *Clin Neurophysiol*. 2002;113(11):1680–1687.

28. Grapperon AM, Verschueren A, Duclos Y, et al. Association between structural and functional corticospinal involvement in amyotrophic lateral sclerosis assessed by diffusion tensor MRI and triple stimulation technique. *Muscle Nerve*. Apr 2014;49(4):551–557. doi:10.1002/mus.23957

29. Hofstadt-van Oy U, Keune PM, Muenssinger J, Hagenburger D, Oschmann P. Normative data and long-term test-retest reliability of the triple stimulation technique (TST) in multiple sclerosis. *Clin Neurophysiol*. Feb 2015;126(2):356–364. doi:10.1016/j.clinph.2014.05.032

30. Giffroy X, Dive D, Kaux JF, et al. Is the triple stimulation technique a better quantification tool of motor dysfunction than motor evoked potentials in multiple sclerosis? *Acta Neurologica Belgica*. Mar 2019;119(1):47–54. doi:10.1007/s13760-018-1001-1

31. Wassermann EM, McShane LM, Hallett M, Cohen LG. Noninvasive mapping of muscle representations in human motor cortex. *Electroencephalogr Clin Neurophysiol*. Feb 1992;85(1):1–8. doi:10.1016/0168-5597(92)90094-r

32. Kleim JA, Kleim ED, Cramer SC. Systematic assessment of training-induced changes in corticospinal output to hand using frameless stereotaxic transcranial magnetic stimulation. *Nature Protocols*. 2007;2(7):1675–1684. doi:10.1038/nprot.2007.206

33. van de Ruit M, Perenboom MJ, Grey MJ. TMS brain mapping in less than two minutes. *Brain Stimul*. Mar-Apr 2015;8(2):231–239. doi:10.1016/j.brs.2014.10.020

34. Jonker ZD, van der Vliet R, Hauwert CM, et al. TMS motor mapping: Comparing the absolute reliability of digital reconstruction methods to the golden standard. *Brain Stimul*. Mar-Apr 2019;12(2):309–313. doi:10.1016/j.brs.2018.11.005

35. Classen J, Knorr U, Werhahn KJ, et al. Multimodal output mapping of human central motor representation on different spatial scales. *J Physiol*. Oct 1 1998;512 (Pt 1)(Pt 1):163–179. doi:10.1111/j.1469-7793.1998.163bf.x

36. Cavaleri R, Schabrun SM, Chipchase LS. The reliability and validity of rapid transcranial magnetic stimulation mapping. *Brain Stimul*. Nov-Dec 2018;11(6):1291–1295. doi:10.1016/j.brs.2018.07.043

37. Wilson SA, Thickbroom GW, Mastaglia FL. Transcranial magnetic stimulation mapping of the motor cortex in normal subjects: The representation of two intrinsic hand muscles. *J Neurol Sci*. Sep 1993;118(2):134–144. doi:10.1016/0022-510x(93)90102-5

38. Uy J, Ridding MC, Miles TS. Stability of maps of human motor cortex made with transcranial magnetic stimulation. *Brain Topogr*. Summer 2002;14(4):293–297. doi:10.1023/a:1015752711146

39. Weiss C, Nettekoven C, Rehme AK, et al. Mapping the hand, foot and face representations in the primary motor cortex: Retest reliability of neuronavigated TMS versus functional MRI. *Neuroimage*. Feb 1 2013;66:531–542. doi:10.1016/j.neuroimage.2012.10.046

40. Raffin E, Pellegrino G, Di Lazzaro V, Thielscher A, Siebner HR. Bringing transcranial mapping into shape: Sulcus-aligned mapping captures motor somatotopy in human primary motor hand area. *Neuroimage*. Oct 15 2015;120:164–175. doi:10.1016/j.neuroimage.2015.07.024

41. Kraus D, Gharabaghi A. Projecting navigated TMS sites on the gyral anatomy decreases inter-subject variability of cortical motor maps. *Brain Stimul*. Jul-Aug 2015;8(4):831–837. doi:10.1016/j.brs.2015.03.006

42. Harquel S, Bacle T, Beynel L, Marendaz C, Chauvin A, David O. Mapping dynamical properties of cortical microcircuits using robotized TMS and EEG: Towards functional cytoarchitectonics. *Neuroimage*. Jul 15 2016;135:115–124. doi:10.1016/j.neuroimage.2016.05.009

43. Kantelhardt SR, Fadini T, Finke M, et al. Robot-assisted image-guided transcranial magnetic stimulation for somatotopic mapping of the motor cortex: A clinical pilot study. *Acta Neurochirurgica*. Feb 2010;152(2):333–343. doi:10.1007/s00701-009-0565-1

44. Giuffre A, Kahl CK, Zewdie E, et al. Reliability of robotic transcranial magnetic stimulation motor mapping. *J Neurophysiol*. Jan 1 2021;125(1):74–85. doi:10.1152/jn.00527.2020

45. Giuffre A, Zewdie E, Carlson HL, et al. Robotic transcranial magnetic stimulation motor maps and hand function in adolescents. *Physiol Rep*. Apr 2021;9(7):e14801. doi:10.14814/phy2.14801

46. Ahdab R, Ayache SS, Brugières P, Farhat WH, Lefaucheur JP. The hand motor hotspot is not always located in the hand knob: A neuronavigated transcranial magnetic stimulation study. *Brain Topogr*. Jul 2016;29(4):590–597. doi:10.1007/s10548-016-0486-2

47. Lotze M, Kaethner RJ, Erb M, Cohen LG, Grodd W, Topka H. Comparison of representational maps using functional magnetic resonance imaging and transcranial magnetic stimulation. *Clin Neurophysiol*. Feb 2003;114(2):306–312. doi:10.1016/s1388-2457(02)00380-2

48. Patton HD, Amassian VE. Single and multiple unit analysis of the cortical stage of pyramdial tract activation. *J Neurophysiol*. 1954;17:345–363.

49. Kaneko K, Kawai S, Fuchigami Y, Morita H, Ofuji A. The effect of current direction induced by transcranial magnetic stimulation on the corticospinal excitability in human brain. *Electroencephalogr Clin Neurophysiol*. Dec 1996;101(6):478–482. doi:10.1016/s0013-4694(96)96021-x

50. Werhahn KJ, Fong JK, Meyer BU, et al. The effect of magnetic coil orientation on the latency of surface EMG and single motor unit responses in the first dorsal interosseous muscle. *Electroencephalogr Clin Neurophysiol*. Apr 1994;93(2):138–146. doi:10.1016/0168-5597(94)90077-9

51. Sakai K, Ugawa Y, Terao Y, Hanajima R, Furubayashi T, Kanazawa I. Preferential activation of different I waves by transcranial magnetic stimulation with a figure-of-eight-shaped coil. *Exp Brain Res*. Jan 1997;113(1):24–32. doi:10.1007/bf02454139

52. Di Lazzaro V, Oliviero A, Saturno E, et al. The effect on corticospinal volleys of reversing the direction of current induced in the motor cortex by transcranial magnetic stimulation. *Exp Brain Res*. May 2001;138(2):268–273. doi:10.1007/s002210100722

53. Ni Z, Charab S, Gunraj C, et al. Transcranial magnetic stimulation in different current directions activates separate cortical circuits. *J Neurophysiol*. Feb 2011;105(2):749–756. doi:10.1152/jn.00640.2010

54. Hamada M, Murase N, Hasan A, Balaratnam M, Rothwell JC. The role of interneuron networks in driving human motor cortical plasticity. *Cerebral Cortex (New York, NY: 1991)*. Jul 2013;23(7):1593–1605. doi:10.1093/cercor/bhs147

55. Di Lazzaro V, Oliviero A, Pilato F, et al. The physiological basis of transcranial motor cortex stimulation in conscious humans. *Clin Neurophysiol*. Feb 2004;115(2):255–266. doi:10.1016/j.clinph.2003.10.009

56. Chen R, Lozano AM, Ashby P. Mechanism of the silent period following transcranial magnetic stimulation: Evidence from epidural recordings. *Exp Brain Res*. Oct 1999;128(4):539–542. doi:10.1007/s002210050878

57. Ni Z, Gunraj C, Wagle-Shukla A, et al. Direct demonstration of inhibitory interactions between long interval intracortical inhibition and short interval intracortical inhibition. *J Physiol*. Jun 15 2011;589(Pt 12):2955–2962. doi:10.1113/jphysiol.2011.207928

58. Paradiso GO, Cunic DI, Gunraj CA, Chen R. Representation of facial muscles in human motor cortex. *J Physiol*. Aug 15 2005;567(Pt 1):323–336. doi:10.1113/jphysiol.2005.088542

59. Sohn YH, Voller B, Dimyan M, et al. Cortical control of voluntary blinking: A transcranial magnetic stimulation study. *Clin Neurophysiol*. Feb 2004;115(2):341–347. doi:10.1016/j.clinph.2003.10.035

60. Triggs WJ, Ghacibeh G, Springer U, Bowers D. Lateralized asymmetry of facial motor evoked potentials. *Neurology*. Aug 23 2005;65(4):541–544. doi:10.1212/01.wnl.0000172916.91302.e7

61. Pilurzi G, Hasan A, Saifee TA, Tolu E, Rothwell JC, Deriu F. Intracortical circuits, sensorimotor integration and plasticity in human motor cortical projections to muscles of the lower face. *J Physiol*. Apr 1 2013;591(7):1889–1906. doi:10.1113/jphysiol.2012.245746

62. Brouwer B, Ashby P. Corticospinal projections to upper and lower limb spinal motoneurons in man. *Electroencephalogr Clin Neurophysiol*. Dec 1990;76(6):509–519. doi:10.1016/0013-4694(90)90002-2

63. Kesar TM, Stinear JW, Wolf SL. The use of transcranial magnetic stimulation to evaluate cortical excitability of lower limb musculature: Challenges and opportunities. *Restorative Neurol Neurosci*. 2018;36(3):333–348. doi:10.3233/rnn-170801

64. Terao Y, Ugawa Y, Hanajima R, et al. Predominant activation of I1-waves from the leg motor area by transcranial magnetic stimulation. *Brain Res*. Mar 17 2000;859(1):137–146. doi:10.1016/s0006-8993(00)01975-2

65. Ziemann U, Ishii K, Borgheresi A, et al. Dissociation of the pathways mediating ipsilateral and contralateral motor-evoked potentials in human hand and arm muscles. *J Physiol*. Aug 1 1999;518(Pt 3)(Pt 3):895–906. doi:10.1111/j.1469-7793.1999.0895p.x

66. Chen R, Yung D, Li JY. Organization of ipsilateral excitatory and inhibitory pathways in the human motor cortex. *J Neurophysiol*. Mar 2003;89(3):1256–1264. doi:10.1152/jn.00950.2002

67. Taga M, Charalambous CC, Raju S, et al. Corticoreticulospinal tract neurophysiology in an arm and hand muscle in healthy and stroke subjects. *J Physiol*. Aug 2021;599(16):3955–3971. doi:10.1113/jp281681

68. Wassermann EM, Pascual-Leone A, Hallett M. Cortical motor representation of the ipsilateral hand and arm. *Exp Brain Res*. 1994;100(1):121–132. doi:10.1007/bf00227284

69. Bawa P, Hamm JD, Dhillon P, Gross PA. Bilateral responses of upper limb muscles to transcranial magnetic stimulation in human subjects. *Exp Brain Res*. Oct 2004;158(3):385–390. doi:10.1007/s00221-004-2031-x

70. Tazoe T, Perez MA. Selective activation of ipsilateral motor pathways in intact humans. *J Neurosci*. Oct 15 2014;34(42):13924–13934. doi:10.1523/jneurosci.1648-14.2014

71. Maitland S, Baker SN. Ipsilateral motor evoked potentials as a measure of the reticulospinal tract in age-related strength changes. *Front Aging Neurosci*. 2021;13:612352. doi:10.3389/fnagi.2021.612352

72. Cantello R, Gianelli M, Civardi C, Mutani R. Magnetic brain stimulation: The silent period after the motor evoked potential. *Neurology*. 1992;42(10):1951–1959.

73. Fuhr P, Agostino R, Hallett M. Spinal motor neuron excitability during the silent period after cortical stimulation. *Electroencephalogr Clin Neurophysiol*. 1991;81:257–262.

74. Inghilleri M, Berardelli A, Cruccu G, Manfredi M. Silent period evoked by transcranial stimulation of the human motor cortex and cervicomedullary junction. *J Physiol*. 1993;466:521–534.

75. Wassermann EM, Pascual-Leone A, Valls-Sole J, Toro C, Cohen LG, Hallett M. Topography of the inhibitory and excitatory responses to transcranial magnetic stimulation in a hand muscle. *Electroencephalogr Clin Neurophysiol*. 1993;89(6):424–433.

76. Triggs WJ, Macdonell RA, Cros D, Chippa KH, Shahani BT, Day BJ. Motor inhibition and excitation are independent effects of magnetic cortical stimulation. *Ann Neurol*. 1992;32:345–351.

77. Davey NJ, Romaiguŝre P, Maskill DW, Ellaway PH. Suppression of voluntary motor activity revealed using transcranial magnetic stimulation of the motor cortex in man. *J Physiol*. 1994;477:223–235.

78. Wilson SA, Lockwood RJ, Thickbroom GW, Mastaglia FL. The muscle silent period following transcranial magnetic cortical stimulation. *J Neurol Sci*. 1993;114(2):216–222.

79. Matsugi A. Changes in the cortical silent period during force control. *Somatosensory Motor Res*. Mar 2019;36(1):8–13. doi:10.1080/08990220.2018.1563536

80. Werhahn KJ, Kunesch E, Noachtar S, Benecke R, Classen J. Differential effects on motorcortical inhibition induced by blockade of GABA uptake in humans. *J Physiol*. 1999;517:591–597.

81. Siebner HR, Dressnandt J, Auer C, Conrad B. Continuous intrathecal baclofen infusions induced a marked increase of the transcranially evoked silent period in a patient with generalized dystonia. *Muscle Nerve.* 1998;21:1209–1212.

82. Connors BW, Malenka RC, Silva LR. Two inhibitory postsynaptic potentials, and GABAA and GABAB receptor-mediated responses in neocortex of rat and cat. *J Physiol (London).* 1988;406:443–468.

83. Ziemann U, Lonnecker S, Paulus W. Inhibition of human motor cortex by ethanol. A transcranial magnetic stimulation study. *Brain.* 1995;118:1437–1446.

84. Ziemann U, Lönnecker S, Steinhoff BJ, Paulus W. The effect of lorazepam on the motor cortical excitability in man. *Exp Brain Res.* 1996;109:127–135.

85. Mohammadi B, Krampfl K, Petri S, et al. Selective and nonselective benzodiazepine agonists have different effects on motor cortex excitability. *Muscle Nerve.* Jun 2006;33(6):778–784. doi:10.1002/mus.20531

86. Lang N, Sueske E, Hasan A, Paulus W, Tergau F. Pregabalin exerts oppositional effects on different inhibitory circuits in human motor cortex: A double-blind, placebo-controlled transcranial magnetic stimulation study. *Epilepsia.* May 2006;47(5):813–819. doi:10.1111/j.1528-1167.2006.00544.x

87. Ni Z, Gunraj CA, Chen R. Short interval intracortical inhibition and facilitation during the silent period in human. *J Physiol (London).* 2007;583:971–982.

88. Kimiskidis VK, Papagiannopoulos S, Sotirakoglou K, Kazis DA, Kazis A, Mills KR. Silent period to transcranial magnetic stimulation: Construction and properties of stimulus-response curves in healthy volunteers. *Exp Brain Res.* 2005;163(1):21–31.

89. Garvey MA, Ziemann U, Becker DA, Barker CA, Bartko JJ. New graphical method to measure silent periods evoked by transcranial magnetic stimulation. *Clin Neurophysiol.* 2001;112(8):1451–1460.

90. Daskalakis ZJ, Molnar GF, Christensen BK, Sailer A, Fitzgerald PB, Chen R. An automated method to determine the transcranial magnetic stimulation-induced contralateral silent period. *Clin Neurophysiol.* 2003;114(5):938–944.

91. King NK, Kuppuswamy A, Strutton PH, Davey NJ. Estimation of cortical silent period following transcranial magnetic stimulation using a computerised cumulative sum method. *J Neurosci Methods.* 2006;150(1):96–104.

92. Rabago CA, Lancaster JL, Narayana S, Zhang W, Fox PT. Automated-parameterization of the motor evoked potential and cortical silent period induced by transcranial magnetic stimulation. *Clin Neurophysiol.* 2009;120(8):1577–1587.

93. Julkunen P, Kallioniemi E, Kononen M, Saisanen L. Feasibility of automated analysis and inter-examiner variability of cortical silent period induced by transcranial magnetic stimulation. *J Neurosci Methods.* 2013;217(1-2):75–81.

94. Wilke S, Groenveld D, Grittner U, List J, Floel A. cSPider: Evaluation of a free and open-source automated tool to analyze corticomotor silent period. *PLoSOne.* 2016;11(6):e0156066.

95. Wilson SA, Thickbroom GW, Mastaglia FL. An investigation of the late excitatory potential in the hand following magnetic stimulation of the motor cortex. *Electroencephalogr Clin Neurophysiol.* 1995;97(1):55–62.

96. Butler JE, Petersen NC, Herbert RD, Gandevia SC, Taylor JL. Origin of the low-level EMG during the silent period following transcranial magnetic stimulation. *Clin Neurophysiol.* Jul 2012;123(7):1409–1414. doi:10.1016/j.clinph.2011.11.034

97. Hupfeld KE, Swanson CW, Fling BW, Seidler RD. TMS-induced silent periods: A review of methods and call for consistency. *J Neurosci Methods.* Dec 1 2020;346:108950. doi:10.1016/j.jneumeth.2020.108950

98. Meyer BU, Roricht S, Grafin von Einsiedel H, Kruggel F, Weindl A. Inhibitory and excitatory interhemispheric transfers between motor cortical areas in normal humans and patients with abnormalities of the corpus callosum. *Brain.* 1995;118:429–440.

99. Meyer BU, Roricht S, Woiciechowsky C. Topography of fibers in the human corpus callosum mediating interhemispheric inhibition between the motor cortices. *Ann Neurol.* 1998;43(3):360–369.

100. Kuhn AA, Brandt SA, Kupsch A, et al. Comparison of motor effects following subcortical electrical stimulation through electrodes in the globus pallidus internus and cortical transcranial magnetic stimulation. *Exp Brain Res.* 2004;155(1):48–55.

101. Compta Y, Valls-Sole J, Valldeoriola F, Kumru H, Rumia J. The silent period of the thenar muscles to contralateral and ipsilateral deep brain stimulation. *Clin Neurophysiol.* 2006;117(11):2512–2520.

102. Lizarraga KJ, Saravanamuttu J, Baarbé JK, Lang AE, Chen R. Interhemispheric pathways in agenesis of the corpus callosum and Parkinson's disease. *Brain Stimul.* Mar-Apr 2020;13(2):360–362. doi:10.1016/j.brs.2019.11.003

103. Perez MA, Butler JE, Taylor JL. Modulation of transcallosal inhibition by bilateral activation of agonist and antagonist proximal arm muscles. *J Neurophysiol.* 2014;111(2):405–414.

104. Giovannelli F, Borgheresi A, Balestrieri F, et al. Modulation of interhemispheric inhibition by volitional motor activity: An ipsilateral silent period study. *J Physiol (London).* 2009;587(Pt 22):5393–5410.

105. Kujirai T, Caramia MD, Rothwell JC, et al. Corticocortical inhibition in human motor cortex. *J Physiol.* 1993;471:501–519.

106. Sanger TD, Garg RR, Chen R. Interactions between two different inhibitory systems in the human motor cortex. *J Physiol.* 2001;530:307–317.

107. Nakamura H, Kitagawa H, Kawaguchi Y, Tsuji H. Intracortical facilitation and inhibition after transcranial magnetic stimulation in conscious humans. *J Physiol.* 1997;498:817–823.

108. Di Lazzaro V, Restuccia D, Oliviero A, et al. Magnetic transcranial stimulation at intensities below active motor threshold activates inhibitory circuits. *Exp Brain Res.* 1998;119:265–268.

109. Fisher J, Nakamura Y, Bestmann S, Rothwell C, Bostock H. Two phases of intracortical inhibition revealed by transcranial magnetic threshold tracking. *Exp Brain Res.* 2002;143(2):240–248.

110. Roshan L, Paradiso GO, Chen R. Two phases of short-interval intracortical inhibition. *Exp Brain Res.* Aug 2003;151(3):330–337. doi:10.1007/s00221-003-1502-9

111. Cengiz B, Murase N, Rothwell JC. Opposite effects of weak transcranial direct current stimulation on different phases of short interval intracortical inhibition (SICI). *Exp Brain Res.* Mar 2013;225(3):321–331. doi:10.1007/s00221-012-3369-0

112. Stagg CJ, Bestmann S, Constantinescu AO, et al. Relationship between physiological measures of excitability and levels of glutamate and GABA in the human motor cortex. *J Physiol.* Dec 1 2011;589(Pt 23):5845–5855. doi:10.1113/jphysiol.2011.216978

113. Demoule A, Verin E, Ross E, et al. Intracortical inhibition and facilitation of the response of the diaphragm to transcranial magnetic stimulation. *J Clin Neurophysiol.* 2003;20(1):59–64.

114. Lefaucheur JP. Excitability of the motor cortical representation of the external anal sphincter. *Exp Brain Res.* 2005;160(2):268–272.

115. Reynolds C, Ashby P. Inhibition in the human motor cortex is reduced just before a voluntary contraction. *Neurology.* 1999;53(4):730–735.

116. Sohn YH, Wiltz K, Hallett M. Effect of volitional inhibition on cortical inhibitory mechanisms. *J Neurophysiol.* 2002;88(1):333–338.

117. Sundby KK, Wagner J, Aron AR. The functional role of response suppression during an urge to relieve pain. *J Cogn Neurosci.* Sep 2019;31(9):1404–1421. doi:10.1162/jocn_a_01423

118. He JL, Fuelscher I, Coxon J, et al. Individual differences in intracortical inhibition predict motor-inhibitory performance. *Exp Brain Res.* Oct 2019;237(10):2715–2727. doi:10.1007/s00221-019-05622-y

119. Ilic TV, Jung P, Ziemann U. Subtle hemispheric asymmetry of motor cortical inhibitory tone. *Clin Neurophysiol.* 2004;115(2):330–340.

120. Tankisi H, Cengiz B, Howells J, Samusyte G, Koltzenburg M, Bostock H. Short-interval intracortical inhibition as a function of inter-stimulus interval: Three methods compared. *Brain Stimul.* Jan-Feb 2021;14(1):22–32. doi:10.1016/j.brs.2020.11.002

121. Lissemore JI, Bhandari A, Mulsant BH, et al. Reduced GABAergic cortical inhibition in aging and depression. *Neuropsychopharmacology.* Oct 2018;43(11):2277–2284. doi:10.1038/s41386-018-0093-x

122. Ridding MC, Taylor JL, Rothwell JC. The effect of voluntary contraction on cortico-cortical inhibition in human motor cortex. *J Physiol.* 1995;487:541–548.

123. Ortu E, Deriu F, Suppa A, Tolu E, Rothwell JC. Effects of volitional contraction on intracortical inhibition and facilitation in the human motor cortex. *J Physiol (London).* 2008;586(21):5147–5159.

124. Awiszus F, Feistner H, Urbach D, Bostock H. Characterisation of paired-pulse transcranial magnetic stimulation conditions yielding intracortical inhibition or I-wave facilitation using a threshold-hunting paradigm. *Exp Brain Res.* 1999;129(2):317–324.

125. Peurala SH, Müller-Dahlhaus JF, Arai N, Ziemann U. Interference of short-interval intracortical inhibition (SICI) and short-interval intracortical facilitation (SICF). *Clin Neurophysiol.* Oct 2008;119(10):2291–2297. doi:10.1016/j.clinph.2008.05.031

126. Ilic TV, Meintzschel F, Cleff U, Ruge D, Kessler KR, Ziemann U. Short-interval paired-pulse inhibition and facilitation of human motor cortex: The dimension of stimulus intensity. *J Physiol.* 2002;545(Pt 1):153–167.

127. Cirillo J, Semmler JG, Mooney RA, Byblow WD. Conventional or threshold-hunting TMS? A tale of two SICIs. *Brain Stimul.* Nov-Dec 2018;11(6):1296–1305. doi:10.1016/j.brs.2018.07.047

128. Sale MV, Lavender AP, Opie GM, Nordstrom MA, Semmler JG. Increased intracortical inhibition in elderly adults with anterior-posterior current flow: A TMS study. *Clin Neurophysiol.* Jan 2016;127(1):635–640. doi:10.1016/j.clinph.2015.04.062

129. Ni Z, Bahl N, Gunraj C, Mazzella F, Chen R. Increased motor cortical facilitation and decreased inhibition in Parkinson's Disease. *Neurology.* 2013;80:1746–1753.

130. Ziemann U, Rothwell JC, Ridding MC. Interaction between intracortical inhibition and facilitation in human motor cortex. *J Physiol.* 1996;496:873–881.

131. Wiegel P, Niemann N, Rothwell JC, Leukel C. Evidence for a subcortical contribution to intracortical facilitation. *Eur J Neurosci.* Jun 2018;47(11):1311–1319. doi:10.1111/ejn.13934

132. Di Lazzaro V, Pilato F, Oliviero A, et al. Origin of facilitation of motor-evoked potentials after paired magnetic stimulation: Direct recording of epidural activity in conscious humans. *J Neurophysiol.* 2006;96(4):1765–1771.

133. Ziemann U, Chen R, Cohen LG, Hallett M. Dextromethorphan decreases the excitability of the human motor cortex. *Neurology.* 1998;51:1320–1324.

134. Gerdelat-Mas A, Loubinoux I, Tombari D, Rascol O, Chollet F, Simonetta-Moreau M. Chronic administration of selective serotonin reuptake inhibitor (SSRI) paroxetine modulates human motor cortex excitability in healthy subjects. *Neuroimage.* 2005;27(2):314–322.

135. Valls-Sole J, Pascual-Leone A, Wassermann EM, Hallett M. Human motor evoked responses to paired transcranial magnetic stimuli. *Electroencephalogr Clin Neurophysiol.* 1992;85(6):355–364.

136. Wassermann EM, Samii A, Mercuri B, et al. Responses to paired transcranial magnetic stimuli in resting, active, and recently activated muscle. *Exp Brain Res.* 1996;109:158–163.

137. Di Lazzaro V, Oliviero A, Mazzone P, et al. Direct demonstration of long latency cortico-cortical inhibition in normal subjects and in a patient with vascular parkinsonism. *Clin Neurophysiol.* 2002;113(11):1673–1679.

138. McNeil CJ, Martin PG, Gandevia SC, Taylor JL. The response to paired motor cortical stimuli is abolished at a spinal level during human muscle fatigue. *J Physiol.* Dec 1 2009;587(Pt 23):5601–5612. doi:10.1113/jphysiol.2009.180968

139. McDonnell MN, Orekhov Y, Ziemann U. The role of GABA(B) receptors in intracortical inhibition in the human motor cortex. *Exp Brain Res.* 2006;173(1):86–93.

140. Berardelli A, Rona S, Inghilleri M, Manfredi M. Cortical inhibition in Parkinson's disease. A study with paired magnetic stimulation. *Brain.* 1996;119:71–77.

141. Opie GM, Semmler JG. Modulation of short- and long-interval intracortical inhibition with increasing motor evoked potential amplitude in a human hand muscle. *Clin Neurophysiol.* Jul 2014;125(7):1440–1450. doi:10.1016/j.clinph.2013.11.015

142. Chen R, Wassermann EM, Caños M, Hallett M. Impaired inhibition in writer's cramp during voluntary muscle activation. *Neurology.* 1997;49:1054–1059.

143. Hammond G, Vallence AM. Modulation of long-interval intracortical inhibition and the silent period by voluntary contraction. *Brain Res.* Jul 16 2007;1158:63–70. doi:10.1016/j.brainres.2007.05.014

144. McNeil CJ, Martin PG, Gandevia SC, Taylor JL. Long-interval intracortical inhibition in a human hand muscle. *Exp Brain Res.* Mar 2011;209(2):287–297. doi:10.1007/s00221-011-2552-z

145. Cash RF, Ziemann U, Murray K, Thickbroom GW. Late cortical disinhibition in human motor cortex: A triple-pulse transcranial magnetic stimulation study. *J Neurophysiol.* 2010;103(1):511–518.

146. Cash RF, Ziemann U, Thickbroom GW. Inhibitory and disinhibitory effects on I-wave facilitation in motor cortex. *J Neurophysiol.* 2011;105(1):100–106.

147. Caux-Dedeystère A, Derambure P, Devanne H. Late cortical disinhibition in relaxed versus active hand muscles. *Neuroscience*. Jul 9 2015;298:52–62. doi:10.1016/j.neuroscience.2015.04.018

148. Ruddy K, Balsters J, Mantini D, et al. Neural activity related to volitional regulation of cortical excitability. *eLife*. Nov 29 2018;7doi:10.7554/eLife.40843

149. Tokimura H, Ridding MC, Tokimura Y, Amassian VE, Rothwell JC. Short latency facilitation between pairs of threshold magnetic stimuli applied to human motor cortex. *Electroencephalogr Clin Neurophysiol*. 1996;103:263–272.

150. Ziemann U, Tergau F, Wassermann EM, Wischer S, Hildebrandt J, Paulus W. Demonstration of facilitatory I wave interaction in the human motor cortex by paired transcranial magnetic stimulation. *J Physiol*. 1998;511:181–190.

151. Chen R, Garg R. Facilitatory I wave interaction in proximal arm and lower limb muscle representations of the human motor cortex. *J Neurophysiol*. 2000;83(3):1426–1434.

152. Chen R. Interactions between inhibitory and excitatory circuits in the human motor cortex. *Exp Brain Res*. 2004;154(1):1–10.

153. Cirillo J, Perez MA. Subcortical contribution to late TMS-induced I-waves in intact humans. *Front Integrat Neurosci*. 2015;9:38. doi:10.3389/fnint.2015.00038

154. Hanajima R, Ugawa Y, Terao Y, et al. Mechanisms of intracortical I-wave facilitation elicited with paired- pulse magnetic stimulation in humans. *J Physiol*. 2002;538(Pt 1):253–261.

155. Di Lazzaro V, Rothwell JC, Oliviero A, et al. Intracortical origin of the short latency facilitation produced by pairs of threshold magnetic stimuli applied to human motor cortex. *Exp Brain Res*. 1999;129(4):494–499.

156. Ziemann U, Tergau F, Wischer S, Hildebrandt J, Paulus W. Pharmacological control of facilitatory I-wave interaction in the human motor cortex: A paired transcranial magnetic stimulation study. *Electroencephalogr Clin Neurophysiol*. 1998;109:321–330.

157. Cash RFH, Udupa K, Gunraj CA, et al. Influence of BDNF Val66Met polymorphism on excitatory-inhibitory balance and plasticity in human motor cortex. *Clin Neurophysiol*. Sep 1 2021;132(11):2827–2839. doi:10.1016/j.clinph.2021.07.029

158. Ugawa Y, Day BL, Rothwell JC, Thompson PD, Merton PA, Marsden CD. Modulation of motor cortical excitability by electrical stimulation over the cerebellum in man. *J Physiol*. 1991;441:57–72.

159. Ugawa Y, Uesaka Y, Terao Y, Hanajima R, Kanazawa I. Magnetic stimulation over the cerebellum in humans. *Ann Neurol*. 1995;37(6):703–713.

160. Pinto AD, Chen R. Suppression of the motor cortex by magnetic stimulation of the cerebellum. *Exp Brain Res*. 2001;140(4):505–510.

161. Spampinato DA, Celnik PA, Rothwell JC. Cerebellar-motor cortex connectivity: One or two different networks? *J Neurosci*. May 20 2020;40(21):4230–4239. doi:10.1523/jneurosci.2397-19.2020

162. Daskalakis ZJ, Paradiso GO, Christensen BK, Fitzgerald PB, Gunraj C, Chen R. Exploring the connectivity between the cerebellum and motor cortex in humans. *J Physiol*. 2004;557(Pt 2):689–700.

163. Rurak BK, Rodrigues JP, Power BD, Drummond PD, Vallence AM. Reduced cerebellar brain inhibition measured using dual-site TMS in older than in younger adults. *Cerebellum (London, England)*. Apr 20 2021;doi:10.1007/s12311-021-01267-2

164. Werhahn KJ, Taylor J, Ridding M, Meyer BU, Rothwell JC. Effect of transcranial magnetic stimulation over the cerebellum on the excitability of human motor cortex. *Electroencephalogr Clin Neurophysiol*. 1996;101(1):58–66.

165. Hardwick RM, Lesage E, Miall RC. Cerebellar transcranial magnetic stimulation: The role of coil geometry and tissue depth. *Brain Stimul*. Sep-Oct 2014;7(5):643–649. doi:10.1016/j.brs.2014.04.009

166. Fisher KM, Lai HM, Baker MR, Baker SN. Corticospinal activation confounds cerebellar effects of posterior fossa stimuli. *Clin Neurophysiol*. Dec 2009;120(12):2109–2113. doi:10.1016/j.clinph.2009.08.021

167. Ugawa Y. Can we see the cerebellar activation effect by TMS over the back of the head? *Clin Neurophysiol*. Dec 2009;120(12):2006–2007. doi:10.1016/j.clinph.2009.09.003

168. Ugawa Y, Terao Y, Hanajima R, et al. Magnetic stimulation over the cerebellum in patients with ataxia. *Electroencephalogr Clin Neurophysiol*. 1997;104(5):453–458.

169. Matsunaga K, Uozumi T, Hashimoto T, Tsuji S. Cerebellar stimulation in acute cerebellar ataxia. *Clin Neurophysiol*. 2001;112(4):619–622.

170. Halko MA, Farzan F, Eldaief MC, Schmahmann JD, Pascual-Leone A. Intermittent theta-burst stimulation of the lateral cerebellum increases functional connectivity of the default network. *J Neurosci.* Sep 3 2014;34(36):12049–12056. doi:10.1523/jneurosci.1776-14.2014

171. Rastogi A, Cash R, Dunlop K, et al. Modulation of cognitive cerebello-cerebral functional connectivity by lateral cerebellar continuous theta burst stimulation. *Neuroimage.* Sep 2017;158:48–57. doi:10.1016/j.neuroimage.2017.06.048

172. Mooney RA, Casamento-Moran A, Celnik PA. The reliability of cerebellar brain inhibition. *Clin Neurophysiol.* Aug 5 2021;132(10):2365–2370. doi:10.1016/j.clinph.2021.06.035

173. Tokimura H, Di Lazzaro V, Tokimura Y, et al. Short latency inhibition of human hand motor cortex by somatosensory input from the hand. *J Physiol.* 2000;523:503–513.

174. Di Lazzaro V, Oliviero A, Profice P, et al. Muscarinic receptor blockade has differential effects on the excitability of intracortical circuits in the human motor cortex. *Exp Brain Res.* 2000;135(4):455–461.

175. Di Lazzaro V, Oliviero A, Saturno E, et al. Effects of lorazepam on short latency afferent inhibition and short latency intracortical inhibition in humans. *J Physiol.* 2005;564(Pt 2):661–668.

176. Turco CV, El-Sayes J, Locke MB, Chen R, Baker S, Nelson AJ. Effects of lorazepam and baclofen on short- and long-latency afferent inhibition. *J Physiol.* Nov 2018;596(21):5267–5280. doi:10.1113/jp276710

177. Bikmullina R, Baumer T, Zittel S, Munchau A. Sensory afferent inhibition within and between limbs in humans. *Clin Neurophysiol.* 2009;120(3):610–618.

178. Dubbioso R, Raffin E, Karabanov A, Thielscher A, Siebner HR. Centre-surround organization of fast sensorimotor integration in human motor hand area. *Neuroimage.* Sep 2017;158:37–47. doi:10.1016/j.neuroimage.2017.06.063

179. Pilurzi G, Ginatempo F, Mercante B, et al. Role of cutaneous and proprioceptive inputs in sensorimotor integration and plasticity occurring in the facial primary motor cortex. *J Physiol.* Feb 2020;598(4):839–851. doi:10.1113/jp278877

180. Wagle-Shukla A, Moro E, Gunraj C, et al. Long-term subthalamic nucleus stimulation improves sensorimotor integration and proprioception. *J Neurol Neurosurg Psychiatry.* 2013;84(9):1020–1028.

181. Hannah R, Rothwell JC. Pulse duration as well as current direction determines the specificity of transcranial magnetic stimulation of motor cortex during contraction. *Brain Stimul.* Jan-Feb 2017;10(1):106–115. doi:10.1016/j.brs.2016.09.008

182. Mirdamadi JL, Suzuki LY, Meehan SK. Attention modulates specific motor cortical circuits recruited by transcranial magnetic stimulation. *Neuroscience.* Sep 17 2017;359:151–158. doi:10.1016/j.neuroscience.2017.07.028

183. Turco CV, Toepp SL, Foglia SD, Dans PW, Nelson AJ. Association of short- and long-latency afferent inhibition with human behavior. *Clin Neurophysiol.* Jul 2021;132(7):1462–1480. doi:10.1016/j.clinph.2021.02.402

184. Roy FD, Gorassini MA. Peripheral sensory activation of cortical circuits in the leg motor cortex of man. *J Physiol.* Sep 1 2008;586(17):4091–4105. doi:10.1113/jphysiol.2008.153726

185. Bikmullina R, Bäumer T, Zittel S, Münchau A. Sensory afferent inhibition within and between limbs in humans. *Clin Neurophysiol.* Mar 2009;120(3):610–618. doi:10.1016/j.clinph.2008.12.003

186. Sailer A, Molnar GF, Cunic DI, Chen R. Effects of peripheral sensory input on cortical inhibition in humans. *J Physiol.* 2002;544:617–629.

187. Chen R, Corwell B, Hallett M. Modulation of motor cortex excitability by median nerve and digit stimulation. *Exp Brain Res.* 1999;129(1):77–86.

188. Turco CV, El-Sayes J, Savoie MJ, Fassett HJ, Locke MB, Nelson AJ. Short- and long-latency afferent inhibition; uses, mechanisms and influencing factors. *Brain Stimul.* Jan-Feb 2018;11(1):59–74. doi:10.1016/j.brs.2017.09.009

189. Civardi C, Cantello R, Asselman P, Rothwell JC. Transcranial magnetic stimulation can be used to test connections to primary motor areas from frontal and medial cortex in humans. *Neuroimage.* 2001;14(6):1444–1453.

190. Koch G, Franca M, Mochizuki H, Marconi B, Caltagirone C, Rothwell JC. Interactions between pairs of transcranial magnetic stimuli over the human left dorsal premotor cortex differ from those seen in primary motor cortex. *J Physiol.* 2007;578(Pt 2):551–562.

191. Bäumer T, Schippling S, Kroeger J, et al. Inhibitory and facilitatory connectivity from ventral premotor to primary motor cortex in healthy humans at rest: A bifocal TMS study. *Clin Neurophysiol*. Sep 2009;120(9):1724–1731. doi:10.1016/j.clinph.2009.07.035

192. Weissbach A, Bäumer T, Brüggemann N, et al. Premotor-motor excitability is altered in dopa-responsive dystonia. *Move Dis*. Oct 2015;30(12):1705–1709. doi:10.1002/mds.26365

193. Ni Z, Isayama R, Castillo G, Gunraj C, Saha U, Chen R. Reduced dorsal premotor cortex and primary motor cortex connectivity in older adults. *Neurobiol Aging*. Jan 2015;36(1):301–303. doi:10.1016/j.neurobiolaging.2014.08.017

194. Groppa S, Schlaak BH, Münchau A, et al. The human dorsal premotor cortex facilitates the excitability of ipsilateral primary motor cortex via a short latency cortico-cortical route. *Hum Brain Mapp*. Feb 2012;33(2):419–430. doi:10.1002/hbm.21221

195. Groppa S, Werner-Petroll N, Münchau A, Deuschl G, Ruschworth MF, Siebner HR. A novel dual-site transcranial magnetic stimulation paradigm to probe fast facilitatory inputs from ipsilateral dorsal premotor cortex to primary motor cortex. *Neuroimage*. Aug 1 2012;62(1):500–509. doi:10.1016/j.neuroimage.2012.05.023

196. Vesia M, Culham JC, Jegatheeswaran G, et al. Functional interaction between human dorsal premotor cortex and the ipsilateral primary motor cortex for grasp plans: A dual-site TMS study. *Neuroreport*. Nov 7 2018;29(16):1355–1359. doi:10.1097/wnr.0000000000001117

197. Davare M, Lemon R, Olivier E. Selective modulation of interactions between ventral premotor cortex and primary motor cortex during precision grasping in humans. *J Physiol*. Jun 1 2008;586(11):2735–2742. doi:10.1113/jphysiol.2008.152603

198. Brown MJN, Goldenkoff ER, Chen R, Gunraj C, Vesia M. Using dual-site transcranial magnetic stimulation to probe connectivity between the dorsolateral prefrontal cortex and ipsilateral primary motor cortex in humans. *Brain Sci*. Jul 26 2019;9(8):177. doi:10.3390/brainsci9080177

199. Wang Y, Cao N, Lin Y, Chen R, Zhang J. Hemispheric differences in functional interactions between the dorsal lateral prefrontal cortex and ipsilateral motor cortex. *Front Hum Neurosci*. 2020;14:202. doi:10.3389/fnhum.2020.00202

200. Hasan A, Galea JM, Casula EP, Falkai P, Bestmann S, Rothwell JC. Muscle and timing-specific functional connectivity between the dorsolateral prefrontal cortex and the primary motor cortex. *J Cogn Neurosci*. Apr 2013;25(4):558–570. doi:10.1162/jocn_a_00338

201. Shirota Y, Hamada M, Terao Y, et al. Increased primary motor cortical excitability by a single-pulse transcranial magnetic stimulation over the supplementary motor area. *Exp Brain Res*. Jun 2012;219(3):339–349. doi:10.1007/s00221-012-3095-7

202. Arai N, Lu MK, Ugawa Y, Ziemann U. Effective connectivity between human supplementary motor area and primary motor cortex: A paired-coil TMS study. *Exp Brain Res*. Jul 2012;220(1):79–87. doi:10.1007/s00221-012-3117-5

203. Mars RB, Klein MC, Neubert FX, et al. Short-latency influence of medial frontal cortex on primary motor cortex during action selection under conflict. *J Neurosci*. May 27 2009;29(21):6926–6931. doi:10.1523/jneurosci.1396-09.2009

204. Green PE, Ridding MC, Hill KD, Semmler JG, Drummond PD, Vallence AM. Supplementary motor area-primary motor cortex facilitation in younger but not older adults. *Neurobiol Aging*. Apr 2018;64:85–91. doi:10.1016/j.neurobiolaging.2017.12.016

205. Koch G, Fernandez DO, Cheeran B, et al. Focal stimulation of the posterior parietal cortex increases the excitability of the ipsilateral motor cortex. *J Neurosci*. 2007;27(25):6815–6822.

206. Karabanov AN, Chao CC, Paine R, Hallett M. Mapping different intra-hemispheric parietal-motor networks using twin Coil TMS. *Brain Stimul*. May 2013;6(3):384–389. doi:10.1016/j.brs.2012.08.002

207. Vesia M, Barnett-Cowan M, Elahi B, et al. Human dorsomedial parieto-motor circuit specifies grasp during the planning of goal-directed hand actions. *Cortex*. Jul 2017;92:175–186. doi:10.1016/j.cortex.2017.04.007

208. Ziluk A, Premji A, Nelson AJ. Functional connectivity from area 5 to primary motor cortex via paired-pulse transcranial magnetic stimulation. *Neurosci Lett*. Oct 22 2010;484(1):81–85. doi:10.1016/j.neulet.2010.08.025

209. Isayama R, Vesia M, Jegatheeswaran G, et al. Rubber hand illusion modulates the influences of somatosensory and parietal inputs to the motor cortex. *J Neurophysiol.* Feb 1 2019;121(2):563–573. doi:10.1152/jn.00345.2018

210. Shields J, Park JE, Srivanitchapoom P, et al. Probing the interaction of the ipsilateral posterior parietal cortex with the premotor cortex using a novel transcranial magnetic stimulation technique. *Clin Neurophysiol.* Feb 2016;127(2):1475–1480. doi:10.1016/j.clinph.2015.06.031

211. Brown MJN, Weissbach A, Pauly MG, et al. Somatosensory-motor cortex interactions measured using dual-site transcranial magnetic stimulation. *Brain Stimul.* Sep-Oct 2019;12(5):1229–1243. doi:10.1016/j.brs.2019.04.009

212. Ferbert A, Priori A, Rothwell JC, Day BL, Colebatch JG, Marsden CD. Interhemispheric inhibition of the human motor cortex. *J Physiol (London).* 1992;453:525–546.

213. Ni Z, Gunraj C, Nelson AJ, et al. Two phases of interhemispheric inhibition between motor related cortical areas and the primary motor cortex in human. *Cerebral Cortex.* 2009;19(7):1654–1665.

214. Ni Z, Leodori G, Vial F, et al. Measuring latency distribution of transcallosal fibers using transcranial magnetic stimulation. *Brain Stimul.* Sep-Oct 2020;13(5):1453–1460. doi:10.1016/j.brs.2020.08.004

215. Belyk M, Banks R, Tendera A, Chen R, Beal DS. Paradoxical facilitation alongside interhemispheric inhibition. *Exp Brain Res.* Sep 2 2021. doi:10.1007/s00221-021-06183-9

216. Lee H, Gunraj C, Chen R. The effects of inhibitory and facilitatory intracortical circuits on interhemispheric inhibition in the human motor cortex. *J Physiol (London).* 2007;580(Pt.3):1021–1032.

217. Nelson AJ, Hoque T, Gunraj C, Ni Z, Chen R. Bi-directional interhemispheric inhibition during unimanual sustained contractions. *BMC Neurosci.* Apr 4 2009;10:31. doi:10.1186/1471-2202-10-31

218. Di Lazzaro V, Oliviero A, Profice P, et al. Direct demonstration of interhemispheric inhibition of the human motor cortex produced by transcranial magnetic stimulation. *Exp Brain Res.* 1999;124(4):520–524.

219. Gerloff C, Cohen LG, Floeter MK, Chen R, Corwell B, Hallett M. Inhibitory influence of the ipsilateral motor cortex on responses to stimulation of the human cortex and pyramidal tract. *J Physiol.* 1998;510:249–259.

220. Wahl M, Lauterbach-Soon B, Hattingen E, et al. Human motor corpus callosum: Topography, somatotopy, and link between microstructure and function. *J Neurosci.* Nov 7 2007;27(45):12132–12138. doi:10.1523/jneurosci.2320-07.2007

221. Netz J, Ziemann U, Homberg V. Hemispheric asymmetry of transcallosal inhibition in man. *Exp Brain Res.* 1995;104(3):527–533.

222. Baumer T, Dammann E, Bock F, Kloppel S, Siebner HR, Munchau A. Laterality of interhemispheric inhibition depends on handedness. *Exp Brain Res.* 2007;180(2):195–203.

223. De Gennaro L, Cristiani R, Bertini M, et al. Handedness is mainly associated with an asymmetry of corticospinal excitability and not of transcallosal inhibition. *Clin Neurophysiol.* 2004;115(6):1305–1312.

224. Irlbacher K, Brocke J, Mechow JV, Brandt SA. Effects of GABA(A) and GABA(B) agonists on interhemispheric inhibition in man. *Clin Neurophysiol.* 2007;118(2):308–316.

225. Mochizuki H, Huang YZ, Rothwell JC. Interhemispheric interaction between human dorsal premotor and contralateral primary motor cortex. *J Physiol.* 2004;561(Pt 1):331–338.

226. Koch G, Franca M, Del Olmo MF, et al. Time course of functional connectivity between dorsal premotor and contralateral motor cortex during movement selection. *J Neurosci.* 2006;26(28):7452–7459.

227. Hinder MR, Fujiyama H, Summers JJ. Premotor-motor interhemispheric inhibition is released during movement initiation in older but not young adults. *PloS One.* 2012;7(12):e52573. doi:10.1371/journal.pone.0052573

228. Koch G, Ruge D, Cheeran B, et al. TMS activation of interhemispheric pathways between the posterior parietal cortex and the contralateral motor cortex. *J Physiol.* Sep 1 2009;587(Pt 17):4281–4292. doi:10.1113/jphysiol.2009.174086

229. Hanajima R, Ugawa Y, Machii K, et al. Interhemispheric facilitation of the hand motor area in humans. *J Physiol.* 2001;531(Pt 3):849–859.

230. Baumer T, Bock F, Koch G, et al. Magnetic stimulation of human premotor or motor cortex produces interhemispheric facilitation through distinct pathways. *J Physiol.* 2006;572(Pt 3):857–868.

231. Baarbé J, Vesia M, Brown MJN, et al. Interhemispheric interactions between the right angular gyrus and the left motor cortex: A transcranial magnetic stimulation study. *J Neurophysiol*. Apr 1 2021;125(4):1236–1250. doi:10.1152/jn.00642.2020

232. Ni Z, Muller-Dahlhaus F, Chen R, Ziemann U. Triple-pulse TMS to study interactions between neural circuits in human cortex. *Brain Stimul*. 2011;4(4):281–293.

233. Merton PA, Morton HB. Stimulation of the cerebral cortex in the intact human subject. *Nature*. 1980;285(5762):227.

234. Day BL, Thompson PD, Dick JP, Nakashima K, Marsden CD. Different sites of action of electrical and magnetic stimulation of the human brain. *Neurosci Lett*. 1987;75:101–106.

235. Chen R, Corwell B, Yaseen Z, Hallett M, Cohen LG. Mechanisms of cortical reorganization in lower-limb amputees. *J Neurosci*. 1998;18:3443–3450.

236. Ugawa Y, Rothwell JC, Day BL, Thompson PD, Marsden CD. Percutaneous electrical-stimulation of corticospinal pathways at the level of the pyramidal decussation in humans. *Ann Neurol*. 1991;29(4):418–427.

237. Taylor JL, Gandevia SC. Noninvasive stimulation of the human corticospinal tract. *J Appl Physiol*. 2004;96(4):1496–1503.

238. Taylor JL, Petersen NT, Butler JE, Gandevia SC. Interaction of transcranial magnetic stimulation and electrical transmastoid stimulation in human subjects. *J Physiol*. 2002;541(3):949–958.

239. Berardelli A, Inghilleri M, Rothwell JC, Cruccu G, Manfredi M. Multiple firing of motoneurones is produced by cortical stimulation but not by direct activation of descending motor tracts. *Electroencephalogr Clin Neurophysiol*. 1991;81(3):240–242.

240. Ugawa Y, Uesaka Y, Terao Y, Hanajima R, Kanazawa I. Magnetic stimulation of corticospinal pathways at the foramen magnum level in humans. *Ann Neurol*. 1994;36(4):618–624.

241. Ugawa Y, Genba-Shimizu K, Kanazawa I. Electrical stimulation of the human descending motor tracts at several levels. *Can J Neurol Sci/Le journal canadien des sciences neurologiques*. Feb 1995;22(1):36–42. doi:10.1017/s0317167100040476

242. Martin PG, Butler JE, Gandevia SC, Taylor JL. Noninvasive stimulation of human corticospinal axons innervating leg muscles. *J Neurophysiol*. Aug 2008;100(2):1080–1086. doi:10.1152/jn.90380.2008

243. Cavaleri R, Schabrun SM, Chipchase LS. The number of stimuli required to reliably assess cortico-motor excitability and primary motor cortical representations using transcranial magnetic stimulation (TMS): A systematic review and meta-analysis. *Syst Rev*. Mar 6 2017;6(1):48. doi:10.1186/s13643-017-0440-8

244. Cuypers K, Thijs H, Meesen RL. Optimization of the transcranial magnetic stimulation protocol by defining a reliable estimate for corticospinal excitability. *PloS One*. 2014;9(1):e86380. doi:10.1371/journal.pone.0086380

245. Chang WH, Fried PJ, Saxena S, et al. Optimal number of pulses as outcome measures of neuronavigated transcranial magnetic stimulation. *Clin Neurophysiol*. Aug 2016;127(8):2892–2897. doi:10.1016/j.clinph.2016.04.001

246. Julkunen P, Säisänen L, Hukkanen T, Danner N, Könönen M. Does second-scale intertrial interval affect motor evoked potentials induced by single-pulse transcranial magnetic stimulation? *Brain Stimul*. Oct 2012;5(4):526–532. doi:10.1016/j.brs.2011.07.006

247. Hassanzahraee M, Zoghi M, Jaberzadeh S. Longer transcranial magnetic stimulation intertrial interval increases size, reduces variability, and improves the reliability of motor evoked potentials. *Brain Connect*. Dec 2019;9(10):770–776. doi:10.1089/brain.2019.0714

248. Möller C, Arai N, Lücke J, Ziemann U. Hysteresis effects on the input-output curve of motor evoked potentials. *Clin Neurophysiol*. May 2009;120(5):1003–1008. doi:10.1016/j.clinph.2009.03.001

249. Snow NJ, Wadden KP, Chaves AR, Ploughman M. Transcranial magnetic stimulation as a potential biomarker in multiple sclerosis: A systematic review with recommendations for future research. *Neural Plast*. 2019;2019:6430596. doi:10.1155/2019/6430596

250. Simpson M, Macdonell R. The use of transcranial magnetic stimulation in diagnosis, prognostication and treatment evaluation in multiple sclerosis. *Multiple Sclerosis Related Dis*. Sep 2015;4(5):430–436. doi:10.1016/j.msard.2015.06.014

251. Neva JL, Lakhani B, Brown KE, et al. Multiple measures of corticospinal excitability are associated with clinical features of multiple sclerosis. *Behav Brain Res.* Jan 15 2016;297:187–195. doi:10.1016/j.bbr.2015.10.015

252. Menon P, Geevasinga N, Yiannikas C, Howells J, Kiernan MC, Vucic S. Sensitivity and specificity of threshold tracking transcranial magnetic stimulation for diagnosis of amyotrophic lateral sclerosis: A prospective study. *Lancet Neurol.* May 2015;14(5):478–484. doi:10.1016/s1474-4422(15)00014-9

253. Shibuya K, Park SB, Geevasinga N, et al. Motor cortical function determines prognosis in sporadic ALS. *Neurology.* Aug 2 2016;87(5):513–520. doi:10.1212/wnl.0000000000002912

254. Dharmadasa T, Howells J, Matamala JM, et al. Cortical inexcitability defines an adverse clinical profile in amyotrophic lateral sclerosis. *Eur J Neurol.* Jan 2021;28(1):90–97. doi:10.1111/ene.14515

255. Lo YL. How has electrophysiology changed the management of cervical spondylotic myelopathy? *Eur J Neurol.* Aug 2008;15(8):781–786. doi:10.1111/j.1468-1331.2008.02199.x

256. Nardone R, Höller Y, Brigo F, et al. The contribution of neurophysiology in the diagnosis and management of cervical spondylotic myelopathy: A review. *Spinal Cord.* Oct 2016;54(10):756–766. doi:10.1038/sc.2016.82

257. Lo YL, Chan LL, Lim W, et al. Transcranial magnetic stimulation screening for cord compression in cervical spondylosis. *J Neurol Sci.* May 15 2006;244(1–2):17–21. doi:10.1016/j.jns.2005.12.002

258. Capone F, Tamburelli FC, Pilato F, et al. The role of motor-evoked potentials in the management of cervical spondylotic myelopathy. *Spine J.* Sep 2013;13(9):1077–1079. doi:10.1016/j.spinee.2013.02.063

259. Lefaucheur JP, Picht T. The value of preoperative functional cortical mapping using navigated TMS. *Neurophysiologie clinique/Clin Neurophysiol.* Apr 2016;46(2):125–133. doi:10.1016/j.neucli.2016.05.001

260. Galloway GM, Dias BR, Brown JL, Henry CM, Brooks DA, 2nd, Buggie EW. Transcranial magnetic stimulation may be useful as a preoperative screen of motor tract function. *J Clin Neurophysiol.* Aug 2013;30(4):386–389. doi:10.1097/WNP.0b013e31829ddeb2

261. Weiss Lucas C, Nettekoven C, Neuschmelting V, et al. Invasive versus non-invasive mapping of the motor cortex. *Hum Brain Mapp.* Oct 1 2020;41(14):3970–3983. doi:10.1002/hbm.25101

262. Krieg SM, Shiban E, Buchmann N, Meyer B, Ringel F. Presurgical navigated transcranial magnetic brain stimulation for recurrent gliomas in motor eloquent areas. *Clin Neurophysiol.* Mar 2013;124(3):522–527. doi:10.1016/j.clinph.2012.08.011

263. Zhang H, Julkunen P, Schröder A, et al. Short-interval intracortical facilitation improves efficacy in nTMS motor mapping of lower extremity muscle representations in patients with supra-tentorial brain tumors. *Cancers.* Nov 2 2020;12(11):3233. doi:10.3390/cancers12113233

264. Picht T, Krieg SM, Sollmann N, et al. A comparison of language mapping by preoperative navigated transcranial magnetic stimulation and direct cortical stimulation during awake surgery. *Neurosurgery.* May 2013;72(5):808–819. doi:10.1227/NEU.0b013e3182889e01

265. Tarapore PE, Findlay AM, Honma SM, et al. Language mapping with navigated repetitive TMS: Proof of technique and validation. *Neuroimage.* Nov 15 2013;82:260–272. doi:10.1016/j.neuroimage.2013.05.018

266. Sollmann N, Zhang H, Fratini A, et al. Risk assessment by presurgical tractography using navigated TMS maps in patients with highly motor- or language-eloquent brain tumors. *Cancers.* May 17 2020;12(5). doi:10.3390/cancers12051264

4

Induction of Motor Cortical Plasticity with Transcranial Magnetic Stimulation

4.1 INTRODUCTION

Plasticity refers to the ability of the neural tissue to modify its structure or functions in response to stimuli, and these changes outlast the stimulation period. Brain plasticity is considered to underlie learning and memory, mediates recovery from brain injury such as trauma and stroke, and is altered in many neurological and psychiatric disorders. Brain plasticity is considered to encompass different possible mechanisms of reorganization, including recruitment of pathways that are functionally homologous but anatomically distinct from the damaged ones, reinforcement of existing synaptic connections, dendritic arborization, and synaptogenesis.[1]

The best-known mechanisms that mediate synaptic plasticity are long-term potentiation (LTP) and long-term depression (LTD). LTP is generally defined as a long-lasting but not necessarily irreversible increase (decrease for LTD) in synaptic strength.[2] Induction of LTP and LTD depends on glutamatergic N-methyl-D-aspartate (NMDA) receptor activation and postsynaptic Ca^{2+} influx.[2,3]

LTP is not a unitary phenomenon, and its mechanisms can differ between different brain regions. Different forms of LTP may occur at the same synapse, and these are designated LTP1, LTP2, and LTP3.[4] LTP1 is rapidly decaying, protein synthesis–independent, and lasts up to 3 hours. LTP2 requires protein synthesis, but is independent of gene transcription, while LTP3 is the most durable and depends on translation and transcription. Different stimulation protocols can produce different phases of LTP, and it has been demonstrated that LTP3 requires stronger induction protocols (e.g., 6–8 theta burst stimulation trains) than does LTP2 (e.g., 2–4 trains).

In vitro and animal studies have used very high-frequency stimulation (e.g., 100–200 Hz for 1 to 4 s) to induce LTP but such frequencies cannot be used with transcranial magnetic stimulation (TMS) in humans because of the risk of inducing seizures and certain machine limitations. Theta burst stimulation (TBS) was devised in an attempt to provide a more physiological paradigm based on animal work. TBS usually involves short 50 Hz bursts of 3–5 pulses repeated at 5 Hz (theta frequency), typically 10 bursts in one train.[4] LTD also involves multiple mechanisms.[3] Homosynaptic LTD is often induced with low-frequency stimulation of 600–900 pulses at 1–5 Hz.

A drawback of these LTP or LTD induction protocols is that the highly synchronous population activities do not occur naturally. Canadian psychologist Donald Hebb made an influential proposal for synaptic plasticity in 1949. He suggested that a memory trace in an ensemble of neurons becomes permanently laid down as changes in synaptic weight when a presynaptic neuron repeatedly takes part in the firing of the postsynaptic cell. The presynaptic activity must precede postsynaptic activity. Subsequent studies confirmed these predictions. In vitro studies found that presynaptic action potentials must be followed by postsynaptic potentials within a narrow time window (~20 ms) for LTP to occur. Importantly, LTD is induced if the postsynaptic potentials occur before the presynaptic potentials.[5–8]

Plasticity inducing TMS protocols in humans are summarized in Table 4.1 and Figure 4.1.

4.2 PAIRED ASSOCIATIVE STIMULATION

LTP- and LTD-like changes can be induced in humans using paired associative stimulation (PAS),[9–12] based on the Hebbian concept of spike-timing–dependent plasticity, with two inputs paired to arrive at a single neuron at approximately the same time. It takes about 20 ms for the sensory impulses from the median nerve to reach the sensory cortex. If the TMS is applied 21–25 ms after median nerve stimulation, primary motor cortex (M1) neurons are synchronously activated by afferent input (presynaptic) and TMS (postsynaptic activation). Thus, repeated pairs of median nerve stimulation and TMS lead to enhanced M1 excitability.[9] Changes in M1 excitability induced by PAS occur rapidly; last at least 60 min; are topographically specific, occurring selectively in median nerve innervated muscles; and are blocked by dextromethorphan (NMDA receptor antagonist) or nimodipine (L-Type voltage-gated Ca^{2+} channel blocker).[12] Thus, the physiological and pharmacological profile of PAS,[13] the effects of motor learning,[14] and how different sessions of PAS interact[15] all suggest that LTP-/LTD-like mechanisms likely underlie cortical plasticity induced by PAS. Cervical epidural recordings showed that PAS25 (TMS applied 25 ms after peripheral nerve stimulation) increased the amplitudes

TABLE 4.1. Summary of plasticity inducing protocols using transcranial magnetic stimulation (TMS)

Protocol	Description of typical procedure	Proposed mechanism of action	Time required for induction (min)
LTP-like protocols			
PAS21.5/ PAS 25	Median or ulnar nerve stimulation at the wrist at 3 times sensory threshold or to produce thumb twitch, paired with TMS to the contralateral M1 delivered ~ 21.5 or 25 ms later, at 0.1 Hz for 30 min (180 pulses)	Spike timing dependent plasticity: Postsynaptic activation (TMS) coincident with presynaptic activation (afferent input)	30
High-frequency rTMS	rTMS applied to M1 at 10 Hz frequency, 100% of resting MT, with 30 stimuli per train, one train every 30 sec and 60 trains (1,800 pulses)	Homosynaptic plasticity: high-frequency stimulation	30
iTBS	3 TMS pulses at 80% active MT is given at 50 Hz, with bursts repeated at a 5 Hz (i.e., 200 ms, theta frequency). Two second trains of TBS applied every 10 s for a total of 190s (600 pulses)	Homosynaptic plasticity: theta burst stimulation	3.2
iTMS1.5	2 identical TMS pulses 1.5 ms apart, adjusted to produce 1 mV MEP in the first dorsal interosseous muscle, repeated every 5 s for 15 min (180 pairs)	Spike timing-dependent plasticity at SICF peak: LTP-like effect	15
DIS	4 pairs of TMS pulses. ISI with each pair 1.3-1.5 ms, time between pairs 200–250 ms. 6 trains of 4 pairs at intertrain interval of 8 s	SICF during late cortical disinhibition	0.75
QPS5	360 trains of 4 pulses at 90% RMT, intertrain interval of 5 s, 5 ms between each pulse. Monophasic pulses are used	Homosynaptic plasticity	30
LTD-like protocols			
PAS10	Stimulation paradigm is identical to PAS21.5 except that time between peripheral nerve stimulation and TMS is 10 ms instead of 21.5 or 25 ms	Spike timing–dependent plasticity: Postsynaptic activation (TMS) preceding the presynaptic activation (afferent input)	30

(continued)

TABLE 4.1. CONTINUED

Protocol	Description of typical procedure	Proposed mechanism of action	Time required for induction (min)
Low frequency rTMS	rTMS applied to M1 at 1 Hz for 1,800 pulses (30 min) at 115% of resting motor threshold (RMT)	Homosynaptic plasticity: low-frequency stimulation	30
cTBS	Similar to iTBS, except that TBS is applied continuously for 40s (600 pulses)	Homosynaptic plasticity: theta burst stimulation	0.7
iTMS2	Similar to iTMS1.5, except that the paired TMS are at interstimulus interval of 2 ms instead of 1.5 ms	Spike timing-dependent plasticity at SICF trough: LTD-like effect	15
QPS30	Similar to QPS5, but the time between pulses are 30 ms instead of 5 ms	Homosynaptic plasticity	30

cTBS, continuous theta burst stimulation; DIS, disinhibition stimulation; iTBS, intermittent theta burst stimulation; iTMS1.5, TMS at I-wave frequency, 1.5 ms; iTMS2, TMS at I-wave frequency, 2 ms; LTD, long term depression; LTP, long term potentiation; MT, motor threshold; PAS, paired associative stimulation; QPS5, quadripulse stimulation, 5 ms; QPS30, quadripulse stimulation, 30 ms; RMT, resting motor threshold; rTMS, repetitive transcranial magnetic stimulation; SICF, short interval intracortical inhibition

of the late descending indirect (I) waves, providing evidence that PAS increased cortical excitability.[16] Interestingly, PAS21.5 did not change the descending volleys, indicating that PAS21.5 and PAS25 affect different cortical circuits.[17]

4.2.1 Typical Setup for PAS

A typical PAS set up is to use median nerve stimulation at the wrist with the cathode positioned proximally to direct the stimulation current centrally. Ulnar nerve stimulation may also be used. The intensity of median nerve stimulation is often set at three times sensory threshold[18] or just sufficient to produce a visible twitch.[19] TMS is applied to the motor cortex, typically with induced current in the posterior-anterior (PA) direction at intensity that induces a motor-evoked potentials (MEP) amplitude of about 1 mV in the abductor pollicis brevis (APB) or the first dorsal interosseous (FDI) muscles or at approximately 1.3 times resting motor threshold (RMT).[9,20] Some studies used a fixed interstimulus interval (ISI) between median nerve stimulation and TMS, such as 21.5 or 25 ms, while other studies set the ISI in relation to the latency of N20 median nerve somatosensory evoked potential (SEP) to account for variations in conduction times from

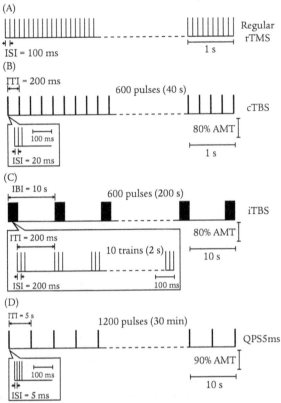

FIGURE 4.1 *(A) Typical stimulus parameters used in four commonly used repetitive transcranial magnetic stimulation protocols. Regular high-frequency repetitive transcranial magnetic stimulation (rTMS) at 10 Hz. Interstimulus interval (ISI) is 100 ms. Stimulus intensity, number of pulses per train, and intertrain intervals (ITIs) are limited for safety reasons. (B) Continuous theta burst stimulation (cTBS). Trains of pulses (600 pulses) are delivered in a continuous pattern with ITI of 200 ms (5 Hz). The bottom frame magnifies one train of stimuli. Each train consists of three pulses with ISI of 20 ms (50 Hz). Stimulus intensity is set at 80% active motor threshold (AMT). (C) Intermittent TBS (iTBS). Trains of pulses (600 pulses) are delivered in an intermittent pattern with interblock interval (IBI) of 10 s (20 blocks in total). The bottom frame magnifies one block of stimuli. Each block consists of 10 trains with ITI of 200 ms (5 Hz). Each train consists of three pulses with ISI of 20 ms (50 Hz). Stimulus intensity is set at 80% AMT. (D) Quadripulse stimulation at 5 ms ISI (QPS5ms). Trains of pulses (1,440 pulses) are delivered in a continuous pattern with ITI of 5 s (0.2 Hz). The bottom frame magnifies one train. Each train consists of four pulses with ISI of 5 ms (200 Hz). Stimulus intensity is set at 90% AMT.*

FROM NI AND CHEN, *J PHYSIOL.* 2008;586:3733–3734, WITH PERMISSION.

peripheral nerve stimulation to the primary somatosensory cortex in different study participants. The range is often N20 + 2 to N2 + 6 ms, which approximately corresponds to 21.5 and 25 ms.[19] In contrast, PAS10 (TMS 10 ms after median nerve stimulation) reduces M1 excitability since the postsynaptic activation (TMS) precedes the presynaptic activation (afferent input).[10]

4.2.2 Effects of PAS Frequency

Different frequencies of peripheral nerve-TMS pairs such as 0.05 Hz,[9] 0.1 Hz,[21] and 0.2 Hz[22] have been used. A study showed that a short duration protocol with 132 stimulus pairs at 0.2 Hz produced greater increase in cortical excitability than a long protocol with 90 stimulus pairs at 0.05 Hz.[23] A meta-analysis suggested that PAS-LTP is most effective at frequencies between 0.05 Hz and 0.2 Hz.[24] A rapid-rate PAS25 protocol with subthreshold median nerve stimulation paired with subthreshold repetitive TMS (rTMS) at 5 Hz increased cortical excitability and decreased short-latency afferent inhibition (SAI).[25] While the same protocol with PAS10 had no effect on cortical excitability,[25] rapid-rate PAS15 decreased cortical excitability and SAI.[26] Thus, rapid-rate PAS also causes spike-timing dependent bidirectional plasticity.

4.2.3 Effects of Interstimulus Interval

A study showed that the plasticity effect of median nerve stimulation followed by TMS at 25 ms (PAS25) was abolished by simultaneous application of anodal or cathodal cerebellar transcranial direct current stimulation (tDCS). In contrast, PAS21.5 was unaffected by anodal cerebellar tDCS.[17,27] These findings suggest that the cerebellum is involved in mediating the effects of PAS25, with sensory input possibly conveyed through the cerebellum, whereas PAS21.5 may be mediated more purely at the cortical level.[27]

While both PAS21.5 and PAS25 produced MEP facilitation, randomly intermixing pairs of median nerve stimulus and TMS at an ISI of 21.5 and 25 ms during plasticity induction produced no facilitation. When anodal cerebellar tDCS was applied simultaneously to cancel the effects of PAS25, plasticity induction was restored. These findings suggest that PAS21.5 and PAS25 are mutually inhibitory.[28]

PAS10[10] adjusted to ISIs of 8.5 or 10 ms based on N20 latency both produced cortical inhibition with LTD-like effects, with a trend for greater inhibition with the adjusted ISI.[20]

4.2.4 Effects of the Number of Stimuli Pairs

One study showed that PAS25 with 50 pairs of ulnar nerve-M1 stimulation at 0.1 Hz had no effect.[29] PAS25 with ulnar nerve stimulation at 0.05 Hz showed dose-dependent progressive increase in M1 excitability when the stimulation duration was increased from 7 to 15 and to 30 min.[30] With PAS25 at delivered at 0.25 Hz, the increase in cortical excitability was higher for 270 pairs of median nerve-M1 stimuli compared to 90 and 180 pairs, demonstrating a dose response relationship between the number of plasticity-inducing stimuli and the plasticity effects.[18]

4.2.5 Effects of TMS Intensity

Using PASN20 + 2 at 0.2 Hz for 180 pairs, and increasing the TMS intensity from producing 1 mV MEP at the APB muscle to producing 1 mV MEP in the presence of median nerve stimulation (SAI), led to greater increase in cortical excitability.[19] Interestingly, pairing median nerve stimulation with subthreshold TMS decreased cortical excitability.[19] These findings suggest that the degree of neural activity induced by stimulation determines the magnitude and direction of the plasticity effects induced by PAS in the motor cortex. Similarly, with PAS10, TMS intensities of 1.3 and 0.95 RMT produced MEP inhibition but not at a lower intensity of 0.8 RMT.[20]

4.2.6 Effects of Current Direction and Voluntary Muscle Contraction

While PAS25 with 50 pairs of ulnar nerve-M1 stimulation at 0.1 Hz inducing current in the PA direction has no effect at rest, the same protocol during slight (5% maximum) voluntary contraction produced MEP facilitation.[29] In addition, PAS with subthreshold TMS at 0.95 active motor threshold (AMT) during voluntary contraction produced facilitation when TMS was applied with induced current in the anterior-posterior (AP) but not in the usual PA direction. No facilitation was observed when digital nerve stimulation was used instead of ulnar nerve stimulation.[29] The greater efficacy of AP compared to PA TMS in inducing plasticity may be due to activation of I3 input. A subsequent study showed that with PAS21.5 at subthreshold intensity of 0.95 AMT during voluntary contraction, MEP facilitation was observed with TMS in the PA but not in the AP direction.[17] These findings suggest that PAS21.5 involves PA input but PAS25 involves AP input.

4.2.7 Effects of Cortical Inhibition

Cortical inhibition is critical for the regulation of excitability and plasticity. Many cellular examples exist in which *disinhibition* (removal of inhibition) is necessary for plasticity to take place. For example, in animal studies, the induction of cortical LTP using theta burst stimulation (TBS)[31–33] or associative plasticity[34] is greatly facilitated by removal of inhibition with pharmacological blockade of gamma aminobutyric acid type A (GABA$_A$) receptors and, conversely, is blocked by GABA$_A$ receptor activation.[35] PAS-induced LTP-like cortical plasticity is pharmacologically blocked by the GABA$_B$ agonist baclofen[36] and by drugs that enhance GABA$_A$ receptor activity.[37]

Short-interval intracortical inhibition (SICI) is a form of cortical inhibition likely mediated by GABA$_A$ receptors. When PAS25 was applied concurrently with SICI by applying double-pulse TMS with a subthreshold conditioning pulse 2 ms before a suprathreshold test pulse instead of a single suprathreshold pulse, PAS plasticity was blocked.[38] Similarly, addition of a subthreshold pulse to induce SICI during plasticity induction with PAS10 blocks the LTD-like effects.[20] Increasing the test stimulus intensity to match the MEP amplitude to that of a single pulse did not restore the plasticity induction effects for both PAS25 and PAS10, indicating blockade of plasticity by SICI could not be explained by the degree of activation of corticospinal neurons and is likely due to intracortical inhibition blocking PAS plasticity.[20,38] However, SICI did not affect the plasticity effects of PAS21.5 from TMS with induced current in the PA direction but blocked the effects of PAS21.5 with induced current in the AP direction.[39] Since AP TMS preferentially evokes the I3 wave while PA TMS evokes the I1 wave, and SICI suppresses the I3 but not the I1 wave, these findings suggest that PAS21.5 (PA direction) may activate circuits involved in the I1 wave which are not affected by SICI whereas PAS25 (PA direction) and PAS21.5 (AP direction) may activate circuits involved in the I3 wave which are inhibited by SICI. Thus, SICI provides a nonpharmacological way to modulate plasticity. On the other hand, engagement of intracortical facilitation (ICF) during PAS25 by adding a subthreshold conditioning pulse 10 ms before the suprathreshold TMS pulse did not alter the LTP-like effects.[38] Similarly, application of ICF with PAS10 did not alter the cortical inhibitory effect.[20]

PAS induction with pairing of median nerve stimulation and TMS between 21.5 and 25 ms induces SAI, which is stronger at an ISI of approximately 21.5 ms than at 25 ms.[19] SAI was unchanged after PAS25.[38] For both PAS(N20 + 2) and PAS(N20 + 6), participants with stronger SAI had weaker plasticity effects, with individual variations of the strength of SAI accounting for about 40% of the variations in PAS effects.[19]

4.2.8 Time of the Day

PAS25 with 90 pairs at 0.05 Hz increased MEP amplitude when the test was conducted in the evening but not in the morning. Administration of corticosteroid prevented MEP facilitation, suggesting this time of day effect could be due to fluctuations in the level of corticosteroids.[40] However, another study found no effect of the time of the day.[41]

4.2.9 Attention and Stimulus Uncertainty

PAS25 effects were larger when the participant's attention was directed to the stimulated hand and was abolished when attention was directed away from the stimulated hand, such as attending to the contralateral hand or performing a competing cognitive task,[22] particularly in those with a high attention load.[42] A study administered PAS25 with 90 paired stimuli and 90 single-pulse TMS. When an auditory clue did not predict (uncertain condition) whether the upcoming stimulus was single or paired, the increase in MEP amplitude was higher than when the auditory clue was predictive of the upcoming stimulus, suggesting that stimulus uncertainty was associated with higher degree of plasticity.[43]

4.2.10 Topographical Specificity

PAS effects are topographically specific, affecting predominately the muscles innervated by the nerve used for PAS and the cortical area stimulated. Using PAS25 with median nerve stimulation, the increase in cortical excitability was much greater for the median nerve-innervated abductor pollicis brevis (APB) than the ulnar nerve-innervated abductor digiti minimi (ADM) muscle.[9] No facilitation was observed for the biceps, tibialis anterior, or APB muscle ipsilateral to cortical stimulation.[9] With a rapid 5 Hz PAS25 and median nerve stimulation, facilitation was observed for APB but not for the ulnar nerve-innervated first dorsal interosseous or the extensor carpi radialis muscle.[25]

4.2.11 Influence of Genetic Variations

Individuals with the rare Met allele single nucleotide polymorphism (SNP) of brain derived neurotrophic factor (BDNF) Val66Met did not have response to PAS25 or metaplasticity when cathodal tDCS was followed by subthreshold 1 Hz rTMS, which was present in the more common val/val genotype.[44] The finding that PAS25 increased cortical excitability in val/val participants but not in Met carriers was confirmed in one study[45] but another found no effect of BDNF genotype.[46] However, among Met homozygotes of the catechol-O-methyltransferase (COMT) Val158Met polymorphism, BDNF Val/Val carriers showed a higher degree of plasticity from PAS25 compared to Met carriers, suggesting that there is an interaction between BDNF and COMT genotypes.[46] A study in 25 children aged 6–18 years found variable responses to PAS25 and no differences among BDNF genotypes.[47]

4.2.12 Effects of Drugs on PAS

The facilitatory effects of PAS25 were blocked by administration of NMDA receptor blocker dextromethorphan and the L-type voltage-gated calcium channel blocker nimodipine and were turned into depression by the T-type voltage-gated calcium channel blocker ethosuximide.[48] These findings are consistent with PAS25 being mediated by synaptic plasticity.

PAS is also affected by dopaminergic neurotransmission. Low-dose (25 mg) dopamine precursor L-dopa abolished the effects of PAS25 and PAS10, while a medium dose

(100 mg) maintains and prolongs the effects of PAS25 and PAS10. High doses (200 mg) reversed PAS25 effects to inhibition but did not change PAS10.[49] Similar effects on PAS25 were obtained by administering the D2 receptor blocker sulpiride together with L-dopa to investigate the effects of dopamine D1 receptor activation.[50] Low (2.5 mg), medium (10 mg), and high (20 mg) doses of the D2 agonist bromocriptine reduced the facilitatory effects of PAS25, but blocked the inhibitory effects of PAS10 at low and high doses but not at the medium dose.[51] These findings are consistent with a nonlinear, inverted U-shaped effect of dosage of dopamine on cortical plasticity.

4.2.13 Interaction Between PAS and Motor Practice

Since LTP and LTD are thought to underlie learning-induced cortical plasticity, the interactions between PAS and motor practice are of considerable interest. To best utilize plasticity-inducing protocols as treatments to enhance rehabilitation for neurological disorders such as stroke, it is crucial to understand their effects on learning.

4.2.13.1 *Effects of Motor Practice on PAS-Induced Plasticity*

A task that involved motor learning with repeated fast thumb abduction was found to change a subsequent PAS LTP protocol (PAS(N20)) from facilitation to inhibition.[52] The same task increased the inhibitory effect of a PAS LTD (PAS(N20-5)) protocol. A task with slow thumb abduction that did not induce motor learning did not change the effects of PAS.[52] These findings are similar to the effects of training in dynamic motor performance (DMP), which involves thumb abduction to a target force window. DMP abolished the effect of PAS25[53] and changed the effects of 90 pulses of PAS25 from weak facilitation to inhibition.[18] However, motor learning was unaffected when the effect of PAS25 was blocked by DMP.[53] The training in DMP had no effect on PAS10. If PAS10 was applied after motor training, the efficacy of PAS25 on cortical excitability was restored.[53] These findings suggest that the mechanisms associated with motor training temporarily suppress associative cortical plasticity and are consistent with animal studies showing that motor learning reduces subsequent LTP but enhances LTD. They are also consistent with the Bienstock-Cooper-Munro (BCM) theory, which states that threshold LTD and LTP depend on the history of cortical activities.[54]

4.2.13.2 *Effects of PAS on Motor Learning*

PAS at an ISI of N20-5 ms, which induced an LTD-like effect, was found to facilitate motor learning that involved rapid thumb flexion when the motor practice began immediately or at 90 min after the PAS protocol. PAS at an ISI of N20 + 2 ms, which induced an LTP-like effect, facilitated motor learning when the practice began immediately after PAS but depressed leaning when practice began 90 min after completion of PAS.[55] Thus, while the findings at 90 min are consistent with homeostatic interaction, non-homeostatic interaction between PAS-LTP and motor learning may occur immediately after PAS. One study examined whether LTP-like induction protocols such as PAS can enhance motor learning. It showed that PAS25 improved motor learning in a rotary pursuit task at 1 week but not at 45 min after the plasticity intervention, whereas PAS10 had no effect.[56] Dynamic motor practice (DMP) that involved thumb abduction to a target force window alone led to increased MEP amplitude. When DMP was applied after PAS with 270 pairs (PAS270), it led to decreased MEP amplitudes, thus indicating homeostatic interaction.[18] Interestingly, PAS90 and PAS180, which had lower plasticity effects, did not change the effects of DMP in cortical excitability. PAS did not change the performance of DMP.[18]

4.2.14 Metaplasticity of PAS Effects

Application of anodal tDCS, which increased cortical excitability, before PAS25 at 0.05 Hz with ulnar nerve stimulation increased the efficacy of PAS. On the other hand, cathodal tDCS, which decreased cortical excitability, decreased the efficacy of subsequent PAS25.[30] This demonstrates a non-homeostatic interaction between tDCS and PAS. However, when anodal tDCS was applied during the same PAS25 induction, the activity turned into inhibition. When cathodal tDCS was applied during PAS25, the period of excitability enhancement was prolonged. Thus, the interactions between tDCS and PAS25 were homeostatic when they were applied simultaneously.[30]

The interactions between two PAS protocols have also been studied. PAS(N20 + 2) with median nerve stimulation at 0.25 Hz with 225 pairs of stimuli was used to induce LTP and PAS(N20-5) was used to induce LTD.[15] Application of PAS(N20 + 2) decreased and PAS(N20-5) increased the MEP facilitation produced by PAS(N20 + 2) applied 30 min after the first protocol. Since the PAS protocol likely activates the same synapses, this demonstrates homosynaptic, homeostatic interactions between two PAS protocols.[15]

PAS is also affected by cortical inputs and shows homeostatic plasticity. After facilitatory 5 Hz rTMS applied to the left dorsal premotor cortex (PMd), PAS(N20 + 2) became inhibitory instead of facilitatory. Conversely, prior administration of inhibitory 1 Hz rTMS to the left PMd turned PAS(N20-5) into facilitation.[57]

4.2.15 Variability in the Effects of PAS

A meta-analysis confirmed that PAS-LTP increased cortical excitability for up to 90 min and PAS-LTD decreased cortical excitability for up to 120 min, with stronger potentiating effects for PAS-LTP than the depression effect of PAS-LTD.[24] However, it is known that there is considerably variability in the effects of PAS. Some studies only included "responder" individuals who had increased corticospinal excitability with PAS-LTP or decreased excitability with PAS-LTD.[53] For example, one study stated that 31 out of 48 participants were "responders".[17] A study that used PAS(N20 + 2) with 225 pairs at 0.25 Hz found 14 participants with LTP-like effects, but 13 participants had LTD-like effects.[58] Moreover, a study with 56 participants using PAS25 at 0.25 Hz with ulnar stimulation and recording from the FDI muscle found no overall plasticity effect, with 61% responder and 39% nonresponders.[41] Another study with 21 participants also found no significant overall effect of PAS25, PAS22, and PAS at individualized intervals between ulnar nerve stimulation and TMS based on MEP and M-wave latencies, although the protocol with individualized intervals had lower interindividual variability.[59] A pooled data analysis from three laboratory studies with 190 participants found no main effect of PAS intervention, with a 53% responder rate.[60] The effects of PAS25 were found to be reproducible but intraindividual reliability was low between two sessions.[61] Reproducibility was found to be greater in the afternoon than the morning.[23] Overall, previous studies indicated that considerable variability in the response to PAS, but the responder rate varied from study to study. This may in part be due to different protocols and varying definitions of "responder."

4.2.16 Other Factors That May Affect the Effects of PAS

Both LTP- and LTD-like effects decreased with age in one study,[58] but another study found no effect of age.[41] Lower RMT correlated with greater LTP-like effects.[58]

Individuals with greater baseline SICI were found to have a greater increase in cortical excitability with PAS25. The authors suggested that individuals in whom TMS predominately evoked late I waves are more susceptible to both SICI and PAS25.[62] However, another study found different results, in that participants with lower baseline SICI were more likely to have increased cortical excitability after PAS, with baseline SICI accounting for approximately 10% of the variability of PAS25.[41]

4.2.17 PAS Involving M1 Leg Area

While most studies tested PAS in the hand area of M1, PAS in the M1 leg area also induced plasticity. Pairing of common peroneal nerve stimulation with TMS using a double-cone coil to activate the tibialis anterior muscle during the last swing phase of walking (0.1 Hz, 120 pairs) increased MEP amplitude in the tibialis anterior muscle when the ISI was set at MEP latency + 5 ms.[63] In contrast, when the ISI was set at MEP latency −10 ms, inhibition was observed.[63] A follow-up study found that MEP facilitation was only observed if the stimuli were applied during the late swing phase, while the same stimulus pairs applied during the mid-swing phase led to MEP inhibition.[64] A study found that pairing common peroneal nerve stimulation with TMS at 0.2 Hz for 30 min (360 pairs) led to MEP facilitation at an ISI of 45–55 ms and MEP inhibition at an ISI of 40 ms.[65] Plasticity induction during ankle dorsiflexion, which activated the target tibialis anterior muscle, produced greater facilitation compared to rest. Optimizing the ISI based on somatosensory evoked potential latency also increased the degree of facilitation.[65] Both monophasic and biphasic TMS at suprathreshold and subthreshold intensities could induce this plasticity at rest.[66] However, another study reported a much wider range of timing between peripheral nerve stimulation and TMS to induce facilitation. With the leg muscles at rest, a PAS protocol pairing the common peroneal nerve at 0.1 Hz for 15 min (90 pairs) surprisingly showed MEP facilitation when the sensory input was timed to arrive at the motor cortex from 15 to 90 ms *after* the TMS pulse.[67] Pairing of three common peroneal pulses with subthreshold TMS also produced MEP facilitation.[67] The authors suggested these findings are due to pairing of sensory input with sustained, subthreshold activation of cortical neurons from a suprathreshold TMS pulse.[67]

A systematic review that examined 12 articles supported the efficacy of a single session of lower limb PAS to modulate corticospinal excitability, but the protocols used in previous studies were highly variable.[68]

4.2.18 Passive Movement Associative Stimulation

This protocol involves pairing of left M1 TMS at 120% RMT with biphasic current targeted to the flexor carpi radialis (FCR) muscle at 1 Hz with 400 stimuli. The participants' wrist was moved passively by a robot and the TMS pulse was timed when the wrist passed from flexion to extension, at the FCR muscle lengthening phase.[69] The protocol resulted in decreased MEP amplitude up to 30 min, which was not observed with TMS alone. However, different timings of passive movements were not tested. The results could be due to the effects of 1 Hz rTMS, and excitability changes could occur at the cortical or spinal level.

A study used beta-band event-related desynchronization of electroencephalogram (EEG) signal from a motor imagery task to trigger peripheral stimulation via passive hand opening by a robotic orthosis combined with TMS for 165 trials. It found increased MEP amplitude when TMS was applied synchronously with the robotic passive hand opening but not when TMS was applied 80 ms after the onset robotic hand opening. The change persisted after a depotentiation task that involved voluntary muscle contraction.[70]

4.2.19 Cortico-Cortical PAS

PAS plasticity can be induced by paired stimulation of two cortical areas at specific intervals, known as cortico-cortical PAS (cc-PAS).

4.2.19.1 Interhemispheric ccPAS

Pairing of left M1 followed by right M1 stimulation at an ISI of 8 ms at 0.05 Hz over 30 min at intensities that produced 1 mV MEP led to increased MEP amplitude from right M1 stimulation and reduction of short-interval interhemispheric inhibition (SIHI) from left to right hemisphere. However, right to left M1 cc-PAS reduced right to left SIHI but did not change left M1 excitability.[71] Another study showed that right to left M1 cc-PAS at an ISI of 15 ms and intensity of 120% RMT at 0.1 Hz with 180 pairs led to increased MEP amplitude and facilitation of fine finger movements.[72]

4.2.19.2 Ventral Premotor Cortex (PMv)-M1 ccPAS

Left PMv (110% RMT)-left M1 (1mV MEP) PAS at an ISI of 8 ms with 90 pairs at 0.1 Hz led to increased inhibitory influence of PMv over M1 when tested at rest. When the participants performed a visuomotor task, the same protocol led to an increased facilitatory influence of PMv over M1. Reversing the order of stimulation, with M1 followed by PMv stimulation at 8 ms, decreased the facilitatory influence of PMv over M1 during the visuomotor task. The effects lasted at least 1 hour.[73] Moreover, PMv-M1 ccPAS improved performance in a nine-hole peg test.[74] A functional magnetic resonance imaging (fMRI) study showed that this intervention led to increased PMv-M1 functional connectivity during task performance but not at rest. This was accompanied by increased influence of PMv input on M1.[75] Another study tested left PMv-M1 ccPAS at a much longer latency of 40 ms with 90 pairs of TMS pulses at 0.1 Hz. PMv to M1 inhibition tested with dual-site TMS at an ISI of 40 ms was increased immediately after the intervention but not at 20 or 40 min afterward.[76]

4.2.19.3 Supplementary Motor Area (SMA)-M1 ccPAS

Repetitive pairing of SMA stimulation (140% AMT, inducing AP current) with bilateral M1 stimulation at an ISI of 6 ms for 150 trials at approximately 0.2 Hz increased M1 excitability, whereas pairing of M1 stimulation followed by SMA stimulation 15 ms later led to decreased M1 excitability. The facilitatory effects required "priming" with a series (150 trials) of near simultaneous bilateral M1 stimulation, with left M1 stimulation at 0.8 ms before right M1 stimulation.[77] Long-latency left SMA-M1 ccPAS at a latency of 40 ms with 90 pairs of TMS pulses at 0.1 Hz was found to increase PMv to M1 inhibition at an ISI of 40 ms at 20 min after the intervention but not at 0 or 40 min.[76]

4.2.19.4 Posterior Parietal Cortex (PPC)-M1 ccPAS

Left PPC (90% RMT) stimulation followed by M1 stimulation (1 mV MEP, induced PA current) at an ISI of 5 ms with 100 pairs at 0.2 Hz while at rest led to decreased M1 excitability, while reversing the pulses with M1 stimulation followed by left PPC stimulation increased M1 excitability. Since the PPC-M1 connection is facilitatory, this is considered anti-Hebbian plasticity.[78] If the participant maintained a slight voluntary contraction during the plasticity induction, the effects were reversed, with pairs of PPC-M1 leading to increased and pairs of M1-PPC stimulation leading to decreased M1 excitability, resulting in Hebbian plasticity. Reversing the current direction of M1 stimulation to AP current with participants at rest during the plasticity induction also led to Hebbian plasticity.[78] These findings suggest that the direction of plasticity induction critically depends on the state of the M1 and the cortical circuits activated. In another study, left PPC (90% RMT) followed by left M1 stimulation (1mV MEP, induced PA current) with 180 pairs at 0.2 Hz and an ISI of 8 ms increased M1 excitability and abolished the facilitatory PPC-M1 interaction observed at baseline assessed with dual-site TMS at 8 ms. Similar increase in right M1 excitability was observed following right PPC-M1 ccPAS.[79] It is possible that pairing PPC with M1 inducing AP current at 5 ms and with M1 inducing PA current at 8 ms activates similar circuits, but further studies are required to examine the mechanisms involved.

4.2.19.5 Cerebellum-M1 PAS

Right cerebellar stimulation with a double-cone coil at 95% AMT (determined with the coil over the inion) paired with left M1 TMS (1 mV MEP) with 120 pairs at 0.25 Hz led to MEP potentiation at an ISI of 2 ms and MEP depression at an ISI of 6 and 10 ms.[80] Since the optimal interval for cerebellar inhibition (CBI) is 5–7 ms,[81,82] M1 activation by TMS precedes M1 disfacilitation from CBI at 2 ms ISI. At an ISI of 6 ms, M1 activation by TMS approximately coincides with disfacilitation from CBI. A study confirmed that cerebellum-M1 PAS at 6 ms reduced M1 excitability but the effects were variable among participants and did not change CBI or PMd-M1 interaction tested with dual-site TMS.[83]

4.2.19.6 Cortico-Motoneuronal (Spinal) PAS

These paradigms are designed to modulate transmission at the corticospinal-motoneuronal synapses in the spinal cord. The initial protocol involves M1 TMS with a circular coil targeted to produce a small MEP from the biceps muscle paired with peripheral nerve stimulation at the supraclavicular fossa. TMS was delivered 3 ms before peripheral stimulation, timed for the corticospinal volley to reach the corticospinal synapse in the spinal cord approximately 1 ms before the antidromic afferent volley. Fifty paired stimuli led to increased cervicomedullary MEPs from electrical transmastoid stimulation and increased voluntary force in the biceps muscle.[84] This change was decreased with administration of dextromethorphan, suggesting that it could involve NMDA receptors.[85]

Pairing of TMS 22 ms before peripheral stimulation or peripheral stimulation delivered 13 ms before TMS led to opposite changes with decreased cervicomedullary MEPs and voluntary force in the biceps muscle.[84]

A modified protocol involves 100 pairings of TMS to the M1 hand area at 100% stimulator output inducing PA current paired with supramaximal (M-Max) ulnar nerve stimulation at the wrist at 0.1 Hz for 17 min. The timing between TMS and ulnar nerve stimulation was adjusted based on MEP latencies from TMS and magnetic stimulation over the cervical spine and M-Max latency. For the spike timing-dependent plasticity (STDP) protocol, the descending corticospinal volley was timed to arrive 1–2 ms before the antidromic volley from ulnar nerve stimulation to produce presynaptic activation before postsynaptic activation at the spinal motoneuron. In the control protocol, the ISI was timed to allow the antidromic volley to reach motoneuron dendrites 5 ms before arrival of the corticospinal volley. The STDP protocol led to increased MEP amplitude from TMS and transcranial electrical stimulation (TES), greater force output from the index finger, and increased dexterity assessed with a nine-hole peg test in spinal cord injury patients but not in healthy controls. The control protocol decreased the size of MEP from TMS and cervicomedullary junction stimulation.[86] These findings demonstrate the possibility of inducing spike timing-dependent plasticity at the synapse between corticospinal neuron and spinal motoneuron with functional consequences. Greater plasticity effect was produced by 100 compared to 50 paired stimuli.[87]

A similar protocol can be used to strengthen the corticospinal synapse for lower limb muscles. TMS was applied with a double-cone coil at 100% stimulator output. It involved 200 paired stimuli delivered at 10 Hz with a corticospinal volley from TMS timed to arrive at the corticomotoneuronal synapse for the tibialis anterior (TA) muscle 2 ms before arrival of antidromic potentials in the motor neuron from common peroneal nerve stimulation.[88] The protocol led to increased MEP amplitude for the TA muscle from both TMS and TES for up to 30 min, together with increased TA electromyogram (EMG) activity and ankle dorsiflexion force. When the timing of TMS and the common peroneal nerve stimulation was changed to the antidromic potential arriving at spinal motor neuron at 15 or 28 ms before the corticospinal volley, the protocol led to decreased MEP amplitude for the TA muscle.[88] Cortico-motoneuronal PAS can also be achieved with motor point stimulation of the target muscle such as the soleus muscle.[89] Motor point stimulation increases the number of target muscle that this paradigm can be applied to.

4.2.19.7 Spinal-Cortical and Cortical-Spinal PAS

Plasticity can be induced by combining cortical and spinal cord stimulation. Cortical stimulation was applied to the left M1 with a double-cone coil targeted to the right tibialis anterior muscle. Spinal stimulation was applied with a cathode at the T11 level. PAS was conducted with 240 pairs of stimuli at 0.1 Hz for 40 min. The ISI was determined from the MEP latencies of the tibialis anterior muscle from TMS and spinal stimulation. In spinal-cortical PAS, spinal stimulation was delivered before TMS, with spinal input serving as presynaptic input to cortical neurons. Spinal-cortical PAS was found to increase MEP amplitude and decrease SICI. With cortical-spinal PAS, TMS was delivered before spinal stimulation and was timed for arrival of corticospinal volleys at the presynaptic terminals of spinal motor neurons before spinal stimulation evoked depolarization of spinal motor neurons. Cortico-spinal PAS decreased MEP amplitudes but did not affect cortical inhibition. Both protocols decreased the M-wave threshold, suggesting that they affect the excitation threshold of motor axons and spinal reflexes. Therefore, both protocols affect cortical, spinal, and peripheral nerve excitability.[90]

4.2.19.8 Basal Ganglia-Cortical PAS

Single-pulse stimulation of the subthalamic nucleus from deep brain stimulation (DBS) electrodes was found to increase M1 excitability at an ISI of about 3 ms, which likely represents antidromic activation of the hyperdirect pathway from M1 to the subthalamic nucleus (STN), and, at approximately 23 ms that may represent transmission along the indirect basal ganglia pathway.[91] Repetitive pairing of STN DBS followed by TMS at an individually determined ISI of about 3 ms for the short interval and at about 23 ms for the medium interval at 0.1 Hz for 180 pairs led to increased MEP amplitude for both interventions, but not with a control protocol at an ISI of 167 ms (Figure 4.2).[92] In cervical dystonia patients treated with internal globus pallidus (GPi) DBS, single-pulse GPi DBS facilitated the M1 at an ISI of approximately 10 ms but inhibited the M1 at approximately 25 ms. Similar to the finding for STN DBS, repeated pairing of GPi DBS at these two time intervals produced LTP-like plasticity of M1.[93] These findings show that pairing of basal ganglia DBS with cortical TMS at suitable intervals can induce associative plasticity in the cortex, and this could be relevant to the mechanisms of DBS.

4.2.19.9 Cortico-Cortical PAS Involving Nonmotor Area

CcPAS involving nonmotor areas can be studied with the technique of TMS-EEG or behavioral measures. Pairing of median nerve stimulation and the TMS of left dorsolateral prefrontal cortex (DLPFC) at an ISI of 25 ms was found to enhance cortical activity, as shown by measurement of TMS evoked potentials (TEP) using the technique of TMS-EEG.[94] Since administration of L-dopa and rivastigmine increased and dextromethorphan decreased the PAS after-effects, dopaminergic, cholinergic, and glutamatergic transmission are likely involved.[95]

ccPAS at an ISI of 10 ms between the right and left lateral prefrontal cortex (LPFC) was used to strengthen interhemispheric frontal connections. Behavioral and TMS-EEG measures suggested that ccPAS strengthened inhibition from the first stimulated to the second stimulated hemisphere.[96]

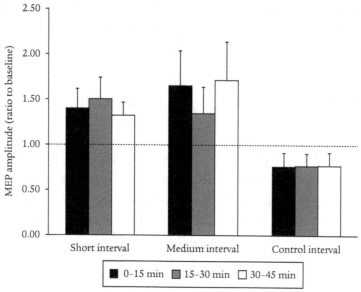

FIGURE 4.2 *Induction of cortical plasticity by repeated pairing of subthalamic deep brain stimulation and transcranial magnetic stimulation (TMS). Effects of 180 pairs of subthalamic nucleus stimulation and motor cortical TMS on cortical excitability. The data are plotted as a ratio to the baseline motor-evoked potential (MEP) amplitude before the plasticity protocol. Ratios >1 indicate facilitation and ratios <1 indicate inhibition. Error bars represent standard error of the mean (SEM). The effects of plasticity protocols on 1mV MEP at the three post-intervention time blocks are shown. The plasticity protocol increased mean MEP amplitudes with short (~3 ms) and medium (~23 ms) intervals from subthalamic nucleus stimulation to motor cortical TMS, but not at the control (167 ms, in the middle of STN pulses delivered at 3 Hz) interval.*
FROM UDUPA ET AL., *J NEUROSCI*. 2016;36(2):396–404, WITH PERMISSION.

A study used cc-PAS to target the right inferior frontal cortex (IFC) and the pre-supplementary motor (pre-SMA).[97] These areas are involved in stopping of movements. When pre-SMA preceded IFC stimulation by 10 ms, younger participants showed impairment in response inhibition in a stop-signal task. In older participants, response inhibition improved when IFC pulse preceded the pre-SMA pulse by 4 ms. The study suggested that cc-PAS modulated cortico-cortical and cortico-subcortical networks.

cc-PAS between frontal and parietal cortices have also been investigated. Right intraparietal sulcus (IPS) to right LPFC ccPAS with 100 paired pulses at an ISI of 10 ms shifted decision-making from a habitual to a more goal-directed strategy.[98] Another study used ccPAS to modify the connection between the left inferior parietal lobule and the middle frontal gyrus with 180 paired pulses at an ISI of 10 ms. Parietal to frontal ccPAS increased logical reasoning while frontal to parietal ccPAS increased relational reasoning.[99] Thus, ccPAS can be used to modulate cortical connectivity and lead to behavior or task performance. A review of ccPAS has been published.[100]

In summary, STDP-like plasticity can be induced with a PAS paradigm targeting the connection between different areas of the central nervous system such as other cortical areas, cerebellum, basal ganglia, and spinal cord. However, the direction of the plasticity is not easily predictable and may change with experimental details such as background muscle activity, involvement in tasks, and induced current directions.

4.3 REGULAR REPETITIVE TRANSCRANIAL MAGNETIC STIMULATION

rTMS involves regularly repeated trains of TMS pulses.[101] By convention, stimulation frequencies of greater than 1 Hz are referred to as high-frequency whereas stimulating frequencies of 1 Hz or less are referred to as low-frequency rTMS.[101] The parameters that affect the effects of regular rTMS include the stimulation frequency, intensity, intertrain intervals, the total number of pulses, and the shape of the pulses (Figure 4.3).

4.3.1 Frequency of rTMS

Low-frequency rTMS decreases corticospinal excitability. Chen et al.[102] demonstrated that a 15-min train of suprathreshold (115% RMT) 0.9 Hz rTMS applied to the M1 reduced MEP size for at least 15 min. Similar results have been reported by others,[103–106] but some studies reported no change in MEP amplitude.[107,108] Epidural recordings showed that the reduced MEP amplitude is associated with reduction of late I-wave amplitude, confirming that it is due to decreased cortical excitability.[109] A review indicated that 13 of 19 studies of low-frequency rTMS showed reduction in MEP amplitude. Some of the variability may occur because the plasticity effects appear to depend on the phase of the

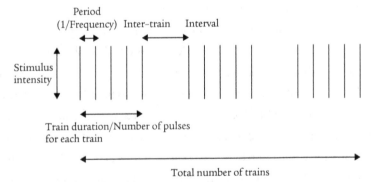

FIGURE 4.3 *Stimulation parameters for regular repetitive transcranial magnetic stimulation (rTMS). Each line represents one pulse. The parameters shown are stimulation frequency, intensity, number of pulses per train, intertrain interval, and the number of trains. Pulse shape and current direction (not shown) should also be considered.*

sensorimotor mu rhythm. One Hz rTMS applied at the positive peak of the mu rhythm led to significant reduction of MEP amplitude, but 1 Hz rTMS applied at the negative peak showed a trend toward a LTP-like effect, while random phase showed a trend toward a LTD-like effect.[110] Five of the six studies that showed no effect used relatively low (85–90% RMT, 90% AMT) stimulus intensities.[111] Most studies reported no change in SICI with low-frequency rTMS.[111]

A fMRI study showed that 1 Hz rTMS to left M1 caused deactivation of the right primary somatosensory cortex (S1) and bilateral posterior parietal and inferior frontal cortices with a finger tapping task that peaked at about 20 min after rTMS.[112] Thus, 1 Hz M1 rTMS caused widespread deactivation of nonmotor networks.

The behavioral effects of 1 Hz rTMS have been investigated. Although it decreased cortical excitability, the peak force and acceleration of the thumb flexion and fifth digit abduction were unaffected.[104] However, when applied immediately after motor practice designed to increase the speed of ballistic pinch between thumb and index finger, 1 Hz rTMS to M1 blocked the retention of behavioral improvement, suggesting that M1 played a role in the consolidation of acquired motor skills.[113]

There are contradictory reports of the effects of low-frequency rTMS on contralateral M1. Three studies found increased MEP amplitude,[114–116] one found decreased,[117] and another found no change.[118]

High-frequency rTMS has opposite effects and increases M1 excitability.[119] With 5 Hz rTMS at 150% RMT, there was clear MEP facilitation. Ten and 20 Hz rTMS with lower intensities (110% RMT) also produced consistent facilitation.[120,121] A review indicated that most studies found an immediate increase in MEP amplitude after 5–20 Hz rTMS, although two studies that used 5 Hz rTMS at relatively low intensity (100% AMT) found no change.[122,123] Six studies reported reduction in SICI following high-frequency rTMS, but four studies reported no change.[111] Epidural recordings following 5 Hz rTMS at 120% RMT found increased amplitudes of late I waves, confirming that the higher MEP amplitude is due to increased cortical excitability.[109]

The mechanisms underlying changes in cortical excitability with regular rTMS are not fully understood. Many investigators suggested that decreased excitability is related to LTD,[102] whereas increased excitability is related to LTP.[124] This is consistent with the observation that D-cycloserine, a NMDA receptor partial agonist, increases the motor cortical plasticity induced by 10 Hz rTMS.[125]

4.3.2 Effects of Stimulus Intensity

A study showed that 1 Hz rTMS for 15 min increased RMT and decreased MEP amplitude when applied at 115% RMT. In contrast, at the intensity of 85% RMT, RMT increased but there was no change in MEP amplitude.[105] Another study reported similar results.[126] Thus, the effects of 1 Hz rTMS appear to be dependent on stimulus intensity.

For high-frequency TMS, the effects of stimulus intensity were demonstrated in a study which showed that 1,500 pulses of 5 Hz rTMS at 90% AMT had no effect, but at 90% RMT increased MEP amplitude.[127]

4.3.3 Number of Pulses

The number of pulses also influences the plasticity effects of rTMS. A study found that 150 pulses of 5 Hz subthreshold (90% RMT) rTMS had no effect on MEP amplitude but 1,800 pulses increased corticospinal excitability for at least 30 min.[128] With subthreshold (80% RMT) 10 Hz rTMS, 20 trains of 5 s (1,000 pulses) led to *decreased* MEP amplitude for up to 90 min with decreased SICI and increased ICF. With 20 trains of 1.5 s (300 pulses) at the same intensity (80% RMT), MEP amplitude increased for up to 120 min.[129] Therefore, the effects of the number of pulses differ depending on the intensity and frequency of stimulation.

4.3.4 Intertrain Interval

High-frequency rTMS is usually applied as trains of pulses with pauses between trains known as *intertrain intervals* (Figure 4.3), in part due to safety considerations and machine limitations. Few studies examined the effects of intertrain intervals. With rTMS at 5 Hz, 90% AMT, and 1,200 biphasic pulses, rTMS in blocks of 200 pulses with intertrain intervals of 60 s and initial induced current in the PA direction induced increased MEP amplitude, as expected. Interestingly, blocks of rTMS with initial current in the AP direction and continuous rTMS without gaps did not produce any change in cortical excitability.[130] This finding showed that breaks in rTMS are important in determining the direction of induced changes. With 20 Hz rTMS at 100% RMT and 2 s trains, intertrain interval between 4 and 32 s all showed increased MEP amplitude with no significant difference among them, although there was a trend for 4 s intertrain interval to show higher MEP amplitude.[131] Reduction in SICI was greater with shorter intertrain intervals. These findings showed that intertrain interval can be shortened to 4 s without loss of rTMS effects, and M1 excitability and intracortical inhibition can be affected differently by rTMS.

4.3.5 Genetic Factors

Subthreshold (90% RMT) and suprathreshold (110% RMT) 10 Hz rTMS increased MEP amplitudes regardless of BDNF genotype. However, MEP amplitudes were higher after suprathreshold compared to subthreshold rTMS in the Val/Val group but not in the Met carriers.[132] Thus, BDNF polymorphism may modulate the effects of rTMS.

4.3.6 Effects of TMS Waveform and Current Directions

With 20 pulses, 2 Hz and 3 Hz rTMS increased MEP amplitudes during rTMS when monophasic pulses were used regardless of whether the induced current was in the anterior-medial or posterior-lateral direction, but no change was observed with biphasic pulses.[133] Monophasic 10 Hz rTMS with 1,000 pulses at 90% RMT produced greater and longer-lasting increases in MEP than did biphasic pulses.[134] Monophasic 1 Hz rTMS was found to produce greater and longer-lasting reduction in corticospinal excitability than did biphasic rTMS.[135,136] The greater effect of monophasic rTMS may be because it targets a more uniform population of axons and neurons, whereas biphasic rTMS affects neuronal populations in different directions.

The importance of pulse shape is further highlighted by studies that used a device with controllable TMS pulse shape. One Hz rTMS with 1,000 pulses at 97.5% RMT was applied to left M1. While conventional sinusoidal bidirectional pulses had no effect, rectangular bidirectional pulses and rectangular unidirectional pulses with the initial AP- or PA-induced current all led to decreased MEP amplitudes.[137] Moreover, monophasic 1 Hz rTMS with pulse widths of 40 μs and 80 μs produced inhibition; pulse width of 120 μs led to facilitation.[138]

4.3.7 Effects of rTMS on Cortical Facilitatory and Inhibitory Circuits

One study showed that 1 Hz rTMS at 85% or 115% RMT had no effect on cSP, SICI, and ICF.[105] This is consistent with a review concluding that low-frequency rTMS had no substantial effect on cortical inhibition.[111] However, high-frequency rTMS appears to reduce cortical inhibition measured with paired-pulse methods.[19,111,127] One study showed that 600 pulses of 5 Hz rTMS at 90% RMT increased short-interval intracortical facilitation (SICF).[127]

4.3.8 Homeostatic Plasticity, Metaplasticity, and Priming of Low-Frequency rTMS

Metaplasticity refers to the modification of plasticity induction by previous neuronal activities of the network. Plasticity needs to be regulated, and homeostatic mechanisms are in place to ensure that activities in the cortical network stay within a useful dynamic range.[54] For example, the induction of LTP is facilitated if a LTP protocol is preceded by a LTD protocol.

Metaplasticity was first demonstrated using TMS with priming stimulation. A priming stimulation with 6 Hz rTMS at a subthreshold intensity of 90% RMT for 10 min enhanced the MEP depression effects of a subsequent 1 Hz rTMS at 115% RMT.[139] This is consistent with priming of LTD observed in vivo[140] and could be a way to increase the effects of low-frequency rTMS.[141]

Another study showed that anodal transcranial direct current stimulation (tDCS), which increased cortical excitability, caused a subsequent subthreshold (85% RMT) 15 min train of 1 Hz rTMS to decrease cortical excitability. In contrast, cathode tDCS, which decreased cortical excitability, caused the same 1 Hz rTMS protocol to increase cortical excitability.[142] This is further demonstration of metaplasticity with low-frequency rTMS.

4.4 THETA BURST STIMULATION

Animal studies have used intermittent TBS (iTBS) to facilitate synaptic transmission[32,143,144] and continuous TBS (cTBS) to produce synaptic suppression.[144,145] Huang and Rothwell applied rTMS in TBS mode.[146,147] Each burst of the TBS protocol consists of 3 weak pulses (80% AMT) at 50 Hz frequency, with the bursts repeated at 5 Hz (theta frequency).[147] iTBS consists of 2 s trains of TBS applied every 10 s for a total of 600 pulses (iTBS600, 190s duration) and produces an approximate 50% increase in MEP amplitude that lasts about 60 min.[147] In contrast, cTBS consists of 40 s of uninterrupted TBS (600 pulses, cTBS600) and produces an approximate 50% decrease in MEP amplitude that lasted about 20 min (Figure 4.1). Epidural recording showed that cTBS reduced the I1 wave, consistent with a cortical origin for the MEP reduction.[148] However, low-frequency rTMS[109] and cortical inhibitory circuits such as SICI and SAI all decreased the late I waves, indicating that different cortical circuits are affected by these protocols. In contrast, iTBS increased late I waves but not the I1 wave.[149] TBS likely involves LTP (iTBS) and LTD (cTBS) based on similarity with induction protocols used in animal studies, and these changes are blocked by NMDA receptor antagonists.[150]

4.4.1 Effects of Test Stimulus Intensity

Most TBS studies used a single stimulus intensity, such as the intensity needed to produce 1 mV MEP before plasticity induction to test changes in cortical excitability. Studies that used an input-output curve found that the MEP depression effect of cTBS600 was most prominent at high stimulus intensities of 150% RMT or higher,[151] whereas the MEP facilitation effect of iTBS600 was greatest and most consistent at a low intensity of 110% RMT.[152]

4.4.2 Effects of Duration of Stimulation and Number of Pulses

A study showed that cTBS with 300 pulses (cTBS300) with the target muscle at rest produced MEP facilitation while 600 pulses (cTBS600) (as in the original protocol) led to MEP inhibition.[153] It appeared that in cTBS600, the initial 300 pulses primed the brain to undergo depression, which changes the effects of the second cTBS300. Moreover, doubling the duration of conventional TBS also reversed the effects of TBS. Thus, cTBS1200 produced MEP facilitation while cTBS600 led to MEP inhibition, as expected. Similarly, iTBS1200 caused MEP inhibition while iTBS600 resulted in MEP inhibition, as previously described.[154] Administration of two TBS600 sessions with breaks of 2, 5, or 20 min found that two cTBS sessions separated by 20 min produced MEP inhibition similar to that of a single cTBS session. Two iTBS sessions separated by 2 min led to MEP facilitation similar to that of a single iTBS session. Two sessions with the other breaks (e.g., 5 min) produced no change in cortical excitability. Thus, prolonging the stimulation protocol or applying two sessions does not increase the plasticity effect but may block or reverse it.[155] However, a study found that iTBS1200 caused MEP facilitation while cTBS1200 led to MEP inhibition.[156] The authors speculated that the effects of TBS are related to voluntary muscle activation (see later discussion) from determination of AMT. They observed the expected effect of TBS with 1,200 pulses because the time between muscle activation for determination of AMT and beginning of TBS was about 30 min, whereas, in the previous study, it was about 5 min.[154] Another study tested iTBS600, 1200, 1800 and found *decreased* motor cortical excitability with iTBS1200. For cTBS600 to 3600, cTBS3600 *increased* excitability.[157]

4.4.3 Effects of Frequency of Bursts

Adjusting the burst frequency according to the individual dominant frequency recorded by EEG between 4 and 16 Hz for iTBS600 produced similar MEP facilitation compared to the conventional frequency of 5 Hz. However, both individualized cTBS600 and 5 Hz cTBS600 produced no significant effect on MEP amplitude.[158] Thus, individualizing the theta component of TBS did not improve its efficacy.

4.4.4 Effects of Muscle Activation

Muscle contractions have a profound effect on the effects of TBS. cTBS300 with target muscle at rest was found to produce MEP facilitation, but, when preceded by tonic voluntary activation of the target muscle 5 min earlier, it led to MEP inhibition.[153] It was suggested that cTBS300 caused MEP inhibition in another study[147] because AMT was determined before cTBS, which required voluntary activation of the target muscle.[153] However, even without prior muscle contraction (such as measurement of AMT), some studies found facilitatory effects of cTBS300[153,159] while others found no overall effects of cTBS300 or cTBS600.[160] Phasic finger movements prior to cTBS600 were found to produce facilitatory effects instead of inhibitory effects, while phasic finger movements before iTBS600 produced MEP inhibition and not facilitation.[161] These results are consistent with the finding that a 2 min contraction of the target muscle at 10% maximum voluntary contraction at 15 min prior to cTBS 600 (0.7 RMT) increased variability and abolished the MEP depressing effect of cTBS.[162] These effects are thought to reflect polarity-reversing metaplasticity. However, muscle contraction may have no effect if it occurs 30 min before TBS.[156]

Contraction of the target muscle *during* application of TBS abolished the effects of both iTBS and cTBS on MEP amplitudes.[163] Muscle contraction immediately *after* iTBS increased the duration of increased MEP amplitude, while, for cTBS, it changed the effect from MEP inhibition to MEP facilitation.[163]

4.4.5 Effect of Drugs

The NMDA receptor antagonist memantine[150] and the dopamine D2 receptor antagonist sulpiride[164] blocked the facilitatory effects of iTBS and the inhibitory effects of cTBS. Moreover, the facilitatory effects of cTBS300 without prior muscle activation was blocked by the NMDA receptor antagonist dextromethorphan and the T-type calcium channel blocker ethosuximide[48] and was turned into depression by the L-type voltage-gated calcium channel blocker nimodipine.[165] These results are consistent with the effects of iTBS being mediated by LTP and cTBS by LTD.

4.4.6 Variability and Predictors of Responses to TBS

The response to TBS has high variability and several studies examined this issue. A meta-analysis of 87 studies concluded that iTBS yielded moderate to large increases in MEP amplitudes up to 30 min, while cTBS reduced MEP amplitudes for up to 60 min, with the largest effects seen at 5 min.[166] A report pooled the data from 22 studies with 430 healthy participants and found that 67.9% of participants showed iTBS induced facilitation and 65.4% showed cTBS induced suppression of MEP. There was moderate within-participant reliability but large between-participant variability.[167]

In contrast, a study with 56 participants found that the effects of cTBS600 and iTBS600 were highly variable with no overall significant effects for either intervention.[168] Another study assessed the response to two sessions of iTBS600, cTBS600, and sham

TBS in 24 participants. Both iTBS600 and cTBS600 were not different from sham stimulation in both TMS-EEG and MEP measurements, and there was high inter- and intra-individual variability.[169]

For iTBS600, a study of 56 participants found no significant overall effect, with 43% of participants classified as "responders."[41] These studies demonstrated high interindividual variability for response to TBS. However, another study found increased MEP amplitude in 22 out of 30 participants tested with iTBS600. The direction and magnitude of the plastic change showed high intraindividual reliability tested with repeat sessions 1–3 weeks apart.[170] In a study with 27 participants, iTBS600 was found to increase MEP amplitudes in two separate sessions, but the increase (23.4%) was greater for Visit 1 than Visit 2 (6.4%), with an average of 7.8 days between visits.[171] There was low correlation and reliability between the results of the two sessions. The study also found high interindividual variability, as previously reported.[168] In 36 older and diabetic participants, iTBS600 (0.8AMT) was found to have low reproducibility, which may be related to the low reproducibility of single-pulse MEP amplitude.[172] Time of the day, age, and baseline SICI did not predict the response to iTBS600.[41]

For cTBS600, a study with 10 participants showed limited test-retest reproducibility and was highest with corticospinal excitability measured at 5 min after cTBS.[173] Another cTBS600 study also found no overall effects in 21 participants, and a cluster analysis showed one cluster of participants with increased MEP amplitude and another cluster with decreased MEP amplitude.[174] Test-retest reliability of two sessions of left M1 cTBS600 was tested in 28 participants. While there was no overall change in MEP amplitude, assessment at 50 min was more reliable than earlier timepoints.[175] However, cTBS600 (0.7 RMT) without preceding voluntary contraction was found to reliably produce MEP inhibition, with 72% of 34 participants showing MEP depression and 0% showing MEP potentiation.[162] The interparticipant variability is much greater if cTBS is preceded by 2 min of weak (10% maximum) target muscle contraction.

Most TBS studies used biphasic TMS machines, and AP was the predominant current direction used for iTBS. Using the difference in MEP latency in the AP and lateral-median (LM) directions as a marker of the ease of recruitment of late I-waves, the expected increase in cortical excitability after iTBS and decrease in excitability after cTBS was observed only in participants with recruitment of late I waves (larger MEP latency differences between with AP and LM stimulation) but not in participants with little difference in MEP latencies between AP and LM directions.[168] Thus, the intracortical circuit activated appears instrumental in determining the plasticity induced by TBS, and this may account for some of the interparticipant variability of response to TBS. Another study of 34 participants confirmed that there was no overall effect of cTBS600, but there was correlation between the differences in the MEP latencies in the AP and LM directions and the MEP depression effect of cTBS600.[176] With a median split, participants with higher baseline MEP variability had greater MEP suppression with cTBS600.[176]

Some studies attempted to predict response to iTBS from neuroimaging data. In 12 participants, iTBS600 (0.7RMT) led to increased MEP amplitude, which negatively correlated with movement-related fMRI activity in the left M1 from a visually cued thumb abduction task, and participants with stronger left SMA-PMv and left PMv-M1 connectivity had greater response to iTBS.[177] Another study reported that nonresponders to iTBS600 had stronger resting state functional connectivity between M1 and the premotor area compared to responders. Three sessions of iTBS600 separated by 15 min did not convert nonresponders to responders.[178]

Connectivity measured with EEG using a phase lag index may also be used to predict response to TBS. Weaker connectivity between C3 and the frontocentral region was associated with greater response to two sessions of left M1 cTBS600 (70% RMT) separated by 10 min.[179]

In summary, it is clear that TBS has high interparticipant variability. Some studies estimated that about two-thirds of participants are "responders" but other studies found even an lower proportion of "responders," and many did not find an overall effect of iTBS or cTBS. The intra-individual variability (test-retest reliability) also appears to be high, but there are different findings from different studies. The results are highly influenced by small differences in the protocol, including voluntary muscle activation before (including measurement of AMT), during, or after TBS; stimulus duration (number of pulses), etc. Recruitment of I waves and genetic factors may also play a role in the variability.

4.4.7 Effect of Genetic Factors on Cortical Plasticity

Several studies tested the influence of SNPs on cortical plasticity induced by TBS. The most extensively studied SNP is that of *BDNF* Val66Met. In one study, participant with the rare *BDNF* met allele had decreased response to iTBS600 and cTBS600,[44] but other studies found no effect of *BDNF* genotype on the overall effects of iTBS600[180–182] or cTBS600.[181,183] However, the expansion in motor maps with motor training followed by iTBS600 occurred only in participants with the val/val genotype but not in met carriers.[182] Intraindividual variability for iTBS600 was higher for *BDNF*-Met carriers than for *BDNF*-Val homozygotes and higher if the time between sessions was less than 7 days.[172]

For cTBS600, one study reported that participants with the Met allele had greater *increase* in cortical excitability; the *BDNF* genotype together with AMT, which determines the intensity of cTBS, accounted for 59% of the variability of the response at 10 min after cTBS600.[174] Moreover, changes in MEP amplitude following cTBS 600 were more reliable in BDNF met⁻ compared to met⁺ participants.[175] Another study reported that participants who required higher stimulus intensities to achieve 1 mV test MEP are more likely to have a paradoxical facilitatory response from cTBS600, and this effect was more pronounced in *BDNF*-Met carriers than in *BDNF*-Val homozygotes, which could lead to more variable response in *BDNF*-Met carriers.[183] A study in stroke patients reported that Val homozygotes had decreased cortical excitability in response to cTBS600, whereas Met carriers exhibited a modest increase in cortical excitability at 20 min post-stimulation followed by inhibition at 30 min.[184] The BDNF genotype did not affect meta-plasticity tested with cTBS600 followed by cTBS600, cTBS600 followed by iTBS600, or iTBS600 followed by iTBS600.[181]

4.4.8 Depotentiation and De-depression of TBS Effects

Depotentiation refers to reversal of LTP effects by a subsequent protocol that has no effect by itself.[185] Similarly, De-Depression refers to reversal of LTD effects. A short train of cTBS150, which had no effect by itself, abolished the LTP-like effect of iTBS600 when it was given 1 min after iTBS600. Moreover, when cTBS600, which caused LTD-like effects, was followed by iTBS150, the LTD-like effects were reversed.[186] These results demonstrated the depotentiation of iTBS effects and the de-depression of cTBS effects in the human motor cortex. Application of depotentiation to the M1 with cTBS150 after motor skill training disrupted the retention of motor skills,[187] indicating that reversal of motor cortical plasticity influences motor learning.

4.4.9 Proximal and Lower Limb Muscle Representations

Most TBS studies tested the hand representation of the motor cortex. A study showed that cTBS600 depressed MEP amplitudes in the FDI muscle when applied to the hand area but resulted in highly variable and overall nonsignificant effect when applied to the biceps representation.[188] In the lower limb representation, iTBS600 increased while cTBS600 decreased cortical excitability. However, there was high variability, and only 27% of participants responded to iTBS while 63% responded to cTBS.[189]

4.4.10 Effects of TBS on S1

cTBS600 applied over the S1 decreased the P25/N33 amplitude of median nerve somatosensory evoked potential while cTBS600 over the M1 increased this amplitude.[190] Thus, cTBS also has suppressive effect over the S1. Moreover, cTBS600 to the S1 increased the temporal discrimination threshold[191] and reduced inhibition of recovery cycle of the N20/P25 component of somatosensory evoked potentials. It was hypothesized that cTBS reduced the inhibitory interactions in the S1 that is normally used to sharpen processing of sensory input.[192] On the other hand, iTBS600 over the S1 improved temporal[191] and tactile discrimination of the fingers, increased the amplitude of the cortical N20/P25 somatosensory evoked potentials,[193] and decreased paired-pulse inhibition of N20/P25.[194]

4.4.11 Interactions Between TBS Protocols

Pairing of iTBS600 followed by iTBS600 15 min later or cTBS600 followed by cTBS600 resulted in suppression of the effects of the second protocol on MEP amplitude.[195] However, pairing of iTBS600 followed by cTBS600 15 min later or cTBS600 followed by iTBS600 resulted in increased effects of the second protocol. Thus, the interaction between TBS protocols appeared to be homeostatic. Interestingly, changes in SICI from the priming protocol correlated with changes in MEP amplitude from the second protocol, suggesting that priming effect on cortical inhibition contributed to the homeostatic regulation of metaplasticity.[195]

4.4.12 Interactions Between PAS and TBS

PAS and TBS involve different synaptic plasticity mechanisms since PAS involves sensory input and suprathreshold TMS pulses which activated more cortical neurons compared to the subthreshold pulses used in TBS. The interaction between cTBS150 and PAS has been examined.[196] As expected, cTBS150 had no effect on cortical excitability, whereas PAS25 increased and PAS10 decreased cortical excitability. Application of cTBS150 before PAS25 increased cortical facilitation, whereas PAS25 followed by cTBS150 led to decreased cortical excitability. Both priming and following cTBS150 changed the effects of PAS10 to facilitation.[196] These findings demonstrated heterosynaptic, homeostatic interaction in the motor cortex. The occurrence of metaplasticity and depotentiation depends on the order of the interventions (Figure 4.4).

   Application of cerebellar cTBS before a rapid-rate PAS25 protocol was reported to convert nonresponders to PAS to responders. Moreover, prior application of iTBS of the cerebellum changed the effects of rapid-rate PAS25 from facilitation to depression. It was suggested that TBS of the cerebellum may prime the effects of PAS of the motor cortex through changes in the cerebellothalamocortical pathway.[197] The effects of rapid-rate PAS25 or cerebellar cTBS followed by rapid-rate PAS25 were depotentiated by application of cTBS150, which had no effect by itself. Moreover, the LTD-like plasticity effects of cerebellar iTBS followed by rapid-rate PAS25 was abolished by cTBS150.[197]

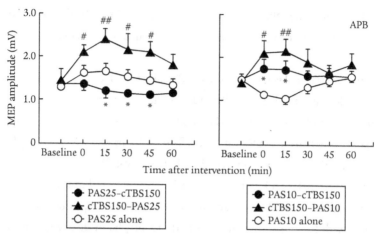

FIGURE 4.4 *Interactions between paired associative stimulation (PAS) and theta burst stimulation (TBS). (Left) PAS25 alone increased cortical excitability. Applying cTBS150, which had no effect by itself, increased the excitatory effects of PAS25, but PAS25 followed by cTBS150 led to decreased cortical excitability. (Right) PAS10 alone decreased cortical excitability. Applying cTBS150 followed by PAS10 or PAS10 followed by cTBS150 both led to increased cortical excitability. These findings demonstrate heterosynaptic, homeostatic interactions in the human motor cortex. Motor-evoked potentials were recorded from the abductor pollicis brevis (APB) muscle.*
FROM NI ET AL., *J NEUROSCI.* 2014;34(21):7314–7321, WITH PERMISSION.

4.5 TMS AT I-WAVE FREQUENCY

The TMS at I-wave frequency (iTMS) protocol refers to repeated delivery of paired TMS at I-wave frequency at 1.5 ms intervals, corresponding to the first peak of SICF. In the initial study, the intensities of two identical TMS pulses were adjusted to produce a MEP of 0.5 to 1 mV delivered at 0.2 Hz for 30 min (360 stimuli pairs).[198] Paired-pulse MEP amplitudes increased during the intervention; single-pulse MEP amplitude increased for 10 min afterward[198] and is associated with increased SICF at all three peaks (1.3, 2.7, 4.3 ms).[199] Fifteen and 30 min of stimulation at 0.2 Hz showed similar effects.[200] Adjusting for the ISI between the two pulses individually to the first peak of SICI produced greater increase in paired-pulse MEP amplitude during the intervention, but single-pulse MEP amplitudes after the intervention was not tested.[201] When the protocol was applied during weak voluntary contraction, with the first pulse generating 1.5 mV in the active FDI muscle and second pulse at 90% AMT, there was increased MEP amplitude, increased first peak of SICF, and emergence of the second and third peaks of SICF after the intervention.[202] The novelty of this protocol is that it directly targets the dynamics of synaptic transmission, which is central to synaptic plasticity. This excitability increase occurs at the cortical level.[203] When the stimuli were paired at an ISI of 2 ms, which resulted in much lower MEP amplitude than an ISI of 1.5 ms, MEP depression was observed.[204]

Carriers of the BDNF met allele were found to have decreased facilitation with iTMS at 1.5 ms and reduced inhibition with iTMS at 2 ms compared to participants with the Val/Val genotype.[205]

An alternative protocol is to target the third peak of SICF or the I3 wave. This involves 180 pairs over 30 min of M1 TMS with induced current in the PA direction at an ISI of 4.3 ms. The first stimulus was 120% RMT, and the second stimulus was at 90% RMT. The protocol leads to increased MEP amplitude from AP current, which elicits I3 wave for 30–110 min, but no change was observed with TMS from PA current. This was accompanied by decreased SICI and increased peak 1 of SICF, tested in the AP but not in the PA direction, and increased F-wave amplitude and persistence. Finger abduction force was also increased. In spinal cord–injured participants, hand dexterity assessed with a nine-hole pegboard test improved.[206] A control protocol at an ISI of 3.5 ms (trough between SICF peaks 2 and 3) had no effect. Thus, this protocol targeting late I waves lead to increased cortical and spinal excitability with behavioral improvement. This is consistent with the suggestion that late I waves receive contribution from subcortical circuits.[206] This protocol also induced MEP facilitation in older participants but required a longer ISI of 4.9 ms compared to 4.1 ms in younger participants, since the third wave of SICF was delayed in older compared to younger participants.[207] A higher degree of SICF at baseline was associated with greater response to this protocol.[208]

4.6 DISINHIBITION STIMULATION

Following a suprathreshold TMS pulse, there is a period of inhibition known as *long-interval intracortical inhibition* (LICI), followed by period of disinhibition termed *late cortical disinhibition* (LCD), also known as *long interval intracortical facilitation* (LICF).[202,209] SICF is increased during LCD.[202] The disinhibition stimulation (DIS) protocol consists of trains of four doublets with an ISI between the two pulses at an individually determined optimal interval for the first peak of SICF (1.3–1.5 ms) with the time between the doublets at the individual optimal disinhibition interval for doublets (200–250 ms) (Figure 4.5). TMS intensity (100–120% RMT) was the minimal intensity to cause an increase in doublet MEP amplitude across the train. Six trains of four doublets were delivered at intertrain intervals of 8 s. Thus, the intervention consisted of 48 stimuli delivered in about 45 s and resulted in increased MEP amplitude during the train of stimuli and for at least 30 min after the intervention.[210] Control protocols with different timing between the doublets or with single stimuli instead of doublets did not lead to increased MEP amplitude. This protocol utilizes LCD, which may be related to presynaptic GABA$_B$ receptor-mediated inhibition, to augment LTP-like plasticity and led to increased cortical excitability with a relatively short

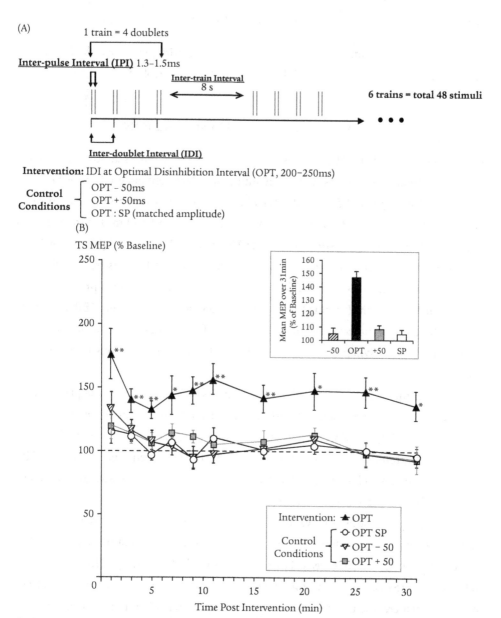

FIGURE 4.5 *Disinhibition stimulation (DIS). Intervention protocol for DIS. The primary transcranial magnetic stimulation (TMS) intervention consisted of 6 trains (intertrain interval, 8 s) of 4 TMS doublets at I-wave frequency (iTMS) (interpulse interval equal to individual peak I-wave facilitation, 1.3–1.5 ms) spaced by the individual optimal disinhibition interval (OPT, 200–250 ms). A total of 48 pulses were applied over ~45 s. Control conditions consisted of decreasing (OPT − 50 ms) or increasing (OPT + 50 ms) the interdoublet interval (IDI) and replacing double-pulse TMS with amplitude-matched single-pulse (SP) TMS. Single pulse motor-evoked potentials (MEPs) were recorded pre- and post-intervention to investigate effects on cortical excitability. (B) Time-course of MEP amplitude changes post-intervention. The primary TMS intervention at OPT resulted in a significant increase in MEP amplitude post-intervention (P <0.001), whereas control experiments did not result in long-term potentiation (LTP)-like plasticity, indicating that late cortical disinhibition facilitates synaptic plasticity in human M1. The average MEP amplitude over 31 min post-intervention relative to pre-intervention baseline was 147% ± 4% at OPT, 105% ± 4% at OPT−50, 108% ± 3% at OPT + 50, and 105% ± 5% in the OPT–SP condition (see inset). *P<0.05, **P<0.01 (post hoc t-tests, significant difference of TS MEP amplitude from baseline).*

FROM CASH ET AL., CEREBRAL CORTEX. 2016;26(1):58–69, WITH PERMISSION.

stimulus train. Motor imagery, which may cause disinhibition, increased the facilitatory effect when applied during the disinhibition stimulation protocol.[211]

4.7 QUADRIPULSE STIMULATION

Quadripulse stimulation (QPS) consists of 360 trains of four pulses at 90% AMT delivered at intertrain interval of 5 s (0.2 Hz, 30 min). The effects depend on the time between the four pulses. QPS at 1.5, 5, and 10 ms between pulses resulted in increased MEP amplitude for more than 30 min, whereas QPS at 30, 50, and 100 ms led to decreased MEP amplitude.[212] Priming stimulation with 10 min of QPS at 5 ms (QPS5), which did not change MEP amplitude by itself, caused a shift of QPS10 effects from facilitation to inhibition and increased the LTD-like effect of QPS30. In contrast, priming stimulation with a short train (10 min) of 5 min of QPS50 led to increased MEP amplitude induced by QPS10 and reversed the QPS30 effect from inhibition to facilitation. This demonstrates homosynaptic, homeostatic plasticity in the interactions between QPS protocols.[212,213]

Reducing the interburst interval of QPS from 5 s to 2.5 s abolished the plasticity effect. Increasing the interburst interval to 7.5 s produced variable response but was similar to conventional PAS.[214] Moreover, while conventional QPS was delivered with monophasic current, biphasic QPS has shorter after effects.[214] Conventional excitatory QPS was reported to have a high responder rate of 80%,[214] although there was no direct comparison with other plasticity induction protocols.

QPS5 applied to the left M1 was found to increase MEP amplitude from the right M1. This increase correlated with the increase in interhemispheric facilitation (IHF) from left M1 to right M1. SIHI also increased from left M1 to right M1. Using fMRI, QPS5 of left M1 was found to decrease the resting state functional connectivity between bilateral M1 while QPS50 increased this connectivity.[215] The effects on resting state connectivity correlated with the effects on MEP. Similar bidirectional modulation of resting state connectivity was also observed with stimulation of prefrontal and parietal association areas.[215] However, how resting state connectivity is affected by inhibitory and excitatory TMS protocols is still unclear.

4.7.1 Interactions Between QPS Protocols Applied to SMA and M1

The supplementary motor area (SMA) was stimulated 3 cm anterior to the optimal site for the tibialis anterior muscle. A short train of priming QPS5 applied to the SMA, which had no effect by itself, reversed the effects of QPS5 and QPS10 applied to M1 from MEP facilitation to inhibition and induced greater MEP inhibition with QPS30. These findings are consistent with homeostatic plasticity and the BCM model. However, the MEP suppression effect of QPS50 and QPS100 was shortened rather than increased, indicating a non-homeostatic interaction.[216]

4.7.2 Effects of QPS on Somatosensory Evoked Potentials

QPS5 applied to the M1 or dorsal premotor cortex increased while QPS50 to the same cortical areas decreased the amplitude of the P25-N33 component of SEP, generated by the somatosensory cortex area 3b and area 1. However, QPS5 or QPS50 applied to S1 had no effect.[217] These findings suggest that QPS to M1 or dorsal premotor cortex changed the excitability of S1.

4.7.3 Other Factors That Influence QPS Effects

The plasticity effect of QPS decreased with age[218] and is unaffected by *BDNF* polymorphism.

4.7.4 Quadripulse Theta Burst Stimulation

The quadripulse theta burst stimulation (qTBS) protocol attempts to merge QPS and TBS. Four pulses at 90% AMT were separated by 200 ms (5 Hz, theta frequency) instead of the 5 s used for QPS. The interstimulus intervals of 1.5 ms (666 Hz) to match I-wave periodicity and 5 ms (200 Hz) were tested. Biphasic pulses with the second pulse in the AP direction at 666 Hz decreased MEP amplitude, while PA qTBS at 666 Hz increased MEP amplitude. Both AP and PA qTBS at 200 Hz increased corticospinal excitability for 60 min.[219] This protocol has not been compared to other plasticity induction protocols.

4.8 COMPARISONS BETWEEN DIFFERENT PLASTICITY PROTOCOLS

Only a few studies compare the effects of different plasticity induction protocols, and the comparisons are limited to assessments of M1 excitability. One study showed that PAS25 increased MEP amplitude while iTBS had no significant effect.[220] Another study found similar effects of PAS25 and iTBS600, but there were no significant effects of 5 Hz rTMS.[106] A study reported increased MEP amplitude with both 5 Hz rTMS and iTBS600, and their effects correlated.[180] Two studies however, found similar efficacy and no overall effects following PAS25 or iTBS.[41,221] Therefore, differences in efficacy between different protocols have not been established.

4.9 SUMMARY OF DIFFERENCES AMONG PLASTICITY PROTOCOLS

PAS utilizes heterosynaptic (involves two synapses), spike-timing–dependent plasticity, whereas regular rTMS, TBS, and QPS involve homosynaptic plasticity with repeated regular (rTMS) or patterned (TBS) stimulation of the same synapses. iTMS targets the dynamics of cortical I waves at the peaks and troughs of SICF, while DIS utilizes SICF during a period of disinhibition. Since these protocols involve different mechanisms, they have different findings in diseases and have different potential therapeutic applications (see Table 4.1).

REFERENCES

1. Rossini PM, Altamura C, Ferreri F, et al. Neuroimaging experimental studies on brain plasticity in recovery from stroke. *Europa Medicophysica.* 2007;43(2):241–254.
2. Malenka RC, Bear MF. LTP and LTD: An embarrassment of riches. *Neuron.* 2004;44(1):5–21.
3. Massey PV, Bashir ZI. Long-term depression: Multiple forms and implications for brain function. *Trends Neurosci.* 2007;30(4):176–184.
4. Raymond CR. LTP forms 1, 2 and 3: Different mechanisms for the "long" in long-term potentiation. *Trends Neurosci.* 2007;30(4):167–175.
5. Debanne D, Gahwiler BH, Thompson SM. Long-term synaptic plasticity between pairs of individual CA3 pyramidal cells in rat hippocampal slice cultures. *J Physiol (London).* 1998;507 (Pt 1):237–247.
6. Bi GQ, Poo MM. Synaptic modifications in cultured hippocampal neurons: Dependence on spike timing, synaptic strength, and postsynaptic cell type. *J Neurosci.* 1998;18(24):10464–10472.
7. Zhang LI, Tao HW, Holt CE, Harris WA, Poo M. A critical window for cooperation and competition among developing retinotectal synapses. *Nature.* 1998;395(6697):37–44.
8. Bi G, Poo M. Distributed synaptic modification in neural networks induced by patterned stimulation. *Nature.* 1999;401(6755):792–796.
9. Stefan K, Kunesch E, Cohen LG, Benecke R, Classen J. Induction of plasticity in the human motor cortex by paired associative stimulation. *Brain.* 2000;123:572–584.
10. Wolters A, Sandbrink F, Schlottmann A, et al. A temporally asymmetric Hebbian rule governing plasticity in the human motor cortex. *J Neurophysiol.* 2003;89(5):2339–2345.
11. Wolters A, Schmidt A, Schramm A, et al. Timing-dependent plasticity in human primary somatosensory cortex. *J Physiol (London).* 2005;565(Pt 3):1039–1052.
12. Stefan K, Kunesch E, Benecke R, Cohen LG, Classen J. Mechanisms of enhancement of human motor cortex excitability induced by interventional paired associative stimulation. *J Physiol.* 2002;543(Pt 2):699–708.
13. Bear MF, Malenka RC. Synaptic plasticity: LTP and LTD. *Curr Opin Neurobiol.* 1994;4:389–399.
14. Ziemann U, Iliac TV, Pauli C, Meintzschel F, Ruge D. Learning modifies subsequent induction of long-term potentiation-like and long-term depression-like plasticity in human motor cortex. *J Neurosci.* 2004;24(7):1666–1672.
15. Muller JF, Orekhov Y, Liu Y, Ziemann U. Homeostatic plasticity in human motor cortex demonstrated by two consecutive sessions of paired associative stimulation. *Eur J Neurosci.* 2007;25(11):3461–3468.
16. Di Lazzaro V, Dileone M, Pilato F, et al. Associative motor cortex plasticity: Direct evidence in humans. *Cerebral Cortex (New York, NY: 1991).* 2009;19(10):2326–2330.
17. Hamada M, Galea JM, Di LV, Mazzone P, Ziemann U, Rothwell JC. Two distinct interneuron circuits in human motor cortex are linked to different subsets of physiological and behavioral plasticity. *J Neurosci.* 2014;34(38):12837–12849.

18. Elahi B, Hutchison WD, Daskalakis ZJ, Gunraj C, Chen R. Dose-response curve of associative plasticity in human motor cortex and interactions with motor practice. *J Neurophysiol.* 2014;111(3):594–601.

19. Cash RFH, Jegatheeswaran G, Ni Z, Chen R. Modulation of the direction and magnitude of Hebbian plasticity in human motor cortex by stimulus intensity and concurrent inhibition. *Brain Stimul.* 2017;10(1):83–90.

20. Weise D, Mann J, Ridding M, et al. Microcircuit mechanisms involved in paired associative stimulation-induced depression of corticospinal excitability. *J Physiol.* 2013;591(19):4903–4920.

21. Morgante F, Espay AJ, Gunraj C, Lang AE, Chen R. Motor cortex plasticity in Parkinson's disease and levodopa-induced dyskinesias. *Brain.* 2006;129(Pt 4):1059–1069.

22. Stefan K, Wycislo M, Classen J. Modulation of associative human motor cortical plasticity by attention. *J Neurophysiol.* 2004;92(1):66–72.

23. Sale MV, Ridding MC, Nordstrom MA. Factors influencing the magnitude and reproducibility of corticomotor excitability changes induced by paired associative stimulation. *Exp Brain Res.* 2007;181(4):615–626.

24. Wischnewski M, Schutter D. Efficacy and time course of paired associative stimulation in cortical plasticity: Implications for neuropsychiatry. *Clin Neurophysiol.* 2016;127(1):732–739.

25. Quartarone A, Rizzo V, Bagnato S, et al. Rapid-rate paired associative stimulation of the median nerve and motor cortex can produce long-lasting changes in motor cortical excitability in humans. *J Physiol.* 2006;575(Pt 2):657–670.

26. Rizzo V, Mastroeni C, Maggio R, et al. Low-intensity repetitive paired associative stimulation targeting the motor hand area at theta frequency causes a lasting reduction in corticospinal excitability. *Clin Neurophysiol.* 2020;131(10):2402–2409.

27. Hamada M, Strigaro G, Murase N, et al. Cerebellar modulation of human associative plasticity. *J Physiol (London).* 2012;590(Pt 10):2365–2374.

28. Strigaro G, Hamada M, Murase N, Cantello R, Rothwell JC. Interaction between different interneuron networks involved in human associative plasticity. *Brain Stimul.* 2014;7(5):658–664.

29. Kujirai K, Kujirai T, Sinkjaer T, Rothwell JC. Associative plasticity in human motor cortex during voluntary muscle contraction. *J Neurophysiol.* 2006;96(3):1337–1346.

30. Nitsche MA, Roth A, Kuo MF, et al. Timing-dependent modulation of associative plasticity by general network excitability in the human motor cortex. *J Neurosci.* 2007;27(14):3807–3812.

31. Hess G, Donoghue JP. Long-term potentiation of horizontal connections provides a mechanism to reorganize cortical maps. *J Neurophysiol.* 1994;71:2543–2547.

32. Hess G, Aizenman CD, Donoghue JP. Conditions for the induction of long-term potentiation in layer II/III horizontal connections of the rat motor cortex. *J Neurophysiol.* 1996;75(5):1765–1778.

33. Castro-Alamancos MA, Donoghue JP, Connors BW. Different forms of synaptic plasticity in somatosensory and motor areas of the neocortex. *J Neurosci.* 1995;15(7 Pt 2):5324–5333.

34. Kanter ED, Haberly LB. Associative long-term potentiation in piriform cortex slices requires GABAA blockade. *J Neurosci.* 1993;13(6):2477–2482.

35. Evans MS, Viola-McCabe KE. Midazolam inhibits long-term potentiation through modulation of GABAA receptors. *Neuropharmacology.* 1996;35(3):347–357.

36. McDonnell MN, Orekhov Y, Ziemann U. Suppression of LTP-like plasticity in human motor cortex by the GABAB receptor agonist baclofen. *Exp Brain Res.* 2007;180(1):181–186.

37. Heidegger T, Krakow K, Ziemann U. Effects of antiepileptic drugs on associative LTP-like plasticity in human motor cortex. *Eur J Neurosci.* 2010;32(7):1215–1222.

38. Elahi B, Gunraj C, Chen R. Short-interval intracortical inhibition blocks long-term potentiation induced by paired associative stimulation. *J Neurophysiol.* 2012;107:1935–1941.

39. Ni Z, Cash RFH, Gunraj C, Bercovici E, Hallett M, Chen R. Involvement of different neuronal components in the induction of cortical plasticity with associative stimulation. *Brain Stimul.* 2019;12(1):84–86.

40. Sale MV, Ridding MC, Nordstrom MA. Cortisol inhibits neuroplasticity induction in human motor cortex. *J Neurosci.* 2008;28(33):8285–8293.

41. Lopez-Alonso V, Cheeran B, Rio-Rodriguez D, Fernandez-Del-Olmo M. Inter-individual variability in response to non-invasive brain stimulation paradigms. *Brain Stimul.* 2014;7(3):372–380.

42. Kamke MR, Hall MG, Lye HF, et al. Visual attentional load influences plasticity in the human motor cortex. *J Neurosci.* 2012;32(20):7001–7008.

43. Sale MV, Nydam AS, Mattingley JB. Stimulus uncertainty enhances long-term potentiation-like plasticity in human motor cortex. *Cortex.* 2017;88:32–41.

44. Cheeran B, Talelli P, Mori F, et al. A common polymorphism in the brain-derived neurotrophic factor gene (BDNF) modulates human cortical plasticity and the response to rTMS. *J Physiol (London).* 2008;586(Pt 23):5717–5725.

45. Cirillo J, Hughes J, Ridding M, Thomas PQ, Semmler JG. Differential modulation of motor cortex excitability in BDNF Met allele carriers following experimentally induced and use-dependent plasticity. *Eur J Neurosci.* 2012.

46. Witte AV, Kurten J, Jansen S, et al. Interaction of BDNF and COMT polymorphisms on paired-associative stimulation-induced cortical plasticity. *J Neurosci.* 2012;32(13):4553–4561.

47. Myers KA, Vecchiarelli HA, Damji O, Hill MN, Kirton A. Significance of BDNF Val66Met polymorphism in brain plasticity of children. *Pediatr Neurol.* 2017;66:e1–e2.

48. Weise D, Mann J, Rumpf JJ, Hallermann S, Classen J. Differential regulation of human paired associative stimulation-induced and theta-burst stimulation-induced plasticity by L-type and T-type Ca2+ channels. *Cerebral Cortex (New York, NY: 1991).* 2017;27(8):4010–4021.

49. Thirugnanasambandam N, Grundey J, Paulus W, Nitsche MA. Dose-dependent nonlinear effect of L-DOPA on paired associative stimulation-induced neuroplasticity in humans. *J Neurosci.* 2011;31(14):5294–5299.

50. Fresnoza S, Paulus W, Nitsche MA, Kuo MF. Nonlinear dose-dependent impact of D1 receptor activation on motor cortex plasticity in humans. *J Neurosci.* 2014;34(7):2744–2753.

51. Fresnoza S, Stiksrud E, Klinker F, et al. Dosage-dependent effect of dopamine D2 receptor activation on motor cortex plasticity in humans. *J Neurosci.* 2014;34(32):10701–10709.

52. Ziemann U, Ilić TV, Pauli C, Meintzschel F, Ruge D. Learning modifies subsequent induction of long-term potentiation-like and long-term depression-like plasticity in human motor cortex. *J Neurosci.* 2004;24(7):1666–1672.

53. Stefan K, Wycislo M, Gentner R, et al. Temporary occlusion of associative motor cortical plasticity by prior dynamic motor training. *Cereb Cortex.* 2006;16(3):376–385.

54. Cooper LN, Bear MF. The BCM theory of synapse modification at 30: Interaction of theory with experiment. *Nature Rev Neurosci.* 2012;13(11):798–810.

55. Jung P, Ziemann U. Homeostatic and nonhomeostatic modulation of learning in human motor cortex. *J Neurosci.* 2009;29(17):5597–5604.

56. Rajji TK, Liu SK, Frantseva MV, et al. Exploring the effect of inducing long-term potentiation in the human motor cortex on motor learning. *Brain Stimul.* 2011;4(3):137–144.

57. Pötter-Nerger M, Fischer S, Mastroeni C, et al. Inducing homeostatic-like plasticity in human motor cortex through converging corticocortical inputs. *J Neurophysiol.* 2009;102(6):3180–3190.

58. Müller-Dahlhaus JF, Orekhov Y, Liu Y, Ziemann U. Interindividual variability and age-dependency of motor cortical plasticity induced by paired associative stimulation. *Exp Brain Res.* 2008;187(3):467–475.

59. Campana M, Papazova I, Pross B, Hasan A, Strube W. Motor-cortex excitability and response variability following paired-associative stimulation: A proof-of-concept study comparing individualized and fixed inter-stimulus intervals. *Exp Brain Res.* 2019;237(7):1727–1734.

60. Lahr J, Passmann S, List J, Vach W, Floel A, Kloppel S. Effects of different analysis strategies on paired associative stimulation: A pooled data analysis from three research labs. *PLo SOne.* 2016;11(5):e0154880.

61. Fratello F, Veniero D, Curcio G, et al. Modulation of corticospinal excitability by paired associative stimulation: Reproducibility of effects and intraindividual reliability. *Clin Neurophysiol.* 2006;117(12):2667–2674.

62. Murase N, Cengiz B, Rothwell JC. Inter-individual variation in the after-effect of paired associative stimulation can be predicted from short-interval intracortical inhibition with the threshold tracking method. *Brain Stimul.* 2015;8(1):105–113.

63. Stinear JW, Hornby TG. Stimulation-induced changes in lower limb corticomotor excitability during treadmill walking in humans. *J Physiol.* 2005;567(Pt 2):701–711.

64. Prior MM, Stinear JW. Phasic spike-timing-dependent plasticity of human motor cortex during walking. *Brain Res.* 2006;1110(1):150–158.

65. Mrachacz-Kersting N, Fong M, Murphy BA, Sinkjaer T. Changes in excitability of the cortical projections to the human tibialis anterior after paired associative stimulation. *J Neurophysiol.* 2007;97(3):1951–1958.

66. Mrachacz-Kersting N, Stevenson AJT. Paired associative stimulation targeting the tibialis anterior muscle using either mono or biphasic transcranial magnetic stimulation. *Front Hum Neurosci.* 2017;11:197.

67. Roy FD, Norton JA, Gorassini MA. Role of sustained excitability of the leg motor cortex after transcranial magnetic stimulation in associative plasticity. *J Neurophysiol.* 2007;98(2):657–667.

68. Alder G, Signal N, Olsen S, Taylor D. A systematic review of paired associative stimulation (PAS) to modulate lower limb corticomotor excitability: Implications for stimulation parameter selection and experimental design. *Front Neurosci.* 2019;13:895.

69. Edwards DJ, Dipietro L, Demirtas-Tatlidede A, et al. Movement-generated afference paired with transcranial magnetic stimulation: An associative stimulation paradigm. *J Neuroengineer Rehab.* 2014;11:31.

70. Kraus D, Naros G, Guggenberger R, Leão MT, Ziemann U, Gharabaghi A. Recruitment of additional corticospinal pathways in the human brain with state-dependent paired associative stimulation. *J Neurosci.* 2018;38(6):1396–1407.

71. Rizzo V, Siebner HS, Morgante F, Mastroeni C, Girlanda P, Quartarone A. Paired associative stimulation of left and right human motor cortex shapes interhemispheric motor inhibition based on a Hebbian mechanism. *Cerebral Cortex (New York, NY: 1991).* 2009;19(4):907–915.

72. Koganemaru S, Mima T, Nakatsuka M, Ueki Y, Fukuyama H, Domen K. Human motor associative plasticity induced by paired bihemispheric stimulation. *J Physiol.* 2009;587(Pt 19):4629–4644.

73. Buch ER, Johnen VM, Nelissen N, O'Shea J, Rushworth MF. Noninvasive associative plasticity induction in a corticocortical pathway of the human brain. *J Neurosci.* 2011;31(48):17669–17679.

74. Fiori F, Chiappini E, Avenanti A. Enhanced action performance following TMS manipulation of associative plasticity in ventral premotor-motor pathway. *Neuroimage.* 2018;183:847–858.

75. Johnen VM, Neubert FX, Buch ER, et al. Causal manipulation of functional connectivity in a specific neural pathway during behaviour and at rest. *eLife.* 2015;4.

76. Chiappini E, Borgomaneri S, Marangon M, Turrini S, Romei V, Avenanti A. Driving associative plasticity in premotor-motor connections through a novel paired associative stimulation based on long-latency cortico-cortical interactions. *Brain Stimul.* 2020;13(5):1461–1463.

77. Arai N, Müller-Dahlhaus F, Murakami T, et al. State-dependent and timing-dependent bidirectional associative plasticity in the human SMA-M1 network. *J Neurosci.* 2011;31(43):15376–15383.

78. Koch G, Ponzo V, Di Lorenzo F, Caltagirone C, Veniero D. Hebbian and anti-Hebbian spike-timing-dependent plasticity of human cortico-cortical connections. *J Neurosci.* 2013;33(23):9725–9733.

79. Chao CC, Karabanov AN, Paine R, et al. Induction of motor associative plasticity in the posterior parietal cortex-primary motor network. *Cerebral Cortex (New York, NY: 1991).* 2015;25(2):365–373.

80. Lu MK, Tsai CH, Ziemann U. Cerebellum to motor cortex paired associative stimulation induces bidirectional STDP-like plasticity in human motor cortex. *Front Hum Neurosci.* 2012;6:260.

81. Ugawa Y, Uesaka Y, Terao Y, Hanajima R, Kanazawa I. Magnetic stimulation over the cerebellum in humans. *Ann Neurol.* 1995;37(6):703–713.

82. Pinto AD, Chen R. Suppression of the motor cortex by magnetic stimulation of the cerebellum. *Exp Brain Res.* 2001;140(4):505–510.

83. Pauly MG, Steinmeier A, Bolte C, et al. Cerebellar rTMS and PAS effectively induce cerebellar plasticity. *Sci Rep.* 2021;11(1):3070.

84. Taylor JL, Martin PG. Voluntary motor output is altered by spike-timing-dependent changes in the human corticospinal pathway. *J Neurosci.* 2009;29(37):11708–11716.

85. Dongés SC, D'Amico JM, Butler JE, Taylor JL. Involvement of N-methyl-d-aspartate receptors in plasticity induced by paired corticospinal-motoneuronal stimulation in humans. *J Neurophysiol.* 2018;119(2):652–661.

86. Bunday KL, Perez MA. Motor recovery after spinal cord injury enhanced by strengthening corticospinal synaptic transmission. *Curr Biol.* 2012;22(24):2355–2361.

87. Fitzpatrick SC, Luu BL, Butler JE, Taylor JL. More conditioning stimuli enhance synaptic plasticity in the human spinal cord. *Clin Neurophysiol.* 2016;127(1):724–731.

88. Urbin MA, Ozdemir RA, Tazoe T, Perez MA. Spike-timing-dependent plasticity in lower-limb moto-neurons after human spinal cord injury. *J Neurophysiol.* 2017;118(4):2171–2180.

89. Fok KL, Kaneko N, Sasaki A, Nakagawa K, Nakazawa K, Masani K. Motor point stimulation in spinal paired associative stimulation can facilitate spinal cord excitability. *Front Hum Neurosci.* 2020;14:593806.

90. Dixon L, Ibrahim MM, Santora D, Knikou M. Paired associative transspinal and transcortical stimulation produces plasticity in human cortical and spinal neuronal circuits. *J Neurophysiol.* 2016;116(2):904–916.

91. Kuriakose R, Saha U, Castillo G, et al. The nature and time course of cortical activation following sub-thalamic stimulation in Parkinson's disease. *Cereb Cortex.* 2010;20(8):1926–1936.

92. Udupa K, Bahl N, Ni Z, et al. Cortical plasticity induction by pairing subthalamic nucleus deep-brain stimulation and primary motor cortical transcranial magnetic stimulation in Parkinson's disease. *J Neurosci.* 2016;36(2):396–404.

93. Ni Z, Kim SJ, Phielipp N, et al. Pallidal deep brain stimulation modulates cortical excitability and plas-ticity. *Ann Neurol.* 2018;83(2):352–362.

94. Rajji TK, Sun Y, Zomorrodi-Moghaddam R, et al. PAS-induced potentiation of cortical-evoked activity in the dorsolateral prefrontal cortex. *Neuropsychopharmacology.* 2013;38(12):2545–2552.

95. Salavati B, Daskalakis ZJ, Zomorrodi R, et al. Pharmacological modulation of long-term potentiation-like activity in the dorsolateral prefrontal cortex. *Front Hum Neurosci.* 2018;12:155.

96. Zibman S, Daniel E, Alyagon U, Etkin A, Zangen A. Interhemispheric cortico-cortical paired associa-tive stimulation of the prefrontal cortex jointly modulates frontal asymmetry and emotional reactivity. *Brain Stimul.* 2019;12(1):139–147.

97. Kohl S, Hannah R, Rocchi L, Nord CL, Rothwell J, Voon V. Cortical paired associative stimulation influences response inhibition: Cortico-cortical and cortico-subcortical networks. *Biol Psychiatry.* 2019;85(4):355–363.

98. Nord CL, Popa T, Smith E, et al. The effect of frontoparietal paired associative stimulation on decision-making and working memory. *Cortex.* 2019;117:266–276.

99. Momi D, Neri F, Coiro G, et al. Cognitive enhancement via network-targeted cortico-cortical associa-tive brain stimulation. *Cerebral Cortex (New York, NY: 1991).* 2020;30(3):1516–1527.

100. Guidali G, Roncoroni C, Bolognini N. Modulating frontal networks' timing-dependent-like plasticity with paired associative stimulation protocols: Recent advances and future perspectives. *Front Hum Neurosci.* 2021;15:658723.

101. Wassermann EM. Risk and safety in repetitive transcranial magnetic stimulation: Report and sug-gested guidelines from the International Workshop on the Safety of Repetitive Transcranial Magnetic Stimulation, June 5–7, 1996. *Electroencephalogr Clin Neurophysiol.* 1998;108:1–16.

102. Chen R, Classen J, Gerloff C, et al. Depression of motor cortex excitability by low-frequency transcra-nial magnetic stimulation. *Neurology.* 1997;48(5):1398–1403.

103. Siebner HR, Tormos JM, Ceballos-Baumann AO, et al. Low-frequency repetitive transcranial magnetic stimulation of the motor cortex in writer's cramp. *Neurology.* 1999;52(3):529–537.

104. Muellbacher W, Ziemann U, Boroojerdi B, Hallett M. Effects of low-frequency transcranial magnetic stimulation on motor excitability and basic motor behavior. *Clin Neurophysiol.* 2000;111(6):1002–1007.

105. Fitzgerald PB, Brown TL, Daskalakis ZJ, Chen R, Kulkarni J. Intensity-dependent effects of 1 Hz rTMS on human corticospinal excitability. *Clin Neurophysiol.* 2002;113(7):1136–1141.

106. Di Lazzaro V, Dileone M, Pilato F, et al. Modulation of motor cortex neuronal networks by rTMS: Comparison of local and remote effects of six different protocols of stimulation. *J Neurophysiol.* 2011;105(5):2150–2156.

107. Brighina F, Giglia G, Scalia S, Francolini M, Palermo A, Fierro B. Facilitatory effects of 1 Hz rTMS in motor cortex of patients affected by migraine with aura. *Exp Brain Res.* 2005;161(1):34–38.

108. Modugno N, Curra A, Conte A, et al. Depressed intracortical inhibition after long trains of subthresh-old repetitive magnetic stimuli at low frequency. *Clin Neurophysiol.* 2003;114(12):2416–2422.

109. Di Lazzaro V, Profice P, Pilato F, Dileone M, Oliviero A, Ziemann U. The effects of motor cortex rTMS on corticospinal descending activity. *Clin Neurophysiol.* 2010;121(4):464–473.

110. Baur D, Galevska D, Hussain S, Cohen LG, Ziemann U, Zrenner C. Induction of LTD-like corticospinal plasticity by low-frequency rTMS depends on pre-stimulus phase of sensorimotor μ-rhythm. *Brain Stimul.* 2020;13(6):1580–1587.

111. Fitzgerald PB, Fountain S, Daskalakis ZJ. A comprehensive review of the effects of rTMS on motor cortical excitability and inhibition. *Clin Neurophysiol.* 2006.

112. Min YS, Park JW, Jin SU, et al. Neuromodulatory effects of offline low-frequency repetitive transcranial magnetic stimulation of the motor cortex: A functional magnetic resonance imaging study. *Sci Rep.* 2016;6:36058.

113. Muellbacher W, Ziemann U, Wissel J, et al. Early consolidation in human primary motor cortex. *Nature.* 2002;415(6872):640–644.

114. Gilio F, Rizzo V, Siebner HR, Rothwell JC. Effects on the right motor hand-area excitability produced by low-frequency rTMS over human contralateral homologous cortex. *J Physiol.* 2003;551(Pt 2):563–573.

115. Schambra HM, Sawaki L, Cohen LG. Modulation of excitability of human motor cortex (M1) by 1 Hz transcranial magnetic stimulation of the contralateral M1. *Clin Neurophysiol.* 2003;114(1):130–133.

116. Heide G, Witte OW, Ziemann U. Physiology of modulation of motor cortex excitability by low-frequency suprathreshold repetitive transcranial magnetic stimulation. *Exp Brain Res.* 2006;171(1):26–34.

117. Wassermann EM, Wedegaertner FR, Ziemann U, George MS, Chen R. Crossed reduction of human motor cortex excitability by 1-Hz transcranial magnetic stimulation. *NeurosciLett.* 1998;250(3):141–144.

118. Plewnia C, Lotze M, Gerloff C. Disinhibition of the contralateral motor cortex by low-frequency rTMS. *Neuroreport.* 2003;14(4):609–612.

119. Pascual-Leone A, Valls-Sol, J, Wassermann EM, Hallett M. Responses to rapid-rate transcranial magnetic stimulation of the human motor cortex. *Brain.* 1994;117:847–858.

120. Jahanshahi M, Ridding MC, Limousin P, et al. Rapid rate transcranial magnetic stimulation--a safety study. *Electroencephalogr Clin Neurophysiol.* 1997;105(6):422–429.

121. Berardelli A, Inghilleri M, Rothwell JC, et al. Facilitation of muscle evoked responses after repetitive cortical stimulation in man. *Exp Brain Res.* 1998;122:79–84.

122. Di Lazzaro V, Oliviero A, Mazzone P, et al. Short-term reduction of intracortical inhibition in the human motor cortex induced by repetitive transcranial magnetic stimulation. *Exp Brain Res.* 2002;147(1):108–113.

123. Lang N, Siebner HR, Ernst D, et al. Preconditioning with transcranial direct current stimulation sensitizes the motor cortex to rapid-rate transcranial magnetic stimulation and controls the direction of after-effects. *Biol Psychiatry.* 2004;56(9):634–639.

124. Wang H, Wang X, Scheich H. LTD and LTP induced by transcranial magnetic stimulation in auditory cortex. *Neuroreport.* 1996;7:521–525.

125. Brown JC, DeVries WH, Korte JE, et al. NMDA receptor partial agonist, d-cycloserine, enhances 10 Hz rTMS-induced motor plasticity, suggesting long-term potentiation (LTP) as underlying mechanism. *Brain Stimul.* 2020;13(3):530–532.

126. Lang N, Harms J, Weyh T, et al. Stimulus intensity and coil characteristics influence the efficacy of rTMS to suppress cortical excitability. *Clin Neurophysiol.* 2006;117(10):2292–2301.

127. Quartarone A, Bagnato S, Rizzo V, et al. Distinct changes in cortical and spinal excitability following high-frequency repetitive TMS to the human motor cortex. *Exp Brain Res.* 2005;161(1):114–124.

128. Peinemann A, Reimer B, Löer C, et al. Long-lasting increase in corticospinal excitability after 1800 pulses of subthreshold 5 Hz repetitive TMS to the primary motor cortex. *Clin Neurophysiol.* 2004;115(7):1519–1526.

129. Jung SH, Shin JE, Jeong YS, Shin HI. Changes in motor cortical excitability induced by high-frequency repetitive transcranial magnetic stimulation of different stimulation durations. *Clin Neurophysiol.* 2008;119(1):71–79.

130. Rothkegel H, Sommer M, Paulus W. Breaks during 5Hz rTMS are essential for facilitatory after effects. *Clin Neurophysiol.* 2010;121(3):426–430.

131. Cash RFH, Dar A, Hui J, et al. Influence of inter-train interval on the plastic effects of rTMS. *Brain Stimul.* 2017;10(3):630–636.

132. Hwang JM, Kim YH, Yoon KJ, Uhm KE, Chang WH. Different responses to facilitatory rTMS according to BDNF genotype. *Clin Neurophysiol.* 2015;126(7):1348–1353.

133. Arai N, Okabe S, Furubayashi T, Terao Y, Yuasa K, Ugawa Y. Comparison between short train, monophasic and biphasic repetitive transcranial magnetic stimulation (rTMS) of the human motor cortex. *Clin Neurophysiol.* 2005;116(3):605–613.

134. Arai N, Okabe S, Furubayashi T, et al. Differences in after-effect between monophasic and biphasic high-frequency rTMS of the human motor cortex. *Clin Neurophysiol.* 2007;118(10):2227–2233.

135. Sommer M, Paulus W. Pulse configuration and rTMS efficacy: A review of clinical studies. *Suppl Clin Neurophysiol.* 2003;56:33–41.

136. Taylor JL, Loo CK. Stimulus waveform influences the efficacy of repetitive transcranial magnetic stimulation. *J Affect Dis.* 2007;97(1-3):271–276.

137. Goetz SM, Luber B, Lisanby SH, et al. Enhancement of neuromodulation with novel pulse shapes generated by controllable pulse parameter transcranial magnetic stimulation. *Brain Stimul.* 2016;9(1):39–47.

138. Halawa I, Shirota Y, Neef A, Sommer M, Paulus W. Neuronal tuning: Selective targeting of neuronal populations via manipulation of pulse width and directionality. *Brain Stimul.* 2019;12(5):1244–1252.

139. Iyer MB, Schleper N, Wassermann EM. Priming stimulation enhances the depressant effect of low-frequency repetitive transcranial magnetic stimulation. *J Neurosci.* 2003;23(34):10867–10872.

140. Abraham WC, Bear MF. Metaplasticity: The plasticity of synaptic plasticity. *Trends Neurosci.* 1996;19(4):126–130.

141. Cho KK, Bear MF. Promoting neurological recovery of function via metaplasticity. *Future Neurol* 2010;5(1):21–26.

142. Siebner HR, Lang N, Rizzo V, et al. Preconditioning of low-frequency repetitive transcranial magnetic stimulation with transcranial direct current stimulation: Evidence for homeostatic plasticity in the human motor cortex. *J Neurosci.* 2004;24(13):3379–3385.

143. Capocchi G, Zampolini M, Larson J. Theta burst stimulation is optimal for induction of LTP at both apical and basal dendritic synapses on hippocampal CA1 neurons. *Brain Res.* 1992;591(2):332–336.

144. Heusler P, Cebulla B, Boehmer G, Dinse HR. A repetitive intracortical microstimulation pattern induces long- lasting synaptic depression in brain slices of the rat primary somatosensory cortex. *Exp Brain Res.* 2000;135(3):300–310.

145. Takita M, Izaki Y, Jay TM, Kaneko H, Suzuki SS. Induction of stable long-term depression in vivo in the hippocampal-prefrontal cortex pathway. *Eur J Neurosci.* 1999;11(11):4145–4148.

146. Huang YZ, Rothwell JC. The effect of short-duration bursts of high-frequency, low-intensity transcranial magnetic stimulation on the human motor cortex. *Clin Neurophysiol.* 2004;115(5):1069–1075.

147. Huang YZ, Edwards MJ, Rounis E, Bhatia KP, Rothwell JC. Theta burst stimulation of the human motor cortex. *Neuron.* 2005;45(2):201–206.

148. Di Lazzaro V, Pilato F, Saturno E, et al. Theta-burst repetitive transcranial magnetic stimulation suppresses specific excitatory circuits in the human motor cortex. *J Physiol.* 2005;565(Pt 3):945–950.

149. Di Lazzaro V, Pilato F, Dileone M, et al. The physiological basis of the effects of intermittent theta burst stimulation of the human motor cortex. *J Physiol.* 2008;586(16):3871–3879.

150. Huang YZ, Chen RS, Rothwell JC, Wen HY. The after-effect of human theta burst stimulation is NMDA receptor dependent. *Clin Neurophysiol.* 2007;118(5):1028–1032.

151. Vallence AM, Goldsworthy MR, Hodyl NA, Semmler JG, Pitcher JB, Ridding MC. Inter- and intra-subject variability of motor cortex plasticity following continuous theta-burst stimulation. *Neuroscience.* 2015;304:266–278.

152. Goldsworthy MR, Vallence AM, Hodyl NA, Semmler JG, Pitcher JB, Ridding MC. Probing changes in corticospinal excitability following theta burst stimulation of the human primary motor cortex. *Clin Neurophysiol.* 2016;127(1):740–747.

153. Gentner R, Wankerl K, Reinsberger C, Zeller D, Classen J. Depression of human corticospinal excitability induced by magnetic theta-burst stimulation: Evidence of rapid polarity-reversing metaplasticity. *Cereb Cortex.* 2008;18(9):2046–2053.

154. Gamboa OL, Antal A, Moliadze V, Paulus W. Simply longer is not better: Reversal of theta burst after-effect with prolonged stimulation. *Exp Brain Res.* 2010;204(2):181–187.

155. Gamboa OL, Antal A, Laczo B, Moliadze V, Nitsche MA, Paulus W. Impact of repetitive theta burst stimulation on motor cortex excitability. *Brain Stimul.* 2011;4(3):145–151.

156. Hsu YF, Liao KK, Lee PL, et al. Intermittent θ burst stimulation over primary motor cortex enhances movement-related β synchronisation. *Clin Neurophysiol.* 2011;122(11):2260–2267.

157. McCalley DM, Lench DH, Doolittle JD, Imperatore JP, Hoffman M, Hanlon CA. Determining the optimal pulse number for theta burst induced change in cortical excitability. *Sci Rep.* 2021;11(1):8726.

158. Brownjohn PW, Reynolds JN, Matheson N, Fox J, Shemmell JB. The effects of individualized theta burst stimulation on the excitability of the human motor system. *Brain Stimul.* 2014;7(2):260–268.

159. Doeltgen SH, Ridding MC. Low-intensity, short-interval theta burst stimulation modulates excitatory but not inhibitory motor networks. *Clin Neurophysiol.* 2011;122(7):1411–1416.

160. Haeckert J, Rothwell J, Hannah R, Hasan A, Strube W. Comparative study of a continuous train of theta-burst stimulation for a duration of 20 s (cTBS 300) versus a duration of 40 s (cTBS 600) in a prestimulation relaxed condition in healthy volunteers. *Brain Sci.* 2021;11(6).

161. Iezzi E, Conte A, Suppa A, et al. Phasic voluntary movements reverse the aftereffects of subsequent theta-burst stimulation in humans. *J Neurophysiol.* 2008;100(4):2070–2076.

162. Goldsworthy MR, Müller-Dahlhaus F, Ridding MC, Ziemann U. Inter-subject variability of LTD-like plasticity in human motor cortex: A matter of preceding motor activation. *Brain Stimul.* 2014;7(6):864–870.

163. Huang YZ, Rothwell JC, Edwards MJ, Chen RS. Effect of physiological activity on an NMDA-dependent form of cortical plasticity in human. *Cerebral Cortex (New York, NY: 1991).* 2008;18(3):563–570.

164. Monte-Silva K, Ruge D, Teo JT, Paulus W, Rothwell JC, Nitsche MA. D2 receptor block abolishes θ burst stimulation-induced neuroplasticity in the human motor cortex. *Neuropsychopharmacology.* 2011;36(10):2097–2102.

165. Wankerl K, Weise D, Gentner R, Rumpf JJ, Classen J. L-type voltage-gated Ca2+ channels: A single molecular switch for long-term potentiation/long-term depression-like plasticity and activity-dependent metaplasticity in humans. *J Neurosci.* 2010;30(18):6197–6204.

166. Chung SW, Hill AT, Rogasch NC, Hoy KE, Fitzgerald PB. Use of theta-burst stimulation in changing excitability of motor cortex: A systematic review and meta-analysis. *Neurosci Biobehav Rev.* 2016;63:43–64.

167. Corp DT, Bereznicki HGK, Clark GM, et al. Large-scale analysis of interindividual variability in theta-burst stimulation data: Results from the "Big TMS Data Collaboration." *Brain Stimul.* 2020;13(5):1476–1488.

168. Hamada M, Murase N, Hasan A, Balaratnam M, Rothwell JC. The role of interneuron networks in driving human motor cortical plasticity. *Cerebral Cortex (New York, NY: 1991).* 2013;23(7):1593–1605.

169. Ozdemir RA, Boucher P, Fried PJ, et al. Reproducibility of cortical response modulation induced by intermittent and continuous theta-burst stimulation of the human motor cortex. *Brain Stimul.* 2021;14(4):949–964.

170. Hinder MR, Goss EL, Fujiyama H, et al. Inter- and intra-individual variability following intermittent theta burst stimulation: Implications for rehabilitation and recovery. *Brain Stimul.* 2014;7(3):365–371.

171. Schilberg L, Schuhmann T, Sack AT. Interindividual variability and intraindividual reliability of intermittent theta burst stimulation-induced neuroplasticity mechanisms in the healthy brain. *J Cogn Neurosci.* 2017;29(6):1022–1032.

172. Fried PJ, Jannati A, Davila-Pérez P, Pascual-Leone A. Reproducibility of single-pulse, paired-pulse, and intermittent theta-burst TMS measures in healthy aging, type-2 diabetes, and Alzheimer's disease. *Front Aging Neurosci.* 2017;9:263.

173. Vernet M, Bashir S, Yoo WK, et al. Reproducibility of the effects of theta burst stimulation on motor cortical plasticity in healthy participants. *Clin Neurophysiol.* 2014;125(2):320–326.

174. Jannati A, Block G, Oberman LM, Rotenberg A, Pascual-Leone A. Interindividual variability in response to continuous theta-burst stimulation in healthy adults. *Clin Neurophysiol.* 2017;128(11):2268–2278.

175. Jannati A, Fried PJ, Block G, Oberman LM, Rotenberg A, Pascual-Leone A. Test-retest reliability of the effects of continuous theta-burst stimulation. *Front Neurosci.* 2019;13:447.

176. Hordacre B, Goldsworthy MR, Vallence AM, et al. Variability in neural excitability and plasticity induction in the human cortex: A brain stimulation study. *Brain Stimul.* 2017;10(3):588–595.

177. Cárdenas-Morales L, Volz LJ, Michely J, et al. Network connectivity and individual responses to brain stimulation in the human motor system. *Cerebral Cortex (New York, NY: 1991).* 2014;24(7):1697–1707.

178. Nettekoven C, Volz LJ, Leimbach M, et al. Inter-individual variability in cortical excitability and motor network connectivity following multiple blocks of rTMS. *Neuroimage.* 2015;118:209–218.

179. Hordacre B, Goldsworthy MR, Graetz L, Ridding MC. Motor network connectivity predicts neuroplastic response following theta burst stimulation in healthy adults. *Brain Structure Function.* 2021;226(6):1893–1907.

180. Li Voti P, Conte A, Suppa A, et al. Correlation between cortical plasticity, motor learning and BDNF genotype in healthy subjects. *Exp Brain Res.* 2011;212(1):91–99.

181. Mastroeni C, Bergmann TO, Rizzo V, et al. Brain-derived neurotrophic factor--a major player in stimulation-induced homeostatic metaplasticity of human motor cortex? *PloS One.* 2013;8(2):e57957.

182. Lee M, Kim SE, Kim WS, et al. Interaction of motor training and intermittent theta burst stimulation in modulating motor cortical plasticity: Influence of BDNF Val66Met polymorphism. *PloS One.* 2013;8(2):e57690.

183. Harvey DY, DeLoretta L, Shah-Basak PP, et al. Variability in cTBS aftereffects attributed to the interaction of stimulus intensity with BDNF Val66Met polymorphism. *Front Hum Neurosci.* 2021;15:585533.

184. Parchure S, Harvey DY, Shah-Basak PP, et al. Brain-derived neurotrophic factor gene polymorphism predicts response to continuous theta burst stimulation in chronic stroke patients. *Neuromodulation.* 2021.

185. Kulla A, Manahan-Vaughan D. Depotentiation in the dentate gyrus of freely moving rats is modulated by D1/D5 dopamine receptors. *Cereb Cortex.* 2000;10(6):614–620.

186. Huang YZ, Rothwell JC, Lu CS, Chuang WL, Lin WY, Chen RS. Reversal of plasticity-like effects in the human motor cortex. *J Physiol (London).* 2010;588:3683–3693.

187. Cantarero G, Lloyd A, Celnik P. Reversal of long-term potentiation-like plasticity processes after motor learning disrupts skill retention. *J Neurosci.* 2013;33(31):12862–12869.

188. Martin PG, Gandevia SC, Taylor JL. Theta burst stimulation does not reliably depress all regions of the human motor cortex. *Clin Neurophysiol.* 2006;117(12):2684–2690.

189. Katagiri N, Yoshida S, Koseki T, et al. Interindividual variability of lower-limb motor cortical plasticity induced by theta burst stimulation. *Front Neurosci.* 2020;14:563293.

190. Ishikawa S, Matsunaga K, Nakanishi R, et al. Effect of theta burst stimulation over the human sensorimotor cortex on motor and somatosensory evoked potentials. *Clin Neurophysiol.* 2007;118(5):1033–1043.

191. Conte A, Rocchi L, Nardella A, et al. Theta-burst stimulation-induced plasticity over primary somatosensory cortex changes somatosensory temporal discrimination in healthy humans. *PloS one.* 2012;7(3):e32979.

192. Rocchi L, Casula E, Tocco P, Berardelli A, Rothwell J. Somatosensory temporal discrimination threshold involves inhibitory mechanisms in the primary somatosensory area. *J Neurosci.* 2016;36(2):325–335.

193. Premji A, Ziluk A, Nelson AJ. Bilateral somatosensory evoked potentials following intermittent theta-burst repetitive transcranial magnetic stimulation. *BMC Neurosci.* 2010;11:91.

194. Ragert P, Franzkowiak S, Schwenkreis P, Tegenthoff M, Dinse HR. Improvement of tactile perception and enhancement of cortical excitability through intermittent theta burst rTMS over human primary somatosensory cortex. *Exp Brain Res.* 2008;184(1):1–11.

195. Murakami T, Müller-Dahlhaus F, Lu MK, Ziemann U. Homeostatic metaplasticity of corticospinal excitatory and intracortical inhibitory neural circuits in human motor cortex. *J Physiol.* 2012;590(22):5765–5781.

196. Ni Z, Gunraj C, Kailey P, Cash RF, Chen R. Heterosynaptic modulation of motor cortical plasticity in human. *J Neurosci.* 2014;34(21):7314–7321.

197. Kishore A, James P, Popa T, et al. Plastic responsiveness of motor cortex to paired associative stimulation depends on cerebellar input. *Clin Neurophysiol.* 2021;132(10):2493–2502.

198. Thickbroom GW, Byrnes ML, Edwards DJ, Mastaglia FL. Repetitive paired-pulse TMS at I-wave periodicity markedly increases corticospinal excitability: A new technique for modulating synaptic plasticity. *Clin Neurophysiol.* 2006;117(1):61–66.

199. Cash RF, Benwell NM, Murray K, Mastaglia FL, Thickbroom GW. Neuromodulation by paired-pulse TMS at an I-wave interval facilitates multiple I-waves. *Exp Brain Res.* 2009;193(1):1–7.

200. Murray LM, Nosaka K, Thickbroom GW. Interventional repetitive I-wave transcranial magnetic stimulation (TMS): The dimension of stimulation duration. *Brain Stimul.* 2011;4(4):261–265.

201. Sewerin S, Taubert M, Vollmann H, Conde V, Villringer A, Ragert P. Enhancing the effect of repetitive I-wave paired-pulse TMS (iTMS) by adjusting for the individual I-wave periodicity. *BMC Neurosci.* 2011;12:45.

202. Cash RF, Ziemann U, Thickbroom GW. Inhibitory and disinhibitory effects on I-wave facilitation in motor cortex. *J Neurophysiol.* 2011;105(1):100–106.

203. Di Lazzaro V, Thickbroom GW, Pilato F, et al. Direct demonstration of the effects of repetitive paired-pulse transcranial magnetic stimulation at I-wave periodicity. *Clin Neurophysiol.* 2007;118(6):1193–1197.

204. Cash RF, Mastaglia FL, Thickbroom GW. Evidence for high-fidelity timing-dependent synaptic plasticity of human motor cortex. *J Neurophysiol.* 2013;109(1):106–112.

205. Cash RFH, Udupa K, Gunraj CA, et al. Influence of BDNF Val66Met polymorphism on excitatory-inhibitory balance and plasticity in human motor cortex. *Clin Neurophysiol.* 2021;132(11):2827–2839.

206. Cirillo J, Perez MA. Subcortical contribution to late TMS-induced I-waves in intact humans. *Front Integrat Neurosci.* 2015;9:38.

207. Opie GM, Cirillo J, Semmler JG. Age-related changes in late I-waves influence motor cortex plasticity induction in older adults. *J Physiol.* 2018;596(13):2597–2609.

208. Opie GM, Sasaki R, Hand BJ, Semmler JG. Modulation of motor cortex plasticity by repetitive paired-pulse TMS at late I-wave intervals is influenced by intracortical excitability. *Brain Sci.* 2021;11(1).

209. Cash RF, Ziemann U, Murray K, Thickbroom GW. Late cortical disinhibition in human motor cortex: A triple-pulse transcranial magnetic stimulation study. *J Neurophysiol.* 2010;103(1):511–518.

210. Cash RF, Murakami T, Chen R, Thickbroom GW, Ziemann U. Augmenting plasticity induction in human motor cortex by disinhibition stimulation. *Cerebral Cortex (New York, NY: 1991).* 2016;26(1):58–69.

211. Ziegler L, Schulte R, Gharabaghi A. Combined endogenous and exogenous disinhibition of intracortical circuits augments plasticity induction in the human motor cortex. *Brain Stimul.* 2019;12(4):1027–1040.

212. Hamada M, Terao Y, Hanajima R, et al. Bidirectional long-term motor cortical plasticity and metaplasticity induced by quadripulse transcranial magnetic stimulation. *J Physiol (London).* 2008;586(16):3927–3947.

213. Matsumoto H, Ugawa Y. Quadripulse stimulation (QPS). *Exp Brain Res.* 2020;238(7-8):1619–1625.

214. Nakamura K, Groiss SJ, Hamada M, et al. Variability in response to quadripulse stimulation of the motor cortex. *Brain Stimul.* 2016;9(6):859–866.

215. Watanabe T, Hanajima R, Shirota Y, et al. Bidirectional effects on interhemispheric resting-state functional connectivity induced by excitatory and inhibitory repetitive transcranial magnetic stimulation. *Hum Brain Mapp.* 2014;35(5):1896–1905.

216. Hamada M, Hanajima R, Terao Y, et al. Primary motor cortical metaplasticity induced by priming over the supplementary motor area. *J Physiol.* 2009;587(Pt 20):4845–4862.

217. Nakatani-Enomoto S, Hanajima R, Hamada M, et al. Bidirectional modulation of sensory cortical excitability by quadripulse transcranial magnetic stimulation (QPS) in humans. *Clin Neurophysiol.* 2012;123(7):1415–1421.

218. Hanajima R, Tanaka N, Tsutsumi R, et al. The effect of age on the homotopic motor cortical long-term potentiation-like effect induced by quadripulse stimulation. *Exp Brain Res.* 2017;235(7):2103–2108.

219. Jung NH, Gleich B, Gattinger N, et al. Quadri-pulse theta burst stimulation using ultra-high frequency bursts: A new protocol to induce changes in cortico-spinal excitability in human motor cortex. *PloS One.* 2016;11(12):e0168410.

220. Player MJ, Taylor JL, Alonzo A, Loo CK. Paired associative stimulation increases motor cortex excitability more effectively than theta-burst stimulation. *Clin Neurophysiol.* 2012;123(11):2220–2226.

221. Vallence AM, Kurylowicz L, Ridding MC. A comparison of neuroplastic responses to non-invasive brain stimulation protocols and motor learning in healthy adults. *Neurosci Lett.* 2013;549:151–156.

TMS in Nonmotor Neurophysiological Studies

5.1 INTRODUCTION

This chapter reviews the use of transcranial magnetic stimulation (TMS) in nonmotor physiological studies. Induction of phosphenes with stimulation of the visual cortex, stimulation of the primary somatosensory cortex (S1), and use of TMS to investigate cortical areas involved in action inhibition are discussed to illustrate how TMS can be used in these types of studies. These studies used single and paired TMS protocols discussed in detail in Chapter 3 and plasticity induction protocols reviewed in Chapter 4. Chapter 6 further discusses the use of TMS in cognitive studies.

5.2 INDUCTION OF PHOSPHENES BY TMS

Phosphenes refer to perceived sensation of flashes of light without visual stimulus. TMS of the occipital cortex leads to the perception of phosphenes in the contralateral hemifield.[1,2] Subjects described the phosphenes as a series of small bright dots or wedge-shaped streaks extending from the foveal region to one hemifield.[3] However, the perception of phosphenes varied considerably among individuals, and, in some study participants, phosphenes cannot be elicited. This is likely related to variations in cortical geometry, representations, and excitability.[3] However, phosphene thresholds are stable and provide a reliable measure within the same individual over time.[4,5] The brightness[6] and the size of the phosphene increases with the intensity of the TMS pulse, and the phosphene area can be used to plot a TMS intensity-recruitment curve.[7]

To elicit phosphenes, participants are usually blindfolded or have eyes closed. A study reported that the phosphene threshold was lower with eyes closed compared with eyes open when the participants were blindfolded.[8] The optimal position to elicit phosphenes is usually 2–4 cm above the inion, and the coil is moved in a grid pattern to obtain the optimal position.[5,9-12] The coil position is lateral to midline and contralateral to the induced phosphene. For example, the optimal position is close to the O1 position (International 10-20 system) when stimulating the left occipital cortex.[13] Many studies placed the coil handle upward with monophasic[5] or biphasic[9,10,12] stimulators, although some used the handle directed horizontally with a biphasic stimulator.[11]

One study found that the phosphene threshold was lower with biphasic than monophasic current.[14] Testing of different current directions with neuronavigation showed that the threshold was lowest when the induced current was perpendicular to the occipital gyrus,[14] similar to the finding in the motor cortex. While most studies used a single pulse, some studies used two pulses at 50 ms[10] or 500 ms[9] apart to be able to elicit phosphenes in more subjects. Phosphene thresholds are generally higher than the motor thresholds. Most studies found no correlation between motor threshold and phosphene threshold,[5,9-11] suggesting that M1 excitability is unrelated to the excitability of the occipital cortex. However, one study testing dark-adapted subjects with eyes open found a correlation between active motor threshold and phosphene threshold.[12] The method of constant stimuli and rapid estimation of phosphene threshold was found to provide a reliable estimate the phosphene threshold.[13]

Stationary phosphenes are most reliability produced by stimulation of the early visual area (V1, V2) and the dorsal visual areas (V3d, V3a) close to the interhemispheric cleft.[15] However, stimulation of the V5/MT+, an extrastriate area in which neurons are tuned to identify direction and velocity of motion, can elicit moving phosphenes.[9,16,17]

5.2.1 Cortical Inhibition and Facilitation of Visual Cortex Tested with Paired-Pulse Method

Paired-pulse TMS, an established technique to test inhibition and facilitation in the motor cortex, can be applied to the visual cortex. At interstimulus intervals (ISIs) of 2–12 ms, conditioning intensity of 90%, and test stimulus intensity of 100% phosphene threshold, there was facilitation of phosphene perception and inhibition was not observed.[18] However, inhibition of phosphene size was observed at an ISI of 2 ms at a low conditioning stimulus intensity of 45% phosphene threshold (Figure 5.1).[7] Furthermore, at this conditioning stimulus intensity, reduction of phosphene area occurred at ISIs from 2 to 200 ms compared to the test stimulus alone. With conditioning intensity at 75% phosphene threshold, no change was found at ISIs of 2–15 ms, and there was inhibition of phosphene area in some subjects at ISIs of 20–500 ms.[19] Thus, inhibition and facilitation

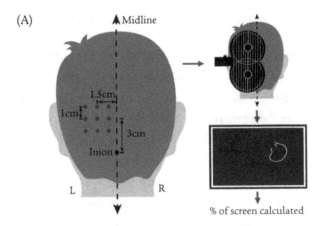

(A) ▲Midline

1.5cm
1cm
3cm
Inion
L   R

% of screen calculated

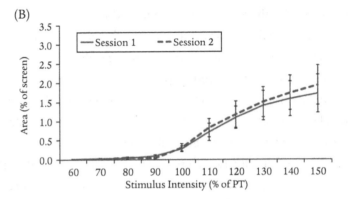

(B)

Area (% of screen)

— Session 1   -- Session 2

Stimulus Intensity (% of PT)

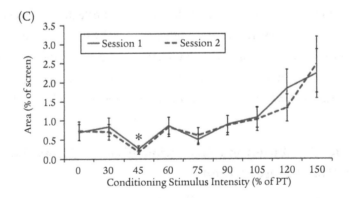

(C)

Area (% of screen)

— Session 1   -- Session 2

Conditioning Stimulus Intensity (% of PT)

FIGURE 5.1 *(A) Short interval intracortical inhibition in the visual cortex. Grid placement over the visual cortex to elicit phosphenes through transcranial magnetic stimulation (TMS). Stimulation targets were spaced 1 cm apart, with the center of the grid 3 cm dorsal and 1.5 cm left-lateral of the inion. Stimulator output was initially set to 60% of maximum stimulator output, and each target was stimulated three times (monophasic, lateral-medial induced current, MagPro X100 with MagOption stimulator and MC-B70 butterfly coil). If no phosphenes were induced, intensity was increased in increments of 10% until phosphenes were reported. If phosphenes were reported at one or more locations, the site reported to generate the brightest, most consistent phosphenes was selected as the target "hot spot." At the hot spot, stimulation intensity was decreased by 2% of stimulator output until no longer reported, then incremented by 1% until the phosphene threshold (PT) was reached. PT was defined as the lowest stimulator output at which at least 5 out of 10 stimuli induced a phosphene. If no phosphenes were reported at any of the 9 locations with 100% of stimulator output, the participant was excluded from further participation (n = 7). The TMS coil was held at 90 degrees to the midline. The BrainSight frameless stereotactic neuronavigation system was used for accuracy of targeting and trajectory. Subjects traced phosphenes on a screen after each trial, and area was calculated. (B) Phosphene area as a function*

FIGURE 5.1 CONTINUED

of stimulator intensity during single-pulse TMS. Error bars indicate standard error of the mean. (C) Phosphene size as a function of conditioning stimulus intensity during paired-pulse TMS. There was inhibition of phosphene area with conditioning stimulus intensity at 45% PT. Error bars indicate standard error of the mean. Asterisk denotes significant inhibition.
FROM KHAMMASH ET AL., *BRAIN STIMUL.* 2019;12(3):702–704, WITH PERMISSION.

can be observed with paired TMS in the occipital cortex, but timing and hence the nature are likely different from those in the motor cortex.

5.3 STIMULATION OF THE PRIMARY SOMATOSENSORY CORTEX

5.3.1 Location for S1 TMS

There are several methods to locate the S1 for TMS. One method is to find the index finger (first dorsal interosseous muscle) representation and move the coil 1–2 cm posteriorly. Some studies confirmed the S1 location by evoking a ticking or prickling sensation in the index finger.[20] The S1 location has also been determined from scalp measurements based on the International 10-20 electrode system.[21] Another method is to use neuronavigation based on individual structural or functional magnetic resonance imaging (MRI),[22] which may be regarded as the gold standard.[23] A meta-analysis found that the S1-hand area is on average 1.5–2 cm posterior but is also lateral to the functionally defined M1-hand area.[23] A study suggested that the S1-index finger representation should be located about 2 cm lateral and 0.5 cm posterior to M1-hand area.[24]

5.3.2 Effects of Single and Paired S1 TMS on Sensory Perception

A single TMS pulse can suppress perception of somatosensory stimuli applied to the contralateral hand about 20 ms earlier.[25–27] With a subthreshold conditioning stimulus followed by a suprathreshold test stimulus, perception of a peripheral electrical stimulus was further attenuated at ISIs of 10 or 15 ms with no effect at shorter ISIs.[26] At ISI of 15 ms, paired TMS further impaired sensorimotor performance compared to the effects of a single test pulse when vibrotactile stimulus was used to guide discrete motor response but not when it was used to continuously guide motor response.[27] Thus, facilitation occurred with paired TMS in S1 but inhibition has not been demonstrated.

5.3.3 Effects of Induction of Plasticity in S1

The effects of different types of repetitive TMS (rTMS) plasticity protocols on S1 has been tested.

5.3.3.1 Regular Frequency Repetitive TMS

Low-frequency (1 Hz) rTMS at 110% RMT decreased tactile acuity, and the duration of the effect increased with duration of the rTMS train.[21] Two studies that applied 5 Hz rTMS to S1 reported improvement in tactile acuity and increased blood oxygen level dependent (BOLD) response to electrical stimulation of the index finger.[20,28]

5.3.3.2 Theta Burst Stimulation

Application of continuous theta burst stimulation (cTBS) to the S1 increased somatosensory temporal discrimination threshold.[29] S1 cTBS decreased pain threshold,[30,31] and the effect lasted for 40 min.[31] S1 cTBS also changes M1 excitability. S1 cTBS in the anterior-posterior followed by posterior-anterior (AP-PA) increased M1 excitability. In contrast, PA-AP cTBS decreased M1 excitability.[32] Moreover, S1 cTBS at 30 Hz instead of the usual 50 Hz increased M1 excitability (Figure 5.2)[33] and decreased short-latency afferent inhibition (SAI),[34] while M1 cTBS at 30 Hz decreased M1 excitability and did not alter SAI. S1 cTBS applied after motor training blocked the consolidation of motor memory, while M1 cTBS had little effect on retention of motor memory.[35]

Intermittent TBS (iTBS) to S1 was found to decrease the somatosensory temporal discrimination threshold.[29] S1 iTBS impaired the effects of rubber hand illusion.[36]

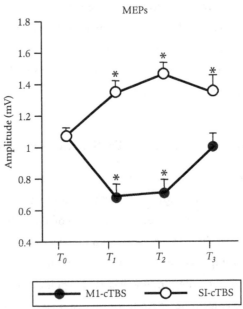

FIGURE 5.2 *Effects of continuous theta burst stimulation (cTBS) of the primary motor cortex (M1) and primary somatosensory cortex (S1) on motor-evoked potential (MEP) amplitude. Group-averaged MEP data (with standard errors) for each time block before and following cTBS over M1 and SI. Following cTBS over M1 (filled circles), MEP amplitudes were significantly decreased at 5 min (T1) and 25 min (T2). In contrast, cTBS over SI (hollow circles) increased MEP amplitudes significantly at 5 (T1), 25 min (T2), and 45 (T3) minutes compared to baseline (T0). Asterisks indicate P < 0.05.*
FROM JACOBS ET AL., BRAIN STIMUL. 2014;7(2):269–274, WITH PERMISSION.

Together, TBS studies on S1 have demonstrated that modulation of S1 can change sensory and pain perception. It also changes the motor system, sensorimotor integration measured by SAI, and motor learning. The effects cannot be explained by spread of stimulation to the M1.

5.3.3.3 Paired Associative Stimulation

Paired associative stimulation (PAS) performed by pairing median nerve stimulation with S1 TMS at 150% RMT at the N20 latency increased the amplitude of the P25 component of median nerve somatosensory evoked potential (SEP). This facilitation occurred when the time between median nerve stimulation and S1 TMS was within a 15 ms range centered at the N20 latency.[37] Using rapid-rate PAS at 5 Hz and TMS at 70% RMT, reduced SEP paired pulse inhibition and SAI occurred when the time between median nerve stimulation and TMS was N20–2.5 ms but not at N20 or N20 + 2.5 ms. However, M1 excitability increased with peripheral nerve stimulation and TMS intervals between N20-2.5 to N20 + 2.5 ms.[38] In a paradigm of cross-modal PAS, participants viewed a hand being touched, and when repeatedly paired with TMS at 150% RMT in 150 trials, it improved tactile acuity assessed with two-point discrimination and increased the amplitude of the P40 component of median nerve SEP.[39] Thus, there is evidence that PAS can be applied to the S1 and leads to changes in physiological and sensory functions.

5.4 USE OF TMS TO INVESTIGATE ACTION INHIBITION

Inhibition of prepared or ongoing responses is an important aspect of voluntary motor control. Commonly used tasks to investigate action inhibition includes the stop-signal task and the go no-go task. Functional imaging studies have implicated many brain areas in response inhibition including the right and left inferior frontal gyrus (IFG), dorso-lateral prefrontal cortex (DLPFC), frontal eye field, supplementary eye field, anterior cingulate area, pre-supplementary motor area (pre-SMA), SMA, superior temporal gyri, parietal cortex, the basal ganglia (particularly the subthalamic nucleus), and the cerebellum.[40,41] TMS, by temporarily interfering with the activity of the stimulated brain region, can be used to investigate the causal role of these areas when applied either during task performance (online effect) or to assess the effects on task performance after application of a plasticity inducing protocol (offline effect). A brief outline is provided here, and the topic has been reviewed in greater detail.[41]

A "offline" study showed that application of 1 Hz rTMS aimed at decreasing cortical excitability to the right IFG impaired the ability to stop, but did not affect response execution.[42] These effects were not observed with 1 Hz rTMS to the medial frontal gyrus or the angular gyrus. Application of cTBS designed to decrease excitability of the right IFG resulted in less efficient action cascading strategy, while iTBS designed to increase excitability had the opposite effect, leading to more efficient strategy.[43] Another study also showed the right IFG cTBS worsened stopping behavior.[44] However, cTBS to the right IFG had no effect on a conditional stop-signal task.[45] cTBS to the right IFG also impaired the ability to withhold movements in no-go trials in a go no-go task.[46]

Several studies investigated the role of the pre-SMA in inhibitory control. In two "online" studies, two TMS pulses applied to the pre-SMA after the go cue increased the stop-signal reaction time (SSRT)[47,48] due to disruption of the implementation of the stopping process.[48] Single-pulse TMS to the pre-SMA after stimulus presentation also worsened response inhibition.[44] In an "offline" study, cTBS to the right pre-SMA decreased SSRT (improved inhibition).[45] In a go no-go task, preSMA cTBS impaired the ability to withhold response in no-go trials.[46] For the parietal cortex, single-pulse TMS applied to the intraparietal sulcus between 0 and 30 ms before stopping resulted in prolongation of SSRT in a stop-signal task, whereas stimulation of the temporoparietal junction had no effect.[49]

Together, these TMS studies have clarified a causal role for the right IFG, pre-SMA, and intraparietal sulcus in action inhibition.

5.5 CONCLUSION

In summary, single-pulse and paired TMS can be used to induce sensations such as phosphenes with visual cortex stimulation or to block perception when applied to the S1. Paired TMS can be used to study inhibition and facilitation in nonmotor areas. Single and paired TMS have the advantage of high temporal resolution, and one can infer causal effects. Repetitive TMS with different plasticity-inducing protocols applied to nonmotor areas can produce behavior changes to investigate the role of different cortical areas.

REFERENCES

1. Marg E, Rudiak D. Phosphenes induced by magnetic stimulation over the occipital brain: Description and probable site of stimulation. *Optometry Vision Sci.* 1994;71(5):301–311.
2. Cowey A, Walsh V. Magnetically induced phosphenes in sighted, blind and blindsighted observers. *Neuroreport.* 2000;11(14):3269–3273.
3. Merabet LB, Theoret H, Pascual-Leone A. Transcranial magnetic stimulation as an investigative tool in the study of visual function. *Optometry Vision Sci.* 2003;80(5):356–368.
4. Kammer T, Beck S. Phosphene thresholds evoked by transcranial magnetic stimulation are insensitive to short-lasting variations in ambient light. *Exp Brain Res.* 2002;145(3):407–410.
5. Stewart LM, Walsh V, Rothwell JC. Motor and phosphene thresholds: A transcranial magnetic stimulation correlation study. *Neuropsychologia.* 2001;39(4):415–419.
6. Meyer BU, Diehl R, Steinmetz H, Britton TC, Benecke R. Magnetic stimuli applied over motor and visual cortex: Influence of coil position and field polarity on motor responses, phosphenes, and eye movements. *Electroencephalogr Clin Neurophysiol Suppl.* 1991;43:121–134.
7. Khammash D, Simmonite M, Polk TA, Taylor SF, Meehan SK. Probing short-latency cortical inhibition in the visual cortex with transcranial magnetic stimulation: A reliability study. *Brain Stimul.* 2019;12(3):702–704.

8. de Graaf TA, Duecker F, Stankevich Y, Ten Oever S, Sack AT. Seeing in the dark: Phosphene thresholds with eyes open versus closed in the absence of visual inputs. *Brain Stimul.* 2017;10(4):828–835.

9. Antal A, Nitsche MA, Kincses TZ, Lampe C, Paulus W. No correlation between moving phosphene and motor thresholds: A transcranial magnetic stimulation study. *Neuroreport.* 2004;15(2):297–302.

10. Boroojerdi B, Meister IG, Foltys H, Sparing R, Cohen LG, Töpper R. Visual and motor cortex excitability: A transcranial magnetic stimulation study. *Clin Neurophysiol.* 2002;113(9):1501–1504.

11. Gerwig M, Kastrup O, Meyer BU, Niehaus L. Evaluation of cortical excitability by motor and phosphene thresholds in transcranial magnetic stimulation. *J Neurol Sci.* 2003;215(1–2):75–78.

12. Deblieck C, Thompson B, Iacoboni M, Wu AD. Correlation between motor and phosphene thresholds: A transcranial magnetic stimulation study. *Hum Brain Mapp.* 2008;29(6):662–670.

13. Mazzi C, Savazzi S, Abrahamyan A, Ruzzoli M. Reliability of TMS phosphene threshold estimation: Toward a standardized protocol. *Brain Stimul.* 2017;10(3):609–617.

14. Kammer T, Vorwerg M, Herrnberger B. Anisotropy in the visual cortex investigated by neuronavigated transcranial magnetic stimulation. *Neuroimage.* 2007;36(2):313–321.

15. Schaeffner LF, Welchman AE. Mapping the visual brain areas susceptible to phosphene induction through brain stimulation. *Exp Brain Res.* 2017;235(1):205–217.

16. Pascual-Leone A, Walsh V. Fast backprojections from the motion to the primary visual area necessary for visual awareness. *Science.* 2001;292(5516):510–512.

17. Stewart L, Battelli L, Walsh V, Cowey A. Motion perception and perceptual learning studied by magnetic stimulation. *Electroencephalogr Clin Neurophysiol Supplement.* 1999;51:334–350.

18. Sparing R, Dambeck N, Stock K, Meister IG, Huetter D, Boroojerdi B. Investigation of the primary visual cortex using short-interval paired-pulse transcranial magnetic stimulation (TMS). *Neurosci Lett.* 2005;382(3):312–316.

19. Khammash D, Simmonite M, Polk TA, Taylor SF, Meehan SK. Temporal dynamics of corticocortical inhibition in human visual cortex: A TMS study. *Neuroscience.* 2019;421:31–38.

20. Tegenthoff M, Ragert P, Pleger B, et al. Improvement of tactile discrimination performance and enlargement of cortical somatosensory maps after 5 Hz rTMS. *PLoS Biol.* 2005;3(11):e362.

21. Knecht S, Ellger T, Breitenstein C, Bernd Ringelstein E, Henningsen H. Changing cortical excitability with low-frequency transcranial magnetic stimulation can induce sustained disruption of tactile perception. *Biol Psychiatry.* 2003;53(2):175–179.

22. Brown MJN, Weissbach A, Pauly MG, et al. Somatosensory-motor cortex interactions measured using dual-site transcranial magnetic stimulation. *Brain Stimul.* 2019;12(5):1229–1243.

23. Holmes NP, Tamè L. Locating primary somatosensory cortex in human brain stimulation studies: Systematic review and meta-analytic evidence. *J Neurophysiol.* 2019;121(1):152–162.

24. Holmes NP, Tamè L, Beeching P, et al. Locating primary somatosensory cortex in human brain stimulation studies: Experimental evidence. *J Neurophysiol.* 2019;121(1):336–344.

25. Cohen LG, Bandinelli S, Sato S, Kufta C, Hallett M. Attenuation in detection of somatosensory stimuli by transcranial magnetic stimulation. *Electroencephalogr Clin Neurophysiol.* 1991;81(5):366–376.

26. Koch G, Franca M, Albrecht UV, Caltagirone C, Rothwell JC. Effects of paired pulse TMS of primary somatosensory cortex on perception of a peripheral electrical stimulus. *Exp Brain Res.* 2006;172(3):416–424.

27. Meehan SK, Legon W, Staines WR. Paired-pulse transcranial magnetic stimulation of primary somatosensory cortex differentially modulates perception and sensorimotor transformations. *Neuroscience.* 2008;157(2):424–431.

28. Pleger B, Blankenburg F, Bestmann S, et al. Repetitive transcranial magnetic stimulation-induced changes in sensorimotor coupling parallel improvements of somatosensation in humans. *J Neurosci.* 2006;26(7):1945–1952.

29. Conte A, Rocchi L, Nardella A, et al. Theta-burst stimulation-induced plasticity over primary somatosensory cortex changes somatosensory temporal discrimination in healthy humans. *PloS One.* 2012;7(3):e32979.

30. Torta DM, Legrain V, Algoet M, Olivier E, Duque J, Mouraux A. Theta burst stimulation applied over primary motor and somatosensory cortices produces analgesia unrelated to the changes in nociceptive event-related potentials. *PloS One.* 2013;8(8):e73263.

31. Rao N, Chen YT, Ramirez R, Tran J, Li S, Parikh PJ. Time-course of pain threshold after continuous theta burst stimulation of primary somatosensory cortex in pain-free subjects. *Neurosci Lett.* 2020;722:134760.

32. Jacobs MF, Zapallow CM, Tsang P, Lee KG, Asmussen MJ, Nelson AJ. Current direction specificity of continuous θ-burst stimulation in modulating human motor cortex excitability when applied to somatosensory cortex. *Neuroreport.* 2012;23(16):927–931.

33. Jacobs MF, Tsang P, Lee KG, Asmussen MJ, Zapallow CM, Nelson AJ. 30 Hz theta-burst stimulation over primary somatosensory cortex modulates corticospinal output to the hand. *Brain Stimul.* 2014;7(2):269–274.

34. Tsang P, Jacobs MF, Lee KGH, Asmussen MJ, Zapallow CM, Nelson AJ. Continuous theta-burst stimulation over primary somatosensory cortex modulates short-latency afferent inhibition. *Clin Neurophysiol.* 2014;125(11):2253–2259.

35. Kumar N, Manning TF, Ostry DJ. Somatosensory cortex participates in the consolidation of human motor memory. *PLoS Biol.* 2019;17(10):e3000469.

36. Frey VN, Butz K, Zimmermann G, et al. Effects of rubber hand illusion and excitatory theta burst stimulation on tactile sensation: A pilot study. *Neural Plasticity.* 2020;2020:3069639.

37. Wolters A, Schmidt A, Schramm A, et al. Timing-dependent plasticity in human primary somatosensory cortex. *J Physiol (London).* 2005;565(Pt 3):1039–1052.

38. Tsang P, Bailey AZ, Nelson AJ. Rapid-rate paired associative stimulation over the primary somatosensory cortex. *PLoS One.* 2015;10(3):e0120731.

39. Zazio A, Guidali G, Maddaluno O, Miniussi C, Bolognini N. Hebbian associative plasticity in the visuotactile domain: A cross-modal paired associative stimulation protocol. *Neuroimage.* 2019;201:116025.

40. Zhang R, Geng X, Lee TMC. Large-scale functional neural network correlates of response inhibition: An fMRI meta-analysis. *Brain Structure Function.* 2017;222(9):3973–3990.

41. Borgomaneri S, Serio G, Battaglia S. Please, don't do it! Fifteen years of progress of non-invasive brain stimulation in action inhibition. *Cortex.* 2020;132:404–422.

42. Chambers CD, Bellgrove MA, Stokes MG, et al. Executive "brake failure" following deactivation of human frontal lobe. *J Cogn Neurosci.* 2006;18(3):444–455.

43. Dippel G, Beste C. A causal role of the right inferior frontal cortex in implementing strategies for multicomponent behaviour. *Nature Communications.* 2015;6:6587.

44. Obeso I, Robles N, Marrón EM, Redolar-Ripoll D. Dissociating the role of the pre-SMA in response inhibition and switching: A combined online and offline TMS approach. *Front Hum Neurosci.* 2013;7:150.

45. Obeso I, Wilkinson L, Teo JT, Talelli P, Rothwell JC, Jahanshahi M. Theta burst magnetic stimulation over the pre-supplementary motor area improves motor inhibition. *Brain Stimul.* 2017;10(5):944–951.

46. Drummond NM, Cressman EK, Carlsen AN. Offline continuous theta burst stimulation over right inferior frontal gyrus and pre-supplementary motor area impairs inhibition during a go/no-go task. *Neuropsychologia.* 2017;99:360–367.

47. Chen CY, Muggleton NG, Tzeng OJ, Hung DL, Juan CH. Control of prepotent responses by the superior medial frontal cortex. *Neuroimage.* 2009;44(2):537–545.

48. Cai W, George JS, Verbruggen F, Chambers CD, Aron AR. The role of the right presupplementary motor area in stopping action: Two studies with event-related transcranial magnetic stimulation. *J Neurophysiol.* 2012;108(2):380–389.

49. Osada T, Ohta S, Ogawa A, et al. An essential role of the intraparietal sulcus in response inhibition predicted by parcellation-based network. *J Neurosci.* 2019;39(13):2509–2521.

TMS in Cognitive Studies

6.1 INTRODUCTION

Over the past few decades, the use of transcranial magnetic stimulation (TMS) as a tool to better understand brain–behavior relationships has grown significantly. TMS studies within the field of cognitive neuroscience have provided evidence for the causal link between the specific brain regions and neuronal networks thought to underly cognitive and behavioral outcomes. Methodological advances in data acquisition and analysis have led to key insights into the temporal and spatial correlates as well as functional and anatomical interactions associated with cognition. In addition to exploratory research applications, TMS has been used for its diagnostic and therapeutic potential, uncovering the mechanisms underlying cognitive impairment in psychiatric and neurological disorders as well as providing potential novel targets for cognitive interventions. In spite of these important insights, the precise mechanisms underlying how TMS may alter cognition are not yet fully understood, and ongoing investigation is needed.[1] As such, this chapter reviews TMS cognitive findings including potential mechanisms and important methodologic considerations and discusses potential applications of TMS cognition research in healthy and clinical populations.

6.1.1 Probing Cognition Circuits and Enhancing Cognitive Functioning

6.1.1.1 Virtual Lesion

In the field of cognitive neuroscience, lesion studies represent an effective approach to studying the link between neuroanatomy and cognitive functioning. Early research viewed the TMS pulses as a transient disruption of cortical functioning, thus generating a "virtual lesion." Examples of virtual lesion TMS studies investigated the effects of single and repetitive TMS (rTMS) of the primary visual cortex on visual imagery and perception,[2] as well as tactile information processing in blind people[3]; premotor and primary motor cortical stimulation on mental rotation,[4] reaction time,[5] and decreased accuracy on a delayed-match-to-sample task[6]; and frontal stimulation on random number generation.[7] However, more recent research suggests that TMS cannot be viewed simply as a disruptive tool because it is capable of producing a range of complex and sometimes subtle neuromodulatory effects.[8]

6.1.1.2 Cognitive Enhancement

In contrast to the virtual lesion studies of TMS, numerous studies have identified enhancement of cognitive functioning as an avenue of exploration. The current understanding of cognitive enhancement following TMS results from inhibiting the activation of extraneous or distracting stimuli, thus allowing task-relevant processing to occur.[9] A meta-analysis identified more than 60 reports of cognitive enhancement following single, paired, or rTMS paradigms.[10] These reports included numerous tasks associated with attention, memory, language, and motor learning, among others.[11-15] However, a more recent meta-analysis examining the cognitive effects of therapeutic rTMS in neuropsychiatric populations failed to find an overall effect for active rTMS compared to sham stimulation across a number of cognitive domains.[16] Whether the effects of TMS results in cognitive enhancement or impairment remains a topic of debate. However, taken together, these results highlight the complex relationship between neuromodulation effects within the brain and cognitive outcomes and suggest that TMS may not be viewed simply as a disruptive or facilitatory mechanism.

6.2 METHODOLOGIC CONSIDERATIONS FOR TMS

The general experimental design for TMS cognition studies commonly includes the administration of single-pulse TMS or short trains of TMS while a study participant is simultaneously completing a cognitive task (i.e., the online approach) or the tasks are completed before and after TMS (i.e., the offline approach). The pulses are delivered to the brain regions thought to underly a specific cognitive process or behavior of interest. It has been suggested that outcomes depend on a number of methodologic factors including the stimulation parameters (i.e., timing, frequency, duration, site of stimulation), brain activation state, cognitive domain, and population of interest.[10] Thus, appropriate study design and transparent methodological reporting are important components in furthering our understanding of the effects of TMS on cognition.

6.2.1 Stimulation Parameters

6.2.1.1 TMS Paradigms

Single-pulse TMS, when applied over different time windows using an online approach, provides key insights into the temporal sequence of cognitive processing. Given its ability to stimulate the cortex with high temporal resolution, single-pulse TMS allows researchers to determine the precise time point in which activation of neural activity modulates task performance. This approach is often referred to as *chronometric TMS*. In contrast to the temporal specificity underlying single-pulse TMS, rTMS offers the ability to stimulate over larger time windows during task execution. Increasing the duration of stimulation is thought to be associated with prolonged and enhanced modulation of cortical activity via temporal summation of the stimulation effects.[17] This approach may therefore be better suited to investigate and induce changes in behavioral/cognitive outcomes. In addition to online approaches, offline rTMS does not interfere with or distract from task execution. This can be especially beneficial when employing more uncomfortable stimulation paradigms, like high-frequency frontal stimulation.[17]

6.2.1.2 Site of Stimulation

Several brain regions have been studied in the context of different cognitive domains using TMS, including the motor, visual, parietal, and prefrontal cortex. As reviewed in Chapter 2, there are a number of approaches to cortical localization. In brief, targeting the motor and visual cortices can be done via recording their signature TMS-induced responses; namely, muscle twitching and phosphenes perception, respectively. Localizing regions without clearly defined responses like the parietal and prefrontal cortices is more challenging; however, recent technological advances, including the use of neuroimaging and frameless stereotaxic systems, have allowed for more accurate and reliable targeting within these regions.

In addition to anatomical information, studies within the field of cognitive neuroscience may use a function-guided approach to TMS targeting. As such, a task with a predictable effect to stimulation may be used as a functional target to coil positioning for subsequent tasks.[17] For example, using what is known as the "hunting procedure,"

Göbel et al. stimulated the area around the P4 electrode in blocks of 20 trials to identify the region that elicited a consistent increase in reaction time on a visual search task. This individualized site was then used as the target location for rTMS stimulation on a subsequent number task.[18] As a limitation, it should be noted that this approach is limited by the availability of predictable TMS responses within certain brain regions, is time-consuming, and generates variability across laboratories based on the criteria used for functional localization. A more reliable method for functional localization is the use of functional magnetic resonance imaging (fMRI). As reviewed in Chapter 2, this method utilizes either functional imaging data or previously identified Talairach coordinates derived from imagining studies investigating similar tasks or cognitive domains.

6.2.2 Brain State

The neurophysiologic effects of TMS depend not only on the characteristics of the stimulation but also on the brain state prior to and during stimulation. Understanding the influence of state-dependency on neuronal activity helps to optimize the effects of TMS on cognitive functioning. Therefore, brain state represents an important factor to consider when designing studies and interpreting results. In response to this, new TMS paradigms were developed including TMS adaptation and TMS priming (for full review see Sandrini et al.[17]). Both paradigms present a stimulus prior to the onset of the test stimulus and TMS, which is thought to differentially activate a subset of functionally distinct neurons to ultimately become more susceptible to the TMS-induced effects. In the adaptation paradigm, a stimulus presented for several seconds is proposed to induce habituation within the neuronal population encoding the features of the adapted stimulus. Studies have shown that adaptation TMS ultimately facilitates the perception or behavior associated with the adapted stimuli's features.[19-21] In contrast, the priming paradigm is based on the principle that repetition of a stimuli's features prior to stimulation leads to facilitation of the detection of the nonprimed stimulus.[22] The selective effects of TMS derived from these paradigms provides insights into the functional specificity of neurons underlying cognition and highlights the importance of controlling for brain state.

6.2.3 Control Conditions

Control conditions provide support that the cognitive effects observed are a direct response to the stimulation rather than to other extraneous variables, such as the somatosensory and auditory effects of TMS. As reviewed in Chapter 7, there are a number of control strategies including, most commonly, sham stimulation. This may be accomplished by tilting or holding the active coil a short distance from the scalp[23-25] or through the use of commercially available sham TMS coils.[26,27]

There are, however, a number of additional control conditions designed specifically for TMS cognitive studies. One such method includes stimulating brain regions which are not thought to underly the cognitive process of interest; for example, the vertex (corresponding to electrode CZ using the 10-20 system).[28-30] Studies investigating the lateralization of cognitive and behavioral processes may also stimulate the same region at both hemispheres as a control measure.[31-33] One limitation to stimulating alternative cortical sites as a control condition is that cortical excitability differs between brain regions[34] making it challenging to ensure that the stimulation parameters are sufficient for cortical activation in both regions.[1] Finally, alternative cognitive or behavioral tasks may be used as a control condition to demonstrate specificity of the effects of TMS on performance of the "active" cognitive task or domain.[1] The difficulty with this approach is determining a viable control task with equivalent difficulty to that of the active task condition.

6.2.4 Combining TMS with Other Methods

Combing TMS with other imaging and brain mapping methods provides a multifocal, whole-brain approach to investigating the neurophysiological effects and mechanisms underlying cognitive functioning. The methods selected can allow for investigation with a high temporal (e.g., electroencephalography [EEG]) or spatial (e.g., fMRI) resolution. Furthermore, as discussed in Chapter 7 on TMS-EEG, nonmotor stimulation, including the prefrontal cortex, a region which is vital for higher order cognitive functioning, relies on the use of additional brain mapping techniques to measure the physiological response to stimulation.[1,35]

Numerous studies have investigated the use single, paired, and rTMS in combination with methods such as EEG, positron emission tomography (PET), or fMRI on several cognitive domains (see Valero-Cabre[1]). Using online approaches, TMS coupled with such methods provides real-time evidence of the spread of activation and dynamic interactions between local and distal networks during cognitive activation. By contrast, offline approaches allow for the investigation of the longer-lasting neuroplastic effects of stimulation.[1,35]

6.3 POTENTIAL MECHANISMS OF COGNITIVE IMPAIRMENT AND ENHANCEMENT

Despite decades of research and the growing popularity of TMS in both research and clinical settings, questions remain regarding the precise mechanisms of action underlying the effects of stimulation on cognitive functioning. In general, it is accepted that the cognitive outcomes (e.g., accuracy, reaction time) depend on physiological properties of the stimulated brain region (e.g., brain state, anatomy, morphology, network connectivity) as well as the specific cognitive demands associated with the task of interest.[36] Thus, our basic understanding of the "excitatory/inhibitory" mechanism of TMS (see Chapters 3 and 4 and Hallet[37]) may represent an oversimplification of the complex, causal relationship between cortical stimulation with TMS and cognitive functioning. Several potential mechanisms have been proposed to account of the cognitive impairing and enhancing effects of TMS, briefly reviewed here.

As mentioned previously, the virtual lesion hypothesis of TMS proposes that the pulse acts to temporarily interfere with neuronal processing and ultimately cognitive functioning. Two main explanations for the inhibitory effects of TMS are that it either suppresses neuronal activity or it amplifies background "noise." Regarding the first hypothesis, TMS has been shown to suppress ongoing neural activity (e.g., Harris et al.[38]) and may interfere with neuronal communication by disrupting the temporal relationship between distant neuronal populations that comprise larger networks.[39] This may result from the induction of intracortical inhibition, via increased levels of the inhibitory neurotransmitter, gamma-aminobutyric acid (GABA). The second hypothesis suggests that TMS may disrupt cognitive functioning by introducing random neuronal activity or noise to ongoing processing.[40] Whether the impairing effects of TMS are due to the suppression of neuronal signal or the introduction of noise remains unknown. However, it has been suggested that it may likely be a combination of the two processes, with varying functionality based on stimulation intensity and neuronal characteristics.[17,36,41]

While the cognitive enhancing effects associated with TMS are still considered to be somewhat paradoxical, one metanalysis identified more than 60 examples of this effect and proposed three general mechanisms underlying these findings.[10] The first mechanism addresses the direct, modulatory effects of TMS on neuronal activity. Studies have shown single-pulse TMS administered prior to the stimulus onset resulted in improved performance,[42,43] which suggests that the stimulation may act to transiently enhance local neuronal activity.[10] Similar findings observed with rTMS are proposed to result from a modulation of cortical oscillatory activity (i.e., the synchronized and repetitive patterns of neural activity).[25,44,45] Additionally, rTMS is thought to induce performance enhancement through the induction of long-term potentiation (LTP)-like neuroplastic changes.[14] Both cortical oscillations[46–48] and LTP[49] are critically implicated in a variety of perceptual, sensorimotor, and cognitive processes.

The second proposed mechanism addresses the nonspecific effects of TMS.[10] As such, it is suggested that the auditory and somatosensory secondary effects of TMS (e.g., clicking, vibrations, activation of fascial muscles, scalp sensations) lead to a psychological response known as *intersensory facilitation*.[50] Both intersensory facilitation[51] and general arousal[52] associated with stimulation may therefore contribute to the cognitive enhancing effects of TMS, rather than true neurophysiological changes in activity.

The final proposed mechanism by Luber et al. is known as the *addition-by-subtraction mechanism*. It is suggested that cognitive enhancement via TMS may be due in part to an inhibition of task-irrelevant or distracting processes. This mechanism is somewhat in line with the virtual lesion hypothesis yet suggests that inhibiting such competing processes or activations lead to a brief reorganization of neuronal networks.[10] Several studies using single-pulse,[53] low-[54] and high-frequency[55] rTMS and theta burst stimulation[56] provide some support for this proposed mechanism.

6.4 POTENTIAL APPLICATIONS: UNDERSTANDING AND IMPROVING COGNITIVE IMPAIRMENTS

Given that TMS provides the ability to directly probe and modulate neuronal activity, applications for the use of TMS both in understanding and potentially treating cognitive impairments are continually growing.

6.4.1 Clinical Populations

Cognitive impairment is a common feature among a number of psychiatric and neurological disorders including Alzheimer's disease, Parkinson's disease, depression, bipolar disorder, and schizophrenia, as well as among aging adults with mild cognitive impairment. These impairments often present across numerous cognitive domains, from executive function, working memory, and attention to information processing and inhibition.[57-60] Furthermore, cognitive impairments are known to have a significant negative impact on quality of life and daily functioning.[58,61,62] While there are several current treatment options targeting cognitive impairment, including cognitive enhancing medication, cognitive training or remediation, and noninvasive brain stimulation,[63-65] the overall clinical efficacy of these treatment options is modest.[65] The benefit of a noninvasive brain stimulation approach like TMS is that it is fairly safe, well-tolerated, and does not necessarily require active participation by the patient.[65]

However, current findings regarding the efficacy of TMS in improving cognitive impairments are inconsistent and are highly dependent on the cognitive domain and population of interest as well as the stimulation parameters.[16,65-67] While individual studies have demonstrated the ability of TMS to improve certain cognitive domains in patients with depression,[68-70] Parkinson's disease,[71] schizophrenia,[72-74] and dementia,[75-77] systematic reviews and meta-analyses challenge the overall strength and reliability of these findings. For example, one meta-analysis specifically examined the cognitive-enhancing effects of high-frequency rTMS in a mixed sample of patients and found that left DLPFC stimulation with 10–15 successive treatment sessions and a treatment intensity of 80–110% of resting motor threshold were most likely to result in cognitive improvement.[67] This review included a number of additional analyses such as low- versus high-frequency, active versus sham stimulation, and clinical versus healthy populations. It is important to note, however, that several of the studies included failed to find a significant cognitive enhancing effect of rTMS, and the subanalyses were limited due in large part to methodical variability among studies.[67] A more recent meta-analysis including 30 randomized, sham-controlled trials studying DLPFC stimulation in patients with various neuropsychiatric conditions did not find an overall association between active rTMS and enhanced cognitive functioning. They did, however, find a moderate effect in a few studies which demonstrated improved working memory following stimulation in patients with schizophrenia.[16] However, a recent large replication attempt at demonstrating working memory enhancement with bilateral HF rTMS to the DLPFC failed to find a difference between active and sham stimulation.[78]

One suggested approach to augmenting the cognitive enhancing potential of TMS is to combine TMS with other interventions like cognitive remediation or training. The goal of cognitive remediation is to improve cognitive processing skills and daily functioning through individualized training of specific impairments.[79] Cognitive remediation alone has shown moderate success in improving cognitive and functional abilities in older healthy individuals[80] and in those with mild cognitive impairment (MCI)[81] and other psychiatric disorders.[63] TMS combined cognitive training using an online approach has been shown to significantly improve cognition in patients with Alzheimer's disease,[82] beyond that of cognitive training alone.[83] Taken together, these findings suggest that TMS represents a potential tool to improve cognitive impairment across clinical populations; however, continued investigation is needed.

6.4.2 Healthy Populations

The possibility of improving cognition with TMS has also been explored in healthy individuals. For example, studies investigating the effects of high-frequency prefrontal rTMS on attentional control have shown improved reaction time on the Stroop interference task[84,85] and fewer commission errors on the Conner's Continuous Performance Task.[86] Similar results have been found in studies investigating episodic memory with paired-pulse TMS[12] and working memory with high-frequency rTMS.[87] Low-frequency rTMS has also shown some promise in improving performance, potentially by inhibiting conflicting or distracting processing,[88,89] in alignment with the addition-by-subtraction mechanism proposed by Luber et al.[10] An alternative application of the cognitive enhancing effects of TMS has been proposed in the context of *neuroergonomics* (i.e., studying the brain at work). As such, it is suggested that TMS may be viewed as a tool to modify behavior in real time to optimize human operator performance in response to the rapid progression of modern technology.[90]

While promising, studies to date have had small sample sizes, and there is little evidence to support the lasting effects of stimulation on cognition; therefore, the use of TMS to enhance cognition in healthy populations remains exploratory. There are several strategies which have been shown to increase the duration and effects of TMS. As discussed earlier with Alzheimer's disease research, priming the stimulated region of interest with a practice or co-occurring task may act to induce Hebbian-like activation within the neuronal network underlying task performance.[91,92] Additionally, increasing the duration and number of rTMS sessions may also prolong the cognitive enhancing effects of TMS.[93] These strategies, in addition to the methodologic considerations described in Section 6.2, are important steps toward optimizing the use of TMS in cognitive neuroscience.

6.5 CONCLUSION

Taken together, the research presented in this chapter outlines the potential role of TMS in better understanding the temporal, spatial, and functional interactions underlying cognitive functioning. Furthermore, the use of TMS as a potential treatment approach across individuals with psychiatric and neurological disorders represents an important direction for future research. In spite of these important insights, there are limitations regarding the role of TMS in cognitive neuroscience, including the paucity of research focusing on the potential long-term effects of TMS. In order to better understand and optimize the use of TMS, appropriate study designs and transparent methodological reporting are vital. As technology advances and the field of TMS moves toward a multimodal, whole-brain approach, advances in our understanding of brain–cognition relationships, discovery of diagnostic biomarkers, and the development of targeted clinical interventions will likely follow.

REFERENCES

1. Valero-Cabre A, Amengual JL, Stengel C, Pascual-Leone A, Coubard OA. Transcranial magnetic stimulation in basic and clinical neuroscience: A comprehensive review of fundamental principles and novel insights. *Neurosci Biobehav Rev.* 2017;83:381–404.
2. Kosslyn SM, Pascual-Leone A, Felician O, Camposano S, Keenan JP, Thompson WL, et al. The role of area 17 in visual imagery: Convergent evidence from PET and rTMS. *Science.* 1999;284(5411):167–170.
3. Cohen LG, Celnik P, Pascual-Leone A, Corwell B, Falz L, Dambrosia J, et al. Functional relevance of cross-modal plasticity in blind humans. *Nature.* 1997;389(6647):180–183.
4. Ganis G, Keenan JP, Kosslyn SM, Pascual-Leone A. Transcranial magnetic stimulation of primary motor cortex affects mental rotation. *Cerebral Cortex.* 2000;10(2):175–180.
5. Schluter ND, Rushworth MF, Passingham RE, Mills KR. Temporary interference in human lateral premotor cortex suggests dominance for the selection of movements. A study using transcranial magnetic stimulation. *Brain.* 1998;121 (Pt 5):785–799.

6. Herwig U, Abler B, Schonfeldt-Lecuona C, Wunderlich A, Grothe J, Spitzer M, et al. Verbal storage in a premotor-parietal network: Evidence from fMRI-guided magnetic stimulation. *NeuroImage.* 2003;20(2):1032–1041.

7. Jahanshahi M, Profice P, Brown RG, Ridding MC, Dirnberger G, Rothwell JC. The effects of transcranial magnetic stimulation over the dorsolateral prefrontal cortex on suppression of habitual counting during random number generation. *Brain.* 1998;121 (Pt 8):1533–1544.

8. Silvanto J, Cattaneo Z. Common framework for "virtual lesion" and state-dependent TMS: The facilitatory/suppressive range model of online TMS effects on behavior. *Brain Cogn.* 2017;119:32–38.

9. Walsh V, Ellison A, Battelli L, Cowey A. Task-specific impairments and enhancements induced by magnetic stimulation of human visual area V5. *Proc Biol Sci.* 1998;265(1395):537–543.

10. Luber B, Lisanby SH. Enhancement of human cognitive performance using transcranial magnetic stimulation (TMS). *NeuroImage.* 2014;85 Pt 3:961–970.

11. Boroojerdi B, Phipps M, Kopylev L, Wharton CM, Cohen LG, Grafman J. Enhancing analogic reasoning with rTMS over the left prefrontal cortex. *Neurology.* 2001;56(4):526–528.

12. Gagnon G, Schneider C, Grondin S, Blanchet S. Enhancement of episodic memory in young and healthy adults: A paired-pulse TMS study on encoding and retrieval performance. *Neurosci Lett.* 2011;488(2):138–142.

13. Boyd LA, Linsdell MA. Excitatory repetitive transcranial magnetic stimulation to left dorsal premotor cortex enhances motor consolidation of new skills. *BMC Neurosci.* 2009;10:72.

14. Butefisch CM, Khurana V, Kopylev L, Cohen LG. Enhancing encoding of a motor memory in the primary motor cortex by cortical stimulation. *J Neurophysiol.* 2004;91(5):2110–2116.

15. Schutter DJ, van Honk J. Increased positive emotional memory after repetitive transcranial magnetic stimulation over the orbitofrontal cortex. *J Psychiatry Neurosci.* 2006;31(2):101–104.

16. Martin DM, McClintock SM, Forster J, Loo CK. Does therapeutic repetitive transcranial magnetic stimulation cause cognitive enhancing effects in patients with neuropsychiatric conditions? A systematic review and meta-analysis of randomised controlled trials. *Neuropsychol Rev.* 2016;26(3):295–309.

17. Sandrini M, Umilta C, Rusconi E. The use of transcranial magnetic stimulation in cognitive neuroscience: A new synthesis of methodological issues. *Neurosci Biobehav Rev.* 2011;35(3):516–536.

18. Gobel S, Walsh V, Rushworth MF. The mental number line and the human angular gyrus. *NeuroImage.* 2001;14(6):1278–1289.

19. Silvanto J, Muggleton NG, Cowey A, Walsh V. Neural adaptation reveals state-dependent effects of transcranial magnetic stimulation. *Eur J Neurosci.* 2007;25(6):1874–1881.

20. Cattaneo Z, Silvanto J. Investigating visual motion perception using the transcranial magnetic stimulation-adaptation paradigm. *Neuroreport.* 2008;19(14):1423–1427.

21. Romei V, Murray MM, Merabet LB, Thut G. Occipital transcranial magnetic stimulation has opposing effects on visual and auditory stimulus detection: Implications for multisensory interactions. *J Neurosci.* 2007;27(43):11465–11472.

22. Cattaneo Z, Rota F, Vecchi T, Silvanto J. Using state-dependency of transcranial magnetic stimulation (TMS) to investigate letter selectivity in the left posterior parietal cortex: A comparison of TMS-priming and TMS-adaptation paradigms. *Eur J Neurosci.* 2008;28(9):1924–1929.

23. Daskalakis ZJ, Farzan F, Barr MS, Maller JJ, Chen R, Fitzgerald PB. Long-interval cortical inhibition from the dorsolateral prefrontal cortex: A TMS-EEG study. *Neuropsychopharmacology.* 2008;33(12):2860–2869.

24. Du X, Choa FS, Summerfelt A, Rowland LM, Chiappelli J, Kochunov P, et al. N100 as a generic cortical electrophysiological marker based on decomposition of TMS-evoked potentials across five anatomic locations. *Exp Brain Res.* 2017;235(1):69–81.

25. Fuggetta G, Pavone EF, Fiaschi A, Manganotti P. Acute modulation of cortical oscillatory activities during short trains of high-frequency repetitive transcranial magnetic stimulation of the human motor cortex: A combined EEG and TMS study. *Hum Brain Mapp.* 2008;29(1):1–13.

26. Bonato C, Miniussi C, Rossini PM. Transcranial magnetic stimulation and cortical evoked potentials: A TMS/EEG co-registration study. *Clin Neurophysiol.* 2006;117(8):1699–1707.

27. Opitz A, Legon W, Mueller J, Barbour A, Paulus W, Tyler WJ. Is sham cTBS real cTBS? The effect on EEG dynamics. *Front Hum Neurosci.* 2014;8:1043.

28. Dormal V, Andres M, Pesenti M. Dissociation of numerosity and duration processing in the left intraparietal sulcus: A transcranial magnetic stimulation study. *Cortex.* 2008;44(4):462–469.
29. Knops A, Nuerk HC, Sparing R, Foltys H, Willmes K. On the functional role of human parietal cortex in number processing: How gender mediates the impact of a "virtual lesion" induced by rTMS. *Neuropsychologia.* 2006;44(12):2270–2283.
30. Rusconi E, Bueti D, Walsh V, Butterworth B. Contribution of frontal cortex to the spatial representation of number. *Cortex.* 2011;47(1):2–13.
31. Cattaneo Z, Silvanto J, Pascual-Leone A, Battelli L. The role of the angular gyrus in the modulation of visuospatial attention by the mental number line. *NeuroImage.* 2009;44(2):563–568.
32. Rusconi E, Turatto M, Umilta C. Two orienting mechanisms in posterior parietal lobule: An rTMS study of the Simon and SNARC effects. *Cogn Neuropsychol.* 2007;24(4):373–392.
33. Rusconi E, Walsh V, Butterworth B. Dexterity with numbers: RTMS over left angular gyrus disrupts finger gnosis and number processing. *Neuropsychologia.* 2005;43(11):1609–1624.
34. Boroojerdi B, Meister IG, Foltys H, Sparing R, Cohen LG, Topper R. Visual and motor cortex excitability: A transcranial magnetic stimulation study. *Clin Neurophysiol.* 2002;113(9):1501–1504.
35. Driver J, Blankenburg F, Bestmann S, Vanduffel W, Ruff CC. Concurrent brain-stimulation and neuroimaging for studies of cognition. *Trends Cogn Sci.* 2009;13(7):319–327.
36. Miniussi C, Ruzzoli M, Walsh V. The mechanism of transcranial magnetic stimulation in cognition. *Cortex.* 2010;46(1):128–130.
37. Hallett M. Transcranial magnetic stimulation: A primer. *Neuron.* 2007;55(2):187–199.
38. Harris JA, Clifford CW, Miniussi C. The functional effect of transcranial magnetic stimulation: Signal suppression or neural noise generation? *J Cogn Neurosci.* 2008;20(4):734–740.
39. Pasley BN, Allen EA, Freeman RD. State-dependent variability of neuronal responses to transcranial magnetic stimulation of the visual cortex. *Neuron.* 2009;62(2):291–303.
40. Ruzzoli M, Marzi CA, Miniussi C. The neural mechanisms of the effects of transcranial magnetic stimulation on perception. *J Neurophysiol.* 2010;103(6):2982–2989.
41. Siebner HR, Hartwigsen G, Kassuba T, Rothwell JC. How does transcranial magnetic stimulation modify neuronal activity in the brain? Implications for studies of cognition. *Cortex.* 2009;45(9):1035–1042.
42. Grosbras MH, Paus T. Transcranial magnetic stimulation of the human frontal eye field: Effects on visual perception and attention. *J Cogn Neurosci.* 2002;14(7):1109–1120.
43. Grosbras MH, Paus T. Transcranial magnetic stimulation of the human frontal eye field facilitates visual awareness. *Eur J Neurosci.* 2003;18(11):3121–3126.
44. Thut G, Veniero D, Romei V, Miniussi C, Schyns P, Gross J. Rhythmic TMS causes local entrainment of natural oscillatory signatures. *Curr Biol.* 2011;21(14):1176–1185.
45. Hamidi M, Slagter HA, Tononi G, Postle BR. Repetitive transcranial magnetic stimulation affects behavior by biasing endogenous cortical oscillations. *Front Integr Neurosci.* 2009;3:14.
46. Basar E, Basar-Eroglu C, Karakas S, Schurmann M. Brain oscillations in perception and memory. *Int J Psychophysiol.* 2000;35(2-3):95–124.
47. Singer W. Neuronal synchrony: A versatile code for the definition of relations? *Neuron.* 1999;24(1):49–65, 111–125.
48. Buzsaki G, Draguhn A. Neuronal oscillations in cortical networks. *Science.* 2004;304(5679):1926–1929.
49. Morris RG. Long-term potentiation and memory. *Philos Trans R Soc Lond B Biol Sci.* 2003;358(1432):643–647.
50. Terao Y, Ugawa Y, Suzuki M, Sakai K, Hanajima R, Gemba-Shimizu K, et al. Shortening of simple reaction time by peripheral electrical and submotor-threshold magnetic cortical stimulation. *Exp Brain Res.* 1997;115(3):541–545.
51. Campana G, Cowey A, Walsh V. Priming of motion direction and area V5/MT: A test of perceptual memory. *Cerebral Cortex.* 2002;12(6):663–669.
52. Drager B, Breitenstein C, Helmke U, Kamping S, Knecht S. Specific and nonspecific effects of transcranial magnetic stimulation on picture-word verification. *Eur J Neurosci.* 2004;20(6):1681–1687.
53. Alford JL, van Donkelaar P, Dassonville P, Marrocco RT. Transcranial magnetic stimulation over MT/MST fails to impair judgments of implied motion. *Cogn Affect Behav Neurosci.* 2007;7(3):225–232.

54. Hodsoll J, Mevorach C, Humphreys GW. Driven to less distraction: RTMS of the right parietal cortex reduces attentional capture in visual search. *Cerebral Cortex.* 2009;19(1):106–114.

55. Harris IM, Benito CT, Ruzzoli M, Miniussi C. Effects of right parietal transcranial magnetic stimulation on object identification and orientation judgments. *J Cogn Neurosci.* 2008;20(5):916–926.

56. Kalla R, Muggleton NG, Cowey A, Walsh V. Human dorsolateral prefrontal cortex is involved in visual search for conjunctions but not features: A theta TMS study. *Cortex.* 2009;45(9):1085–1090.

57. Medalia A, Lim R. Treatment of cognitive dysfunction in psychiatric disorders. *J Psychiatr Pract.* 2004;10(1):17–25.

58. Millan MJ, Agid Y, Brune M, Bullmore ET, Carter CS, Clayton NS, et al. Cognitive dysfunction in psychiatric disorders: Characteristics, causes and the quest for improved therapy. *Nat Rev Drug Discov.* 2012;11(2):141–168.

59. Simen AA, Bordner KA, Martin MP, Moy LA, Barry LC. Cognitive dysfunction with aging and the role of inflammation. *Ther Adv Chronic Dis.* 2011;2(3):175–195.

60. Douglas KM, Gallagher P, Robinson LJ, Carter JD, McIntosh VV, Frampton CM, et al. Prevalence of cognitive impairment in major depression and bipolar disorder. *Bipolar Disord.* 2018;20(3):260–274.

61. Papakostas GI, Petersen T, Mahal Y, Mischoulon D, Nierenberg AA, Fava M. Quality of life assessments in major depressive disorder: A review of the literature. *Gen Hosp Psychiatry.* 2004;26(1):13–17.

62. Schrag A, Jahanshahi M, Quinn N. What contributes to quality of life in patients with Parkinson's disease? *J Neurol Neurosurg Psychiatry.* 2000;69(3):308–312.

63. Kim EJ, Bahk YC, Oh H, Lee WH, Lee JS, Choi KH. Current status of cognitive remediation for psychiatric disorders: A review. *Front Psychiatry.* 2018;9:461.

64. Wallace TL, Ballard TM, Pouzet B, Riedel WJ, Wettstein JG. Drug targets for cognitive enhancement in neuropsychiatric disorders. *Pharmacol Biochem Behav.* 2011;99(2):130–145.

65. Begemann MJ, Brand BA, Curcic-Blake B, Aleman A, Sommer IE. Efficacy of non-invasive brain stimulation on cognitive functioning in brain disorders: A meta-analysis. *Psychol Med.* 2020;50(15):2465–2486.

66. Kim TD, Hong G, Kim J, Yoon S. Cognitive enhancement in neurological and psychiatric disorders using transcranial magnetic stimulation (TMS): A review of modalities, potential mechanisms and future implications. *Exp Neurobiol.* 2019;28(1):1–16.

67. Guse B, Falkai P, Wobrock T. Cognitive effects of high-frequency repetitive transcranial magnetic stimulation: A systematic review. *J Neural Transm (Vienna).* 2010;117(1):105–122.

68. Cheng CM, Juan CH, Chen MH, Chang CF, Lu HJ, Su TP, et al. Different forms of prefrontal theta burst stimulation for executive function of medication-resistant depression: Evidence from a randomized sham-controlled study. *Prog Neuro-Psychopharmacol Biol Psychiatry.* 2016;66:35–40.

69. Vanderhasselt MA, De Raedt R, Baeken C, Leyman L, D'Haenen H. A single session of rTMS over the left dorsolateral prefrontal cortex influences attentional control in depressed patients. *World J Biol Psychiatry.* 2009;10(1):34–42.

70. Moser DJ, Jorge RE, Manes F, Paradiso S, Benjamin ML, Robinson RG. Improved executive functioning following repetitive transcranial magnetic stimulation. *Neurology.* 2002;58(8):1288–1290.

71. Srovnalova H, Marecek R, Rektorova I. The role of the inferior frontal gyri in cognitive processing of patients with Parkinson's disease: A pilot rTMS study. *Movem Dis.* 2011;26(8):1545–1548.

72. Zheng LN, Guo Q, Li H, Li CB, Wang JJ. [Effects of repetitive transcranial magnetic stimulation with different paradigms on the cognitive function and psychotic symptoms of schizophrenia patients]. Beijing *Da Xue Xue Bao Yi Xue Ban.* 2012;44(5):732–736.

73. Barr MS, Farzan F, Rajji TK, Voineskos AN, Blumberger DM, Arenovich T, et al. Can repetitive magnetic stimulation improve cognition in schizophrenia? Pilot data from a randomized controlled trial. *Biol Psychiatry.* 2013;73(6):510–517.

74. Wolwer W, Lowe A, Brinkmeyer J, Streit M, Habakuck M, Agelink MW, et al. Repetitive transcranial magnetic stimulation (rTMS) improves facial affect recognition in schizophrenia. *Brain Stimul.* 2014;7(4):559–563.

75. Eliasova I, Anderkova L, Marecek R, Rektorova I. Non-invasive brain stimulation of the right inferior frontal gyrus may improve attention in early Alzheimer's disease: A pilot study. *J Neurol Sci.* 2014;346(1–2):318–322.

76. Zhao J, Li Z, Cong Y, Zhang J, Tan M, Zhang H, et al. Repetitive transcranial magnetic stimulation improves cognitive function of Alzheimer's disease patients. *Oncotarget.* 2017;8(20):33864–33871.

77. Koch G, Bonni S, Pellicciari MC, Casula EP, Mancini M, Esposito R, et al. Transcranial magnetic stimulation of the precuneus enhances memory and neural activity in prodromal Alzheimer's disease. *NeuroImage.* 2018;169:302–311.

78. Voineskos AN, Blumberger DM, Schifani C, Hawco C, Dickie EW, Rajji TK, et al. Effects of repetitive transcranial magnetic stimulation on working memory performance and brain structure in people with schizophrenia spectrum disorders: A double-blind, randomized, sham-controlled trial. *Biol Psychiatry Cogn Neurosci Neuroimaging.* 2021;6(4):449–458.

79. Clare L, Woods RT, Moniz Cook ED, Orrell M, Spector A. Cognitive rehabilitation and cognitive training for early-stage Alzheimer's disease and vascular dementia. *Cochrane Database Syst Rev.* 2003(4):CD003260.

80. Willis SL, Tennstedt SL, Marsiske M, Ball K, Elias J, Koepke KM, et al. Long-term effects of cognitive training on everyday functional outcomes in older adults. *JAMA.* 2006;296(23):2805–2814.

81. Li H, Li J, Li N, Li B, Wang P, Zhou T. Cognitive intervention for persons with mild cognitive impairment: A meta-analysis. *Ageing Res Rev.* 2011;10(2):285–296.

82. Rabey JM, Dobronevsky E, Aichenbaum S, Gonen O, Marton RG, Khaigrekht M. Repetitive transcranial magnetic stimulation combined with cognitive training is a safe and effective modality for the treatment of Alzheimer's disease: A randomized, double-blind study. *J Neural Transm (Vienna).* 2013;120(5):813–819.

83. Bagattini C, Zanni M, Barocco F, Caffarra P, Brignani D, Miniussi C, et al. Enhancing cognitive training effects in Alzheimer's disease: RTMS as an add-on treatment. *Brain Stimul.* 2020;13(6):1655–1664.

84. Vanderhasselt MA, De Raedt R, Baeken C, Leyman L, D'Haenen H. The influence of rTMS over the left dorsolateral prefrontal cortex on Stroop task performance. *Exp Brain Res.* 2006;169(2):279–282.

85. Vanderhasselt MA, De Raedt R, Baeken C, Leyman L, Clerinx P, D'Haenen H. The influence of rTMS over the right dorsolateral prefrontal cortex on top-down attentional processes. *Brain Res.* 2007;1137(1):111–116.

86. Hwang JH, Kim SH, Park CS, Bang SA, Kim SE. Acute high-frequency rTMS of the left dorsolateral prefrontal cortex and attentional control in healthy young men. *Brain Res.* 2010;1329:152–158.

87. Bagherzadeh Y, Khorrami A, Zarrindast MR, Shariat SV, Pantazis D. Repetitive transcranial magnetic stimulation of the dorsolateral prefrontal cortex enhances working memory. *Exp Brain Res.* 2016;234(7):1807–1818.

88. Snyder A, Bahramali H, Hawker T, Mitchell DJ. Savant-like numerosity skills revealed in normal people by magnetic pulses. *Perception.* 2006;35(6):837–845.

89. Oliveri M, Zhaoping L, Mangano GR, Turriziani P, Smirni D, Cipolotti L. Facilitation of bottom-up feature detection following rTMS-interference of the right parietal cortex. *Neuropsychologia.* 2010;48(4):1003–1010.

90. McKinley RA, Bridges N, Walters CM, Nelson J. Modulating the brain at work using noninvasive transcranial stimulation. *NeuroImage.* 2012;59(1):129–137.

91. Ragert P, Dinse HR, Pleger B, Wilimzig C, Frombach E, Schwenkreis P, et al. Combination of 5 Hz repetitive transcranial magnetic stimulation (rTMS) and tactile coactivation boosts tactile discrimination in humans. *Neurosci Lett.* 2003;348(2):105–108.

92. Thickbroom GW. Transcranial magnetic stimulation and synaptic plasticity: Experimental framework and human models. *Exp Brain Res.* 2007;180(4):583–593.

93. Thut G, Pascual-Leone A. A review of combined TMS-EEG studies to characterize lasting effects of repetitive TMS and assess their usefulness in cognitive and clinical neuroscience. *Brain Topogr.* 2010;22(4):219–232.

TMS with EEG

7.1 INTRODUCTION

As reviewed in previous chapters, transcranial magnetic stimulation (TMS) represents a reliable, noninvasive brain stimulation method that can be used to measure neurophysiological processes in healthy and clinical populations in vivo. However, one clear limitation of TMS-electromyogram (EMG) paradigms is associated with the reliance on gathering neurophysiological information from motor cortex. This has been due, in large part, to methodologic challenges associated with measuring responses to stimulation from nonmotor brain regions.[1] TMS combined with electroencephalography (EEG) directly addresses this limitation by enabling a recording of electrical activity at the level of the cortex through scalp electrodes, rather than through peripheral motor responses. As such, TMS-EEG can provide insights into cortico-cortical interactions, aberrant neuroplasticity, and excitation/inhibition imbalances from brain regions more closely linked to pathophysiologic and therapeutic targets of various disorders.[2] In this context, this chapter provides an overview of TMS-EEG research with a focus on the basic principles of data acquisition, processing, and analysis as well as the application of TMS-EEG in healthy and clinical populations.

7.1.1 Basic Principles of TMS-EEG

Much of what we know about human brain activity originated from early EEG studies conducted by Hans Berger in the 1930s. This ground-breaking research revealed that groups of neurons form complex, transiently linked networks with an innate ability to oscillate across various frequency ranges. This unique neuronal feature is now understood to underly local and long-range neuronal communication and represents a critical link between the activity of single neurons and behavior.[3] Neuronal synchrony, as is seen in response to a stimulus for example, results in relatively large fluctuations in electrical potentials, primarily generated from the summation of excitatory or inhibitory postsynaptic potentials.[4-6] This summation depends on the spatial and temporal contiguity of thousands or hundreds of thousands of synapses to produce electrical potentials that are measurable at the level of the scalp.[7] Additionally, the synchronous pattern of firing recorded by EEG electrodes is thought to be a result of several co-occurring factors, including the structural properties of neurons, the functional properties of neurotransmitter systems, and the interaction of various neuronal networks.[8] Over the years, EEG recordings have provided key insights into the functioning and timing of neuronal activity implicated in a variety of perceptual, sensory, and cognitive processes.

As outlined in previous chapters, TMS generates time-varying magnetic fields surrounding the coil that result in the induction of an electrical current in underlying brain tissue when the coil is held over the scalp. When applied to the motor region, the TMS-induced current results in neuronal depolarization and the propagation of action potentials, ultimately leading to activation of the targeted muscle. Using these principles applied to TMS-EEG, the TMS coil held directly over the EEG electrodes induces changes in electrical activity referred to as *TMS-evoked potentials* (TEP)s. Similar to motor evoked potentials (MEPs) associated with TMS-EMG, TEPs represent a measure of cortical reactivity and are indexed by changes in amplitude and the latency of electrical activity in response to the TMS pulse (Figure 7.1).

The first successful co-registration of TMS and EEG was conducted by Cracco et al. (1989) using a one-electrode system to measure TMS responses at the contralateral cortical area.[10] It was not until several years later that the field was able to progress, due in large part to the development of the multichannel TMS-compatible EEG systems.[11,12] Using high-resolution EEG along with TMS, Ilmoniemi was able to record the initial cortical TMS response a few milliseconds after the TMS pulse, as well as characterize the spread of activation across the brain.[11] This study, for the first time, illustrated the pattern of TMS-induced neuronal responses within the motor and occipital cortices. Taken together, these initial studies highlight the potential of TMS-EEG as a method to probe neuronal processes across the brain (Figure 7.2).

7.2 OUTCOME MEASURES OF TMS–EEG

The TMS-induced features captured by the EEG recording vary based on the analytic method, the region and time window of interest, and number of electrodes included, among other issues. EEG components are commonly represented in terms of amplitude

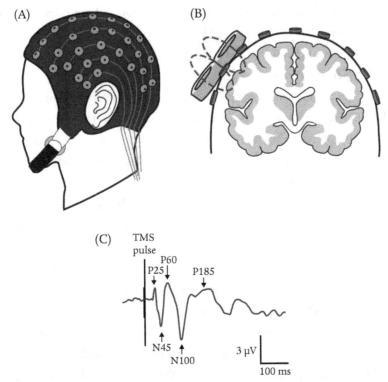

FIGURE 7.1 *A schematic diagram of transcranial magnetic stimulation (TMS) and electroenceph-alogram (EEG) and the resulting TMS-evoked potentials (TEPs). (A) A standard 62-channel EEG cap which can record changes in electrical activity evoked by TMS stimulation. (B) The magnetic field (red dotted lines) generated by the TMS coil, which in turn induces electrical stimulation in the targeted brain region. (C) The resulting TEP associated with single-pulse TMS. The negative and pos-itive TEP components depicted in this figure are measured over different latencies relative to the onset of TMS pulse.*

FROM HUI ET AL., *CLIN PHARMACOL THER.* 2019;106(4):734–746.

(i.e., the peak value of a sinusoidal signal, measured in μV), frequency (i.e., the number of cycles per second, measured in Hz), and phase (i.e., the position on the cycle of a waveform during a point in time, measured in degrees or radians).[7] Combining EEG with TMS provides the opportunity to investigate cortical reactivity and connectivity directly evoked by the TMS pulse and can ultimately provide a better understanding of the dy-namic nature of neuronal networks.[13,14]

7.2.1 Reactivity

Reactivity is a measure of the localized or global response of the brain to an event. Analytic methods for EEG signals are commonly categorized into (1) the *time domain*, characterizing latency and amplitude of event related potentials or evoked potentials and

(A)

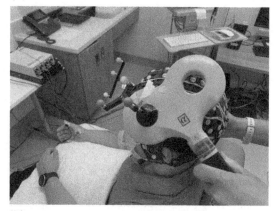

(B)

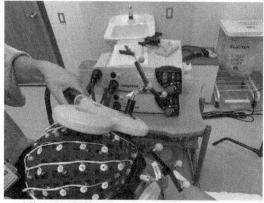

(C)

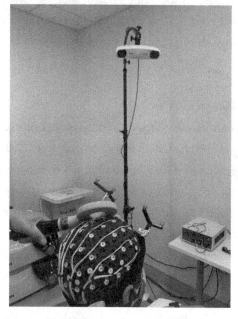

FIGURE 7.2 CONTINUED

(D)

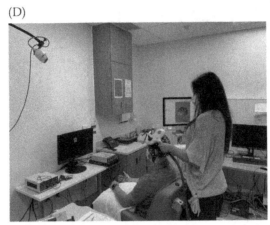

FIGURE 7.2 *Transcranial magnetic stimulation (TMS) and electroencephalogram (EEG) laboratory setup. Basic setup and equipment required to carry about a TMS-EEG study. The images on the left demonstrate the placement of the TMS coil over top of the EEG electrodes over the left dorsolateral prefrontal cortex (DLPFC). The images on the right include the use of neuronavigation (reviewed in Chapter 2). Neuronavigation works by precisely monitoring the position and orientation of trackers attached to the participant's head and to the coil.*

global mean field amplitude; (2) the *frequency domain*, decomposing the signal into specific frequency bands to measure outcomes such as evoked and induced power, relative and absolute power, or event-related synchronization/desynchronization; (3) the *time-frequency domain*, a measure of the change in power within each frequency as a function of time, with outcome measures including event-related spectral perturbation; and (4) the *phase domain*, measuring the phase of a signal in response to a stimulus at a specific time point. For a thorough description of these methods see Farzan et al.,[8] Pellicciari et al.,[15] and Hill et al.[16]

7.2.1.1 TMS-Evoked Potentials

The TEP represents a complex waveform comprised of a reliable set of time-locked peaks and troughs, occurring at specific latencies and lasting up to 300 ms or longer.[16] These peaks and troughs are generated via the summation of excitatory and inhibitory postsynaptic potentials[13] and are understood to reflect cortical excitatory/inhibitory processes. Importantly, TEPs have been shown to be a robust and reliable measure.[17]

The most studied region using TMS-EEG is the primary motor cortex (M1). In general, this region is characterized by several peaks, including N15, P30, N45, P55, N100, P180, and N280.[17,18] Pharmacological studies and those employing paired-pulse TMS paradigms have shed light on the physiological underpinnings of TEPs, suggesting that early peaks (i.e., N15–P30) likely reflect cortical excitability, while later peaks (i.e., N45–N100) reflect cortical inhibition.[19] Second to the M1 region, TEPs from the dorsolateral prefrontal cortex (DLPFC) have been well-characterized. DLPFC stimulation generates peaks including P25, N40, P60, N100, and P185.[20] Similar to the M1 distribution, a large spread of activity over bilateral central sites is observed with the later peaks (i.e., N100 and P180),[21] whereas DLPFC stimulation is associated with generally smaller peak responses compared to the M1 region. Furthermore, the distribution of the early peak (i.e., N40) is observed over the stimulated electrodes followed by a spread over central and contralateral frontal sites (P60). Importantly, TEPs associated with both M1 and DLPFC stimulation have been shown to be highly reproducible.[17,22]

Several methods have been developed to evaluate TEPs recorded both locally and globally, each with its own strengths and limitations. Regarding local TEP measures, region-of-interest (ROI) analyses represent the most commonly studied approaches. For this approach, waveform features such as amplitude and latency are averaged across neighboring electrodes[16] and are displayed as a waveform of varying amplitude over time. An additional method to analyzing local TEPs is called *local mean field power* (LMFP)[23] or cortical evoked activity (CEA).[24] This represents a measure of the standard deviation of the signal or rectified area under the curve (AUC), respectively, for a specific region and timepoint. Of note, the LMFP/CEA methods do not require a clear peak to be present given that the signal is rectified, and thus potentially important information regarding the polarity is not considered.[21] These methods do require that the electrodes comprising the region of interest are selected a priori; therefore, ROI, LMFP, and CEA analyses are best suited for studies where such hypotheses are possible.

In contrast to the methods which focus on local brain activation, an alternative approach known as *global mean field amplitude* (GMFA) measures the global TMS response. This is accomplished by averaging the evoked activity or standard deviation across all electrodes at a specific timepoint.[25,26] This approach is best suited for studies that do not have an a priori hypothesis regarding a region-specific TMS response and are interested instead in global activation.[21] Regardless of the selected method, the analysis of TEPs provides important insights into the functional dynamics of neuronal networks across the cortex (Figure 7.3).

7.2.1.2 Cortical Oscillations

Reactivity analyses may also be considered in terms of cortical oscillations. Cortical oscillations represent synchronous fluctuations in excitability of large groups of neurons, resulting in common target cells receiving neural inputs simultaneously. Measuring changes in oscillatory activity provides important insight regarding the structure, properties, and state of the underlying neuronal networks. Research has begun to uncover the role that neural oscillations play in neuroplasticity in healthy humans as well as in pathophysiology and treatment associations in clinical populations.[27]

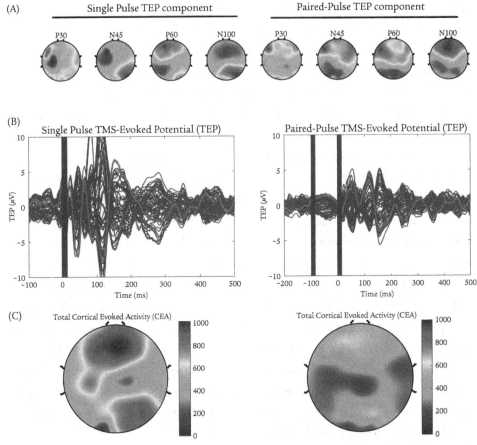

FIGURE 7.3 *Diagram of transcranial magnetic stimulation (TMS) and cortical evoked potentials. (A) A topographical representation of TMS-evoked potential (TEP) activity recorded using electroen-cephalogram (EEG) following single-pulse (left) and paired-pulse (right) stimulation. The negative and positive TEP components are measured over different latencies relative to the onset of TMS pulse. For example, the P30, N45, P60, and N100 components are depicted in this figure. (B) Butterfly plots of the TEPs across each EEG channel. The purple lines represent data removed due to TMS pulse artifact, while the red line represents the selected electrode of interest. (C) A topographical representation of the total cortical evoked activity measured across sample data from a standard 62-electrode recording.*

Neuronal populations naturally oscillate at frequencies ranging from approximately 0.05 Hz to more than 500 Hz, and are typically divided into five frequency bands, each underlying different brain states and neuronal processes. In humans, delta activity (0.5–3.5 Hz) is most prominent during slower-wave sleep[28] and is associated with auto-nomic functions and motivational processes.[29] Theta activity (4–7 Hz) is associated with memory and navigational processes, emotional arousal, and fear conditioning.[30-34] Alpha activity (8–12 Hz) is dominant during relaxed wakefulness[35-37] and is thought to underly active inhibition.[36] Beta activity (13–30 Hz) is associated with motor functions.[38-40] Finally, gamma activity (>30 Hz) has been implicated in a range of processes including input selection, feature integration, attention, and memory.[41-43] Changes in oscillatory activity across different brain regions and frequencies evoked by TMS have been characterized in recent research. For example, studies have shown that TMS evokes alpha oscillations in occipital and frontal regions, beta oscillations in parietal and premotor areas, and gamma oscillations in occipital, premotor areas, and frontal regions.[21]

Regarding TMS-EEG time-frequency analyses, such as Fourier TRANSFORM methods or wavelet decomposition, a sliding time window is employed to quantify oscillatory changes in power over time and frequency directly associated with the TMS event.[8,15] The analysis of TMS-evoked changes in oscillatory activity can be categorized into two approaches, an evoked oscillatory response (EOR) or total oscillatory response (TOR). Regarding EOR, time-frequency decomposition is performed once the data have been averaged across trials, which is phase-locked (i.e., evoked) to the TMS event.[44] Averaging the data first increases the signal-to-noise ratio of EEG responses that are directly related to TMS pulse. Thus, persistent latency and phase information will survive the averaging process and be represented in the final time-frequency analysis.[15] In contrast with TOR, the time-frequency decomposition is applied to each individual trial before being averaged, therefore capturing both phase-locked (i.e., evoked) and non–phase-locked (i.e., induced) oscillatory responses to the TMS event.[45] Given this, the TOR approach may be able to capture more complex oscillatory responses.

7.2.2 Connectivity

In addition to reactivity, TMS-EEG analyses may also be approached from the perspective of connectivity. *Connectivity* is a measure of the interaction between two or more features, such as brain regions or network nodes, that generate a dynamical system underlying neuronal communication. The combination of TMS with EEG can assess the temporal sequence of neuronal activation and propagation of the signal over time. This information provides insight into the structural, anatomical, and functional basis of neuronal communication underlying cognitive functioning and the etiological relationship between dysfunctional connectivity and neuropsychiatric disorders.

Connectivity analyses can be classified into two general categories: undirected and directed. Undirected or "functional" connectivity methods, including correlation, coherence, phase-locking value, mutual information, or synchrony, do not allow for conclusions regarding causal interactions. Rather, this approach quantifies the relationship between EEG features across electrodes or epochs. In contrast, "effective" connectivity, such as directed transfer function and dynamic causal modeling, describes the directional interaction between features (e.g., Does the node lead or lag in the interaction?). Therefore it requires a priori assumptions regarding the involved neuronal network and a hypothesis-driven experimental design.[8,46,47] An important consideration regarding some connectivity approaches is the potential confound of volume conduction, which may re-sult in spurious correlations between signals recorded from neighboring electrodes.

7.3 ARTIFACTS

In addition to the standard artifacts commonly observed with EEG recordings, there are a number of TMS-related artifacts that further contaminate the EEG signal. EEG artifacts can be categorized into environmental (e.g., powerline) and physiological noise (e.g., car-diac rhythms, eye blinks and head movements, facial/scalp muscle contraction). These artifacts are commonly removed offline via digital filters; however, filtering procedures have the potential to also remove important physiological information.

One of the most significant artifacts associated with TMS-EEG is related to the voltage spike at the EEG sensors produced by the electromagnetic field generated by the TMS coil. In earlier studies, this artifact resulted in the saturation of EEG amplifiers and made analysis of the initial TMS induced brain response (i.e., the first 50 ms) difficult. Several additional TMS-related artifacts arising from various sources are detailed in several review papers.[8,13,48] These artifacts include but are not limited to TMS-induced eyeblinks and ac-tivation of cranial muscles and peripheral nerves beneath the coil, movement of EEG elec-trodes caused by the electromagnetic field and coil vibration, the electrode–skin interface, the capacitor recharge in TMS stimulator, and both auditory and somatosensory evoked potentials (SEPs) due to the click and tactile sensation of the TMS pulse. Several of these factors contribute to what is known as the *TMS decay artifact*, a large shift in the signal that impedes the correct realignment of the signal to baseline for several milliseconds following the TMS pulse.[49,50] Advances in technology and our understanding of the nature of these artifacts have led to numerous strategies to prevent or correct these artifacts.

7.3.1 How to Prevent Artifacts

While offline artifact removal techniques can successfully reduce the presence of TMS-induced artifact, there are a number of strategies available to reduce noise induction during the EEG recording.

7.3.1.1 Sensors

First, TMS-compatible EEG electrodes can minimize the electrical artifacts generated by movement of the electrodes and enhance safety associated with heating caused by the TMS pulse.[51] To further reduce artifacts associated with coil movements or electrical interference, placement of the electrodes and orientation of their wires should be consid-ered. It is recommended that, if possible, the reference and ground electrodes should not be located near the TMS coil. Additionally, EEG wires should be kept loop free, grouped together, and oriented perpendicular to the TMS-induced current orientation (i.e., the handle of the coil).[51,52] Finally, ensuring that sensor–skin impedance is relatively low (i.e., <5 KΩ) [53] and that the skin is appropriately prepared by cleaning with alcohol before applying the electrode gel can help to minimize noise.

7.3.1.2 *Auditory and Somatosensory Potentials*

The delivery of the TMS pulse is followed by a loud clicking sound (100–120 dB), which is associated with a time-locked auditory-evoked potential (AEP).[49,54] Given that the onset of the resultant evoked potential is observed during the N100-P180 complex (i.e., negativity at 100 ms and positivity at 180 ms), the "true" TMS cortical response may be masked.[54] A number of proposed strategies are aimed at attenuating AEPs, including using earplugs or headphones or white noise cancellation through earphones.[55,56]

The delivery of the TMS pulse is also associated with SEPs, leading to activation of sensory afferents, scalp tactile receptors, and scalp and facial muscles. It is recommended that a thin layer of foam be placed between the coil and the scalp to dampen bone conduction and scalp sensations caused by coil vibration.[57] The artifacts associated with facial muscle activation and time-locked eye-blinks commonly observed during frontal/lateral stimulation[58] can be removed through offline analyses.

7.3.2 How to Remove Artifacts Offline

Despite advances in TMS-EEG–compatible technologies and the numerous strategies developed to minimize noise during data acquisition, the need for offline artifact removal processes is almost unavoidable. There are several approaches to offline processing that can generally be categorized into two approaches: removal of the contaminated section of data entirely or disentangling and selectively removing the artifacts from the brain response through mathematical techniques. Each approach presents its own benefits and challenges.

The deletion approach can be accomplished most simply by excluding data collected from the noisy electrodes. Given that the electrodes closest to the site of stimulation are often the most contaminated, this approach may introduce bias into the analytic process. An alternative approach is to exclude contaminated trials within each electrode. While this method conserves data collected across more electrodes, it, too, is associated with bias as more trials are likely to be deleted close to the site of stimulation.[8] A similar approach to these methods involves excluding contaminated time periods. This can be accomplished by using a fixed time window equal to the length of the TMS artifact averaged across study participants or trials[59] or conducted based on an individual electrode's, trial's, or participant's data. To account for the missing data associated with each of these three methods, data interpolation can be employed. One important strategy to minimize bias in data removal uses predetermined thresholds, excluding electrodes if a certain number of trials are too noisy (e.g., >60%) or excluding trials if a certain number of electrodes are noisy (e.g., >20%).[8]

The data preservation methods use various mathematical procedures and follow several assumptions, with this approach aiming to preserve brain responses by isolating and removing only the TMS-induced artifacts. For example, the *template subtraction method* attempts to model the TMS artifact by applying TMS pulses under various parameters to a phantom head.[51] Information regarding the amplitude and duration of the TMS pulse are then used to develop a TMS artifact profile that can be identified and eliminated from the EEG recording. Of course, this method is not entirely accurate as phantom head and human experiments are not identical.[8] A similar template subtraction method has been applied primarily in task-based studies using what is known as a *calibration trial*. Here, the TMS-induced artifact is identified for each electrode during a trial during which no task is administered, and the template is then used to remove the artifact from the task condition.[60,61] One key flaw with this approach is that it relies on the assumption that the TMS-induced artifact is stationary. To address the limitation of the template subtraction model, others have attempted to remove the TMS artifact through the use of Bayesian modeling with linear Kalman filters.[62]

Another commonly used offline processing technique is the application of *blind source separation methods*. This approach is used to identify and decompose the EEG signal into component parts. For example, independent component analysis (ICA) identifies temporally independent components from a linearly mixed signal of cortical and noncortical sources. Once identified, the components which represent noise, based on their spatial and temporal features, are removed and the remaining physiological components are combined to reconstruct the EEG signal. In contrast to ICA, *principal component analysis* (PCA) identifies scalp topographies with maximally orthogonalized components (i.e., describing the variability of the observed data).[63,64] An important consideration when using the blind source separation method is that it follows the assumption that EEG signals are composed of brain signals and TMS artifact sources that are temporally and spatially independent. Thus, if the assumption of independence is not met (e.g., in the overlap of the TMS-induced eye blink with the N100 TEP component), ICA may not be able to accurately separate these components.

Despite the growing interest in TMS-EEG, challenges associated with signal processing and the lack of standardized analysis methods have hindered its widespread use. Over the past several years, there has been a rise in the number of TMS-EEG analysis programs, including Fieldtrip[65] and EEGLAB.[66] Recently, two open-source, user-friendly, preprocessing toolboxes were published (i.e., TESA software[64] and TMS-EEG toolbox[67]) with functions including targeted removal of general EEG- and TMS-induced artifacts, data interpolation, and quality control check points with visual displays. These novel approaches provide users with easy access to current analysis methods and ultimately a means to promote consistency and transparency across the field of TMS-EEG.

7.4 TESTING PARAMETERS AND CONSIDERATIONS

7.4.1 The Influence of Testing Parameters

7.4.1.1 Site of Stimulation

Targeting the motor cortex by positioning the coil over the area that produces the largest MEP amplitude in the peripheral target muscle (i.e., the "hot spot") is fairly straight-forward; however, targeting nonmotor regions is more challenging given the lack of the EMG output. Coil placement strategies for nonmotor regions include anatomical or functional landmarks (e.g., the "5 cm method": 5 cm anterior to the motor hot spot for the DLPFC), individual or group average MRI coordinates, electrode placement using the EEG 10-20 system (e.g., over the F3 and F4 electrode for left or right DLPFC), and rest- or task-based fMRI or EEG outcomes.[68] Each method has its advantages and limitations related to precision, price, and accessibility. For example, the 5 cm method is easy to execute and is inexpensive, but it fails to consider cortex morphology and often results in coil positioning that falls outside of the DLPFC region (i.e., Broadman area 9).[69] Similarly, while the 10-20 method is relatively easy to perform and does not require additional neuronavigation equipment, this approach does not take into account head shape or the morphology of the underlying cortex. While expensive and more time-consuming, localizing the DLPFC through the use of online neuronavigation with functional standardized coordinates (e.g., Talairach or MNI stereotaxic coordinates) to determine the ideal scalp location likely optimizes accuracy and reduces interindividual variability.[68]

While the implementation of these methods for targeting nonmotor regions enhances the likelihood that the intended cortical region is stimulated, there are additional morphological, physiological, and technical factors that introduce other sources of variability.[8] To further enhance reliability across participants, stimuli, and protocols, it has been suggested to place the coil by fixing the angle relative to the gyrification of the underlying cortex for each participant.[8] Additionally, the implementation of a robotic arm system instead of manual coil handling reduces the variability associated with administrator movement (see Chapter 2 for further descriptions of this approach).

7.4.1.2 TMS Protocols

Numerous TMS protocols have been developed to measure cortical excitation and inhibition, neuroplasticity, and connectivity. TMS protocols include but are not limited to single-pulse measures, such as cortical silent period and motor threshold; paired-pulse measures, such as intracortical facilitation (ICF), short-latency intracortical inhibition (SICI), long-latency intracortical inhibition (LICI), interhemispheric inhibition, and short-latency afferent inhibition; and measures to induce neuroplasticity, such as repetitive TMS (rTMS), theta burst protocols, and paired associative stimulation (PAS). (Refer to Chapters 3 and 4 for detailed descriptions of these protocols.) Several of these protocols have been adapted from TMS-EMG to be used in TMS-EEG research to index excitatory or inhibitory processes by measuring changes in EEG activity via TEPs. Furthermore, the use of different TMS-EEG protocols can be combined with pharmacological or other brain stimulation interventions, like electroconvulsive therapy (ECT) or magnetic seizure therapy (MST), whereby TEPs are recorded before and after the administration of the intervention. This field of research has the potential to provide key insights into the impact of these interventions on neuronal functioning as well as uncover potential mechanisms contributing to TMS-evoked EEG activity.

7.4.1.3 Stimulus Intensity

We know from EMG outcomes of paired-pulse paradigms that stimulus intensity impacts the muscle response. For example, the LICI protocol consists of two suprathreshold TMS pulses (i.e., 110–120% of resting motor threshold [RMT]) while the SICI protocol consists of a subthreshold (i.e., 80% RMT) conditioning stimulus followed by a suprathreshold test pulse. These two protocols are understood to activate gamma aminobutyric acid (GABA) receptor-mediated cortical inhibition differentially, whereby LICI probes $GABA_B$ activity and SICI probes $GABA_A$ activity.[70,71] This is due in part to the differences in the stimulus intensities as well as the intervals between the TMS pulses. As such, modifying the intensity within these protocols has been shown to have differential effects on the TMS evoked responses.[72]

Intensities for nonmotor regions are often based on those determined from the M1 regions, regardless of the region of interest. However, additional factors and methods should be considered when determining stimulation intensities for TMS-EEG experiments. It is recommended that intensities be measured with the EEG cap on the participant, given the potential variability introduced by the electrodes on the coil–scalp distance. A more specialized approach to determining intensity is through the use of a brain-navigated tool. This method adjusts the stimulation intensity based on the predicted E-field (V/m) generated by TMS in the region of interest and in real time. While this method may be a more accurate measure of stimulus intensities, it is also more expensive and therefore not as accessible. An additional approach uses EEG outcome measures as a means to determine intensity; however, this method requires artifact correction and data processing to be done online.[8]

7.4.2 The Influence of Brain State

TMS-EEG represents one of the very few techniques currently available that can noninvasively infer relationships between brain states and cortical network dynamics. Using TMS to directly probe and monitor brain state–dependent influences on cortical excitability has important functional implications for connectivity, neuroplasticity, and cognitive functions. Brain state can be defined based on age, behavioral state (i.e., unconsciousness, sleep, rest, cognitive processing), and healthy versus diseased state,[8] each of which in known to impact TMS outcomes differently.[73,74]

In addition to the above-mentioned factors, TMS-EEG outcomes are known to be sensitive to changes in attention. To account for potential interindividual variability associated with attention, participants may be asked to orient toward a simple task like an oddball task or counting of stimuli. This is especially true for TMS protocols thought to be associated with neuroplasticity, including rTMS and PAS.[75,76] However, it should be noted that such attentional tasks likely influence the brain state and connectivity and thus may also influence the outcomes.[77] Furthermore, the time of day at which EEG experiments are conducted is known to not only affect one's alertness and cognitive abilities, but also impact neuronal activity as assessed by EEG.[78,79] As such, studies involving repeated TMS-EEG assessments should consider standardizing the time of day at which data are collected if possible.

Of course, one must also consider the complex and reciprocal relationship between TMS-EEG outcomes and medications. Studies have shown that drugs with a known mode of action can provide insights into the underlying mechanisms of TMS responses and vice versa, where a TMS protocol can provide insight into acute drug effects.[80] However, one must also consider the potentially confounding effects of medication on TMS-evoked responses. This is especially important when interpreting findings within clinical populations compared to control participants.[21] Chronic medication use has been shown to alter brain function and structure; therefore, special attention must be paid to studies that aim to evaluate anatomical or physiological changes longitudinally in clinical populations.[81] In addition to medication use, several other interventions including cognitive behavioral therapy,[82] exercise,[83] and brain stimulation[84] have been shown to alter brain state and therefore may impact TMS outcomes.

7.4.3 The Importance of Control Conditions

As mentioned in Section 7.2.1, TMS stimulation leads to co-occurring and complex cortical responses that results from sources beyond direct transcranial activation. The presence of such co-activations, including somatosensory and auditory evoked potentials, are dependent on a number of factors, including intensity, site of stimulation, and coil type.

Given that the EEG activity associated with sensory-evoked potentials and direct TMS-evoked responses can occur simultaneously, removing the unintended activation can be challenging, and may mask the true TMS response.

In addition to implementing effective strategies for preventing or removing such artifacts, control/sham conditions may enhance the reliability and validity of TMS-EEG findings. Sham stimulation can be accomplished in a number of ways including tilting or holding the active coil a short distance from the scalp.[59,85,86] This approach reduces the induced electric field below threshold. Furthermore, this method maintains the airborne "click" sound but minimizes the somatosensory responses associated with bone conduction[87] and therefore may not accurately simulate the sensations of active TMS.[88] To account for these limitations, device manufacturers have developed sham TMS coils which induce a small electric field in the cortex while maintaining reduced contributions of the auditory and somatosensory responses.[89,90]

One recent study aimed to identify the impact that multisensory co-stimulation has on the TEP using a number of the above-mentioned strategies, including different coil orientations and stimulation at different locations.[91] The sham condition for each experiment generated a subthreshold electric field while attempting to mimic the somatosensory and auditory features of active TMS. Their results demonstrated that multisensory co-stimulation has a significant impact on TEP outcome, which is often misinterpreted as direct TMS-evoked response. Their findings also suggest that the use of current strategies to prevent such co-activations, like noise masking and foam padding, do not completely eliminate their presence. The authors suggest a number of important strategies to consider and report in future TMS-EEG studies to ensure the more accurate and reliable results.[91] These include but are not limited to (1) demonstrating that multisensory co-stimulation is suppressed completely or controlled for, (2) employing a sham condition that matches the sensory experience of active TMS as closely as possible, (3) including a psychophysical assessment of the participants' experienced sensory perception of active and sham conditions, and (4) developing data analyses that can be used to compare the spatiotemporal characteristics of the active and sham conditions.

7.5 TMS-EEG APPLICATIONS

Drawing from basic science and translational research, single-cell recordings and in vitro approaches in animals probe the effects of TMS on cellular and subcellular functioning while animal models of diseases in combination with TMS provide insights into mechanisms underlying disordered brain functioning. Furthermore, clinical research in humans highlights the enormous potential of TMS-EEG in terms of predictive, diagnostic, and prognostic utility.[21] The following section reviews TMS-EEG research on markers of healthy brain function as well as clinical applications of TMS-EEG.

7.5.1 TMS-EEG Insights on Healthy Brain Functioning

7.5.1.1 *Cortical Inhibition/Excitation*

Numerous single-pulse and paired-pulse TMS protocols have been adapted for the study of excitatory and inhibitory processes across the cortex. The most commonly studied protocol is LICI (described in Chapter 3). Using TMS-EEG, several studies have outlined the time course of LICI-induced suppression of the EEG signal across the cortex including the M1, parietal, and DLPFC regions[59,92] and across specific TEP time points.[93,94] Furthermore, TMS-EEG studies have also investigated a number of other EEG features. For example, LICI has been shown to suppress gamma and beta oscillations in the DLPFC.[94,95]

Other TMS protocols including SICI and ICF (described in Chapter 3) highlight the bidirectional effect of these two protocols on TMS-evoked EEG responses, whereby SICI reduced early TEP amplitudes (i.e., P30 and P60), while ICF enhanced them.[96] Furthermore, studies have shown that paired-pulse TMS-EEG responses are modulated by age,[97] stimulation intensity,[98] and, importantly, interstimulus interval.[99] Finally, less commonly studied TMS protocols including cortical silent period (CSP) and short-latency afferent inhibition (SAI) have also been investigated using TMS-EEG.[21] However, further research is needed to substantiate current findings.

7.5.1.2 *Neuroplasticity*

While several TMS protocols have been developed to index neuroplasticity, the majority of what we know about these paradigms is derived from the M1 region. Only recently have researchers been able to determine if our current findings are replicated in other brain regions. For example, PAS, which involves the pairing of suprathreshold TMS pulses (commonly to the M1 region) with an appropriately timed peripheral nerve stimulation (commonly the median nerve), is thought to induce spike timing–dependent plasticity.[100] Research has reliably shown that interstimulus intervals ranging from 21.5 to 25 ms are facilitatory, whereas shorter intervals of around 10 ms are inhibitory.[100,101] Similar results have been found in TMS-evoked EEG activity from the M1 region.[102]

Using a modified PAS protocol with an interstimulus interval of 24 ms, researchers have also been able to induce potentiation of cortical activity from the DLPFC. This specific interval was selected given that median nerve stimulation results in a somatosensory-evoked potential over the contralateral frontal brain region with a latency of 24 ms in animals. One such study demonstrated a potentiation of cortical-evoked activity in the DLPFC region that was frequency-specific within the gamma and theta bands.[24] Similarly, modified PAS protocols that pair TMS across two brain regions including the posterior parietal cortex (PPC) and M1 region,[103] as well as PPC and DLPFC[104] have revealed frequency, order of stimulation, and site-specific changes in EEG activity.

In a therapeutic context, plasticity-inducing protocols including rTMS and theta burst stimulation (TBS) modulate aberrant cortical activity thought to underly the pathophysiology of neuropsychiatric disorders. During rTMS, multiple trains of magnetic pulses are administered using a variety of protocols (i.e., frequencies, patterns, locations, intensities), resulting in an enhancement or suppression of cortical activity lasting beyond the period of stimulation (see Chapter 4 for a more detailed description). It is generally accepted that low-frequency stimulation (i.e., 1 Hz) results in a suppression of activity while higher frequencies (i.e., 5–20 Hz) lead to facilitation.[105] While the number of rTMS studies employing TMS-EEG are limited, results suggest that low-frequency stimulation may lead to a reduction in M1 activity, as indexed by TEP-specific reductions in amplitude.[106] However, continued investigation is needed to validate current findings.

TBS protocols involve the accelerated administration of rTMS via short bursts of three stimuli at 30–50 Hz, applied over a carrier frequency of 5 Hz. The pattern of stimulation can be delivered intermittently (iTBS with 2 s trains every 10 s for 190 s total) or continuously (cTBS for a total of 20–40 s) in its traditional administration. Studies suggest that iTBS is associated with an increase in corticospinal excitability (i.e., MEP facilitation) whereas cTBS is associated with an inhibitory effect.[107] TMS-EEG studies have demonstrated decreased TMS-evoked activity at specific timepoints as well as a modulation of cortical oscillatory activity following cTBS delivered to the M1 region.[108,109] Results in iTBS are less clear as very few TMS-EEG studies in the M1 region exist. Similarly, while few studies have examined the effects of iTBS in the DLPFC, findings have demonstrated the presence of short-term plasticity as indexed by increases in TEP amplitudes and oscillatory activity.[110,111]

7.5.1.3 Pharmaco-TMS Studies

Pharmacological interventions, when used in combination with TMS protocols, provides important insights into the contribution of neurotransmitter mechanisms underlying specific TMS-evoked EEG responses. One of the most well-studied neurotransmitter systems in pharmaco-TMS research is GABA. Results consistently indicate that $GABA_A$ and $GABA_B$ receptor subunits differentially modulate TEP components, namely N45 and N100, as well as induced and evoked oscillatory activity.[112,113] Furthermore, it is suggested that early synchronization (30–200 ms) and late desynchronization (200–400 ms) of oscillatory activity following the TMS pulse may be controlled by separate inhibitory mechanisms associated with different GABAergic subunits.[114]

Using paired-pulse paradigms in combination with GABAergic drugs has similarly demonstrated that the $GABA_B$ receptor agonist baclofen enhances the inhibitory effects of LICI with M1[93] and DLPFC[115] stimulation. Conversely, diazepam, a $GABA_A$ receptor agonist, has been shown to decrease the amplitude of late TEP components.[93] This bidirectional modulation of cortical activity observed with baclofen and diazepam was replicated using SICI in the M1 region.[116] Several other neurotransmitter systems have been studied through the use of different pharmacological interventions in combination with TMS-EEG, including but not limited to L-DOPA, a precursor of dopamine; rivastigmine, an acetylcholinesterase inhibitor; and lamotrigine and levetiracetam, antiepileptic drugs; as well as several drugs which induce loss of consciousness (see Tremblay et al.[21] for an in-depth review of the findings).

7.5.2 TMS-EEG Insights into Brain Function in Clinical Populations

Previous TMS-EMG studies have clearly demonstrated changes in motor cortical excitability across a range of psychiatric and neurological disorders, providing preliminary insights into the pathophysiology and therapeutic efficacy of interventions in these populations.[2] Given that previous findings are limited to the motor cortex, and brain regions are known to differ in their cortical architecture and neuronal compositions, these findings are not necessarily translatable across the whole brain.[2] Thus, TMS-EEG offers a unique ability to investigate nonmotor regions that are more relevant to clinical disorders, like the DLPFC. The following section reviews the general applications of TMS-EEG in clinical populations, namely its diagnostic and prognostic potential as well as its use in guiding treatment approaches.

7.5.2.1 *Diagnostic Applications*

TMS-EEG has been used to characterize the neurophysiological underpinnings of several psychiatric disorders. For example, in schizophrenia, studies have provided evidence of impaired prefrontal cholinergic cortical inhibition in patients.[97] Alterations in the generation and modulation of LICI-induced gamma activity in frontal regions[117,118] and an excessive spread of neural excitation[119] have also been identified. Studies aimed at investigating the neurobiological impact of substance abuse on cortical activity revealed impairments in frontal cortical inhibition in patients with alcohol dependence post-detoxification.[120] In contrast, acute alcohol consumption was associated with changes in functional connectivity and TMS-evoked EEG activity.[121] In mood disorders, altered prefrontal plasticity was observed in patients with major depressive disorder (MDD) as indexed by PAS with DLPFC stimulation.[122] A lower main natural frequency within frontal regions in both MDD and those with bipolar disorder was also observed.[123] TMS-EEG studies have also been conducted in children and adolescents with autism spectrum disorder and those with attention deficit hyperactivity disorder (ADHD)[21]; however, continued investigation is needed given the preliminary nature of this research.

TMS-EEG studies have investigated the integrity of cortical functioning and brain circuitries in a number of neurological disorders. Several small TMS-EEG studies have revealed altered cortical reactivity and connectivity in patients with Alzheimer's disease (AD) across the sensorimotor cortex[124,125] Furthermore, a study conducted in pre-symptomatic carriers of the Huntington's disease genetic mutation displayed altered phase synchronization and TMS-evoked cortical activity compared to healthy controls.[126]

In addition to neurodegenerative disorders, TMS-EEG studies have also provided preliminary insights into neurological disorders associated with acquired brain injury. Disorders of consciousness resulting from severe brain injury have been fairly well studies using TMS-EEG, given that this method is able to probe cortical functioning independent of patient participation. TMS-EEG measures of cortical reactivity, connectivity, and TMS-induced oscillatory activity have been used to effectively differentiate unresponsive patients from those showing minimal signs of consciousness.[127] Finally, TMS-EEG studies used to compare different psychiatric or neurological disorders[117,123,128] represent an important future direction for this field of research as it has the potential to identify potential biomarkers of specific diseases or disease states, as well as certain endophenotypes or risk factors that are common across different disorders.

7.5.2.2 Predictors of Prognosis and Treatment Response

In addition to providing novel diagnostic insights, TMS-EEG also provides a unique opportunity to identify potential predictors of prognosis and therapeutic outcomes. With respect to prognostic predictors, TMS-EEG measures may be used to identify preexisting neuronal characteristics or vulnerabilities that are associated with certain disease courses. For example, one recent study aimed to determine if alterations in prefrontal connectivity could predict disease severity in patients with Alzheimer's disease. Their results indicated that higher P30 amplitudes in the superior parietal cortex predicted poorer cognitive and memory performance, suggestive of an excitation–inhibition imbalance between anterior and posterior regions. Longitudinal studies assessing long-term changes are needed to validate these findings.[129] TMS-EEG research has also been used to better understand the mechanisms underlying motor recovery following stroke. One study found that a better prognosis was associated with a reliable N100 component elicited from the affected hemisphere in acute post-stroke individuals. Of note, combining MEP and TEP responses was found to provide a better predictor than either measure alone given that they probe different circuits.[130]

TMS-EEG features measured prior to an intervention also represent potential predicative markers of therapeutic response. For example, one study revealed that greater baseline cortical inhibition predicted remission of suicide ideation following magnetic seizure therapy in treatment-resistant depression.[131] Similarly, in patients with bipolar disorder, baseline measures of cortical excitability predicted response to chronotherapy (i.e., the combination of sleep deprivation and light therapy). A pharmacological study showed that two commonly prescribed antiepileptic drugs, lamotrigine and levetiracetam, both similarly modulated TMS-evoked activity (i.e., enhanced N445 and suppressed P180), leading authors to propose that these features may represent candidate predictive markers of treatment response.[132] Taken together, these promising studies highlight the potential of TMS-EEG to aid in the clinical decision-making process by selecting the most suitable treatment for each individual patient in the future.

7.5.2.3 *Assessing Treatment Efficacy and Guiding Treatment Approaches*
TMS-EEG represents a reliable tool to objectively quantify dynamic changes in brain activity directly linked to numerous interventions from pharmacotherapy and brain stimulation therapies to cognitive training and psychotherapy. TMS findings in mood disorders, for example, have provided insights into potential markers of the effects of certain interventions on cortical activity, including ECT and TBS.[133,134] TMS studies may also help to optimize therapeutic neuromodulation by guiding the development of novel treatment parameters. For example, aberrant frequency- and region-specific oscillatory activity in schizophrenia[117] may represent potential targets for interventions.

In addition to monitoring the efficacy of treatments, EEG measures can also be used to guide the delivery of TMS and ultimately optimize clinical or behavioral outcomes.[135] Using this approach, research combining TMS-EEG with a brain–computer interface, known as *closed-loop neuroscience*, enables a stimulus to be applied in response to a simultaneously measured brain state. Thus, the neuronal "output" of the brain directly influences the delivery of the stimulus or input to the brain, thereby closing the loop. Relevant EEG features representing a brain state of interest, such as a certain phase within an oscillatory cycle or a change in spectral power within a frequency band, could be used to trigger the delivery of the TMS pulse, thereby modifying the brain state.[136] The therapeutic implications of this closed-loop approach have only begun to be explored in a number of populations, including in monitoring epileptiform EEG activity and preventing seizures in patients with epilepsy.[137] Additionally, studies have investigated the use of brain–computer interface–based prosthetic devices in rehabilitating motor function in patients following stroke.[138] While numerous technical challenges currently exist, including the presence of TMS-induced artifacts in the EEG recording and the need for real-time EEG analysis, it is clear that closed-loop neuroscience has significant therapeutic potential.

7.6 CONCLUSION

The research presented in this chapter highlights the potential of TMS-EEG to improve our understanding of the brain, from uncovering cortical features of healthy brain functioning to identifying potential biomarkers for specific disease states and predictors of clinical response to a variety of interventions. However, continued investigation is necessary if we are to utilize TMS-EEG to its full potential. One important direction of future research is to continue to improve on current methods to standardize data acquisition and analysis, allowing for an integration of findings across the field of TMS-EEG research. Future investigations would also benefit from transparency in reporting and controlling the numerous elements which are known to impact the quality of the EEG signal and overall findings. Recent advancements in technology and our understanding of TMS protocols through the use of EEG have led the field closer to the goal of developing targeted and individualized therapies for clinical populations.

REFERENCES

1. Fitzgerald PB. TMS-EEG: A technique that has come of age? *Clin Neurophysiol.* 2010;121(3):265–267.
2. Bunse T, Wobrock T, Strube W, Padberg F, Palm U, Falkai P, et al. Motor cortical excitability assessed by transcranial magnetic stimulation in psychiatric disorders: A systematic review. *Brain Stimul.* 2014;7(2):158–169.
3. Buzsaki G, Draguhn A. Neuronal oscillations in cortical networks. *Science.* 2004;304(5679):1926–1929.
4. Olejniczak P. Neurophysiologic basis of EEG. *J Clin Neurophysiol.* 2006;23(3):186–189.
5. Murakami S, Okada Y. Contributions of principal neocortical neurons to magnetoencephalography and electroencephalography signals. *J Physiol.* 2006;575(Pt 3):925–936.
6. Buzsaki G, Anastassiou CA, Koch C. The origin of extracellular fields and currents: EEG, ECoG, LFP and spikes. *Nat Rev Neurosci.* 2012;13(6):407–420.
7. Dickter CLK, PD. *EEG Methods for the Psychological Sciences.* Los Angelas: SAGE; 2014.
8. Farzan F, Vernet M, Shafi MM, Rotenberg A, Daskalakis ZJ, Pascual-Leone A. Characterizing and modulating brain circuitry through transcranial magnetic stimulation combined with electroencephalography. *Front Neural Circuits.* 2016;10:73.
9. Hui J, Tremblay S, Daskalakis ZJ. The current and future potential of transcranial magnetic stimulation with electroencephalography in psychiatry. *Clin Pharmacol Ther.* 2019;106(4):734–746.
10. Cracco RQ, Amassian VE, Maccabee PJ, Cracco JB. Comparison of human transcallosal responses evoked by magnetic coil and electrical stimulation. Electroencephalogr *Clin Neurophysiol.* 1989;74(6):417–424.
11. Ilmoniemi RJ, Virtanen J, Ruohonen J, Karhu J, Aronen HJ, Naatanen R, et al. Neuronal responses to magnetic stimulation reveal cortical reactivity and connectivity. *Neuroreport.* 1997;8(16):3537–3540.
12. Virtanen J, Ruohonen J, Naatanen R, Ilmoniemi RJ. Instrumentation for the measurement of electric brain responses to transcranial magnetic stimulation. *Med Biol Eng Comput.* 1999;37(3):322–326.
13. Rogasch NC, Fitzgerald PB. Assessing cortical network properties using TMS-EEG. *Hum Brain Mapp.* 2013;34(7):1652–1669.
14. Miniussi C, Thut G. Combining TMS and EEG offers new prospects in cognitive neuroscience. *Brain Topogr.* 2010;22(4):249–256.
15. Pellicciari MC, Veniero D, Miniussi C. Characterizing the cortical oscillatory response to TMS pulse. *Front Cell Neurosci.* 2017;11:38.
16. Hill AT, Rogasch NC, Fitzgerald PB, Hoy KE. TMS-EEG: A window into the neurophysiological effects of transcranial electrical stimulation in non-motor brain regions. *Neurosci Biobehav Rev.* 2016;64:175–184.
17. Lioumis P, Kicic D, Savolainen P, Makela JP, Kahkonen S. Reproducibility of TMS-Evoked EEG responses. *Hum Brain Mapp.* 2009;30(4):1387–1396.
18. Komssi S, Kahkonen S. The novelty value of the combined use of electroencephalography and transcranial magnetic stimulation for neuroscience research. *Brain Res Rev.* 2006;52(1):183–192.
19. Darmani G, Ziemann U. Pharmacophysiology of TMS-evoked EEG potentials: A mini-review. *Brain Stimul.* 2019;12(3):829–831.

20. Kahkonen S, Komssi S, Wilenius J, Ilmoniemi RJ. Prefrontal transcranial magnetic stimulation produces intensity-dependent EEG responses in humans. *NeuroImage*. 2005;24(4):955–960.

21. Tremblay S, Rogasch NC, Premoli I, Blumberger DM, Casarotto S, Chen R, et al. Clinical utility and prospective of TMS-EEG. *Clin Neurophysiol*. 2019;130(5):802–844.

22. Kerwin LJ, Keller CJ, Wu W, Narayan M, Etkin A. Test-retest reliability of transcranial magnetic stimulation EEG evoked potentials. *Brain Stimul*. 2018;11(3):536–544.

23. Pellicciari MC, Brignani D, Miniussi C. Excitability modulation of the motor system induced by transcranial direct current stimulation: A multimodal approach. *NeuroImage*. 2013;83:569–580.

24. Rajji TK, Sun Y, Zomorrodi-Moghaddam R, Farzan F, Blumberger DM, Mulsant BH, et al. PAS-induced potentiation of cortical-evoked activity in the dorsolateral prefrontal cortex. *Neuropsychopharmacology*. 2013;38(12):2545–2552.

25. Komssi S, Kahkonen S, Ilmoniemi RJ. The effect of stimulus intensity on brain responses evoked by transcranial magnetic stimulation. *Hum Brain Mapp*. 2004;21(3):154–164.

26. Esser SK, Huber R, Massimini M, Peterson MJ, Ferrarelli F, Tononi G. A direct demonstration of cortical LTP in humans: A combined TMS/EEG study. *Brain Res Bull*. 2006;69(1):86–94.

27. Assenza G, Capone F, di Biase L, Ferreri F, Florio L, Guerra A, et al. Corrigendum: Oscillatory activities in neurological disorders of elderly: Biomarkers to target for neuromodulation. *Front Aging Neurosci*. 2017;9:252.

28. Steriade MM, RW. *Brain Control of Wakefulness and Sleep*. New York: Springer; 2005.

29. Knyazev GG. EEG delta oscillations as a correlate of basic homeostatic and motivational processes. *Neurosci Biobehav Rev*. 2012;36(1):677–695.

30. Sederberg PB, Kahana MJ, Howard MW, Donner EJ, Madsen JR. Theta and gamma oscillations during encoding predict subsequent recall. *J Neurosci*. 2003;23(34):10809–10814.

31. Raghavachari S, Lisman JE, Tully M, Madsen JR, Bromfield EB, Kahana MJ. Theta oscillations in human cortex during a working-memory task: Evidence for local generators. *J Neurophysiol*. 2006;95(3):1630–1638.

32. Sammer G, Blecker C, Gebhardt H, Bischoff M, Stark R, Morgen K, et al. Relationship between regional hemodynamic activity and simultaneously recorded EEG-theta associated with mental arithmetic-induced workload. *Hum Brain Mapp*. 2007;28(8):793–803.

33. Onton J, Delorme A, Makeig S. Frontal midline EEG dynamics during working memory. *Neuroimage*. 2005;27(2):341–356.

34. Knyazev GG. Motivation, emotion, and their inhibitory control mirrored in brain oscillations. *Neurosci Biobehav Rev*. 2007;31(3):377–395.

35. Klimesch W. EEG alpha and theta oscillations reflect cognitive and memory performance: A review and analysis. *Brain Res Brain Res Rev*. 1999;29(2-3):169–195.

36. Jensen O, Mazaheri A. Shaping functional architecture by oscillatory alpha activity: Gating by inhibition. *Front Hum Neurosci*. 2010;4:186.

37. Klimesch W. EEG-alpha rhythms and memory processes. *Int J Psychophysiol*. 1997;26(1-3):319–340.

38. Baker SN. Oscillatory interactions between sensorimotor cortex and the periphery. *Curr Opin Neurobiol*. 2007;17(6):649–655.

39. Sanes JN, Donoghue JP. Oscillations in local field potentials of the primate motor cortex during voluntary movement. *Proc Natl Acad Sci U S A*. 1993;90(10):4470–4474.

40. Klostermann F, Nikulin VV, Kuhn AA, Marzinzik F, Wahl M, Pogosyan A, et al. Task-related differential dynamics of EEG alpha- and beta-band synchronization in cortico-basal motor structures. *Eur J Neurosci*. 2007;25(5):1604–1615.

41. Fries P. Neuronal gamma-band synchronization as a fundamental process in cortical computation. *Annu Rev Neurosci*. 2009;32:209–224.

42. Jensen O, Kaiser J, Lachaux JP. Human gamma-frequency oscillations associated with attention and memory. *Trends Neurosci*. 2007;30(7):317–324.

43. Senkowski D, Schneider TR, Foxe JJ, Engel AK. Crossmodal binding through neural coherence: Implications for multisensory processing. *Trends Neurosci*. 2008;31(8):401–409.

44. Mouraux A, Iannetti GD. Across-trial averaging of event-related EEG responses and beyond. *Magn Reson Imaging*. 2008;26(7):1041–1054.

45. Herrmann CS, Rach S, Vosskuhl J, Struber D. Time-frequency analysis of event-related potentials: A brief tutorial. *Brain Topogr.* 2014;27(4):438–450.

46. Rossini PM, Di Iorio R, Bentivoglio M, Bertini G, Ferreri F, Gerloff C, et al. Methods for analysis of brain connectivity: An IFCN-sponsored review. *Clin Neurophysiol.* 2019;130(10):1833–1858.

47. Bortoletto M, Veniero D, Thut G, Miniussi C. The contribution of TMS-EEG coregistration in the exploration of the human cortical connectome. *Neurosci Biobehav Rev.* 2015;49:114–124.

48. Ilmoniemi RJ, Hernandez-Pavon JC, Makela NN, Metsomaa J, Mutanen TP, Stenroos M, et al. Dealing with artifacts in TMS-evoked EEG. *Annu Int Conf IEEE Eng Med Biol Soc.* 2015;2015:230–233.

49. Rogasch NC, Thomson RH, Farzan F, Fitzgibbon BM, Bailey NW, Hernandez-Pavon JC, et al. Removing artefacts from TMS-EEG recordings using independent component analysis: Importance for assessing prefrontal and motor cortex network properties. *NeuroImage.* 2014;101:425–439.

50. Hernandez-Pavon JC, Metsomaa J, Mutanen T, Stenroos M, Maki H, Ilmoniemi RJ, et al. Uncovering neural independent components from highly artifactual TMS-evoked EEG data. *J Neurosci Methods.* 2012;209(1):144–157.

51. Veniero D, Bortoletto M, Miniussi C. TMS-EEG co-registration: On TMS-induced artifact. *Clin Neurophysiol.* 2009;120(7):1392–1399.

52. Sekiguchi H, Takeuchi S, Kadota H, Kohno Y, Nakajima Y. TMS-induced artifacts on EEG can be reduced by rearrangement of the electrode's lead wire before recording. *Clin Neurophysiol.* 2011;122(5):984–990.

53. Julkunen P, Paakkonen A, Hukkanen T, Kononen M, Tiihonen P, Vanhatalo S, et al. Efficient reduction of stimulus artefact in TMS-EEG by epithelial short-circuiting by mini-punctures. *Clinical Neurophysiol.* 2008;119(2):475–481.

54. Nikouline V, Ruohonen J, Ilmoniemi RJ. The role of the coil click in TMS assessed with simultaneous EEG. *Clinical Neurophysiol.* 1999;110(8):1325–1328.

55. Paus T, Sipila PK, Strafella AP. Synchronization of neuronal activity in the human primary motor cortex by transcranial magnetic stimulation: An EEG study. *J Neurophysiol.* 2001;86(4):1983–1990.

56. Fuggetta G, Fiaschi A, Manganotti P. Modulation of cortical oscillatory activities induced by varying single-pulse transcranial magnetic stimulation intensity over the left primary motor area: A combined EEG and TMS study. *NeuroImage.* 2005;27(4):896–908.

57. Massimini M, Ferrarelli F, Huber R, Esser SK, Singh H, Tononi G. Breakdown of cortical effective connectivity during sleep. *Science.* 2005;309(5744):2228–2232.

58. Mutanen T, Maki H, Ilmoniemi RJ. The effect of stimulus parameters on TMS-EEG muscle artifacts. *Brain Stimul.* 2013;6(3):371–376.

59. Daskalakis ZJ, Farzan F, Barr MS, Maller JJ, Chen R, Fitzgerald PB. Long-interval cortical inhibition from the dorsolateral prefrontal cortex: A TMS-EEG study. *Neuropsychopharmacology.* 2008;33(12):2860–2869.

60. Thut G, Northoff G, Ives JR, Kamitani Y, Pfennig A, Kampmann F, et al. Effects of single-pulse transcranial magnetic stimulation (TMS) on functional brain activity: A combined event-related TMS and evoked potential study. *Clin Neurophysiol.* 2003;114(11):2071–2080.

61. Reichenbach A, Whittingstall K, Thielscher A. Effects of transcranial magnetic stimulation on visual evoked potentials in a visual suppression task. *NeuroImage.* 2011;54(2):1375–1384.

62. Morbidi F, Garulli A, Prattichizzo D, Rizzo C, Manganotti P, Rossi S. Off-line removal of TMS-induced artifacts on human electroencephalography by Kalman filter. *J Neurosci Methods.* 2007;162(1–2):293–302.

63. Onton J, Westerfield M, Townsend J, Makeig S. Imaging human EEG dynamics using independent component analysis. *Neurosci Biobehav Rev.* 2006;30(6):808–822.

64. Rogasch NC, Sullivan C, Thomson RH, Rose NS, Bailey NW, Fitzgerald PB, et al. Analysing concurrent transcranial magnetic stimulation and electroencephalographic data: A review and introduction to the open-source TESA software. *NeuroImage.* 2017;147:934–951.

65. Oostenveld R, Fries P, Maris E, Schoffelen JM. FieldTrip: Open source software for advanced analysis of MEG, EEG, and invasive electrophysiological data. *Comput Intell Neurosci.* 2011;2011:156869.

66. Delorme A, Makeig S. EEGLAB: An open source toolbox for analysis of single-trial EEG dynamics including independent component analysis. *J Neurosci Methods.* 2004;134(1):9–21.

67. Atluri S, Frehlich M, Mei Y, Garcia Dominguez L, Rogasch NC, Wong W, et al. TMSEEG: A MATLAB-based graphical user interface for processing electrophysiological signals during transcranial magnetic stimulation. *Front Neural Circuits.* 2016;10:78.

68. Rusjan PM, Barr MS, Farzan F, Arenovich T, Maller JJ, Fitzgerald PB, et al. Optimal transcranial magnetic stimulation coil placement for targeting the dorsolateral prefrontal cortex using novel magnetic resonance image-guided neuronavigation. *Hum Brain Mapp.* 2010;31(11):1643–1652.

69. Herwig U, Padberg F, Unger J, Spitzer M, Schonfeldt-Lecuona C. Transcranial magnetic stimulation in therapy studies: Examination of the reliability of "standard" coil positioning by neuronavigation. *Biol Psychiatry.* 2001;50(1):58–61.

70. Kujirai T, Caramia MD, Rothwell JC, Day BL, Thompson PD, Ferbert A, et al. Corticocortical inhibition in human motor cortex. *J Physiol.* 1993;471:501–519.

71. Valls-Sole J, Pascual-Leone A, Wassermann EM, Hallett M. Human motor evoked responses to paired transcranial magnetic stimuli. *Electroencephalogr Clin Neurophysiol.* 1992;85(6):355–364.

72. Sanger TD, Garg RR, Chen R. Interactions between two different inhibitory systems in the human motor cortex. *J Physiol.* 2001;530(Pt 2):307–317.

73. Pascual-Leone A, Freitas C, Oberman L, Horvath JC, Halko M, Eldaief M, et al. Characterizing brain cortical plasticity and network dynamics across the age-span in health and disease with TMS-EEG and TMS-fMRI. *Brain Topogr.* 2011;24(3-4):302–315.

74. Bertini M, Ferrara M, De Gennaro L, Curcio G, Fratello F, Romei V, et al. Corticospinal excitability and sleep: A motor threshold assessment by transcranial magnetic stimulation after awakenings from REM and NREM sleep. *J Sleep Res.* 2004;13(1):31–36.

75. Stefan K, Wycislo M, Classen J. Modulation of associative human motor cortical plasticity by attention. *J Neurophysiol.* 2004;92(1):66–72.

76. Conte A, Gilio F, Iezzi E, Frasca V, Inghilleri M, Berardelli A. Attention influences the excitability of cortical motor areas in healthy humans. *Exp Brain Res.* 2007;182(1):109–117.

77. Morishima Y, Akaishi R, Yamada Y, Okuda J, Toma K, Sakai K. Task-specific signal transmission from prefrontal cortex in visual selective attention. *Nature Neurosci.* 2009;12(1):85–91.

78. Croce P, Quercia A, Costa S, Zappasodi F. Circadian rhythms in fractal features of EEG signals. *Front Physiol.* 2018;9:1567.

79. Cummings L, Dane A, Rhodes J, Lynch P, Hughes AM. Diurnal variation in the quantitative EEG in healthy adult volunteers. *Br J Clin Pharmacol.* 2000;50(1):21–26.

80. Ziemann U. TMS and drugs. *Clin Neurophysiol.* 2004;115(8):1717–1729.

81. Fusar-Poli P, Smieskova R, Kempton MJ, Ho BC, Andreasen NC, Borgwardt S. Progressive brain changes in schizophrenia related to antipsychotic treatment? A meta-analysis of longitudinal MRI studies. *Neurosci Biobehav Rev.* 2013;37(8):1680–1691.

82. Radhu N, Daskalakis ZJ, Guglietti CL, Farzan F, Barr MS, Arpin-Cribbie CA, et al. Cognitive behavioral therapy-related increases in cortical inhibition in problematic perfectionists. *Brain Stimul.* 2012;5(1):44–54.

83. Fowler DE, Tok MI, Colakoglu M, Bademkiran F, Colakoglu Z. Exercise with vibration dumb-bell enhances neuromuscular excitability measured using TMS. *J Sports Med Phys Fitness.* 2010;50(3):336–342.

84. Farzan F, Pascual-Leone A, Schmahmann JD, Halko M. Enhancing the temporal complexity of distributed brain networks with patterned cerebellar stimulation. *Sci Rep.* 2016;6:23599.

85. Du X, Choa FS, Summerfelt A, Rowland LM, Chiappelli J, Kochunov P, et al. N100 as a generic cortical electrophysiological marker based on decomposition of TMS-evoked potentials across five anatomic locations. *Exp Brain Res.* 2017;235(1):69–81.

86. Fuggetta G, Pavone EF, Fiaschi A, Manganotti P. Acute modulation of cortical oscillatory activities during short trains of high-frequency repetitive transcranial magnetic stimulation of the human motor cortex: A combined EEG and TMS study. *Hum Brain Mapp.* 2008;29(1):1–13.

87. ter Braack EM, de Vos CC, van Putten MJ. Masking the auditory evoked potential in TMS-EEG: A comparison of various methods. *Brain Topogr.* 2015;28(3):520–528.

88. Davis NJ, Gold E, Pascual-Leone A, Bracewell RM. Challenges of proper placebo control for non-invasive brain stimulation in clinical and experimental applications. *Eur J Neurosci.* 2013;38(7):2973–2977.

89. Bonato C, Miniussi C, Rossini PM. Transcranial magnetic stimulation and cortical evoked potentials: A TMS/EEG co-registration study. *Clin Neurophysiol.* 2006;117(8):1699–1707.

90. Opitz A, Legon W, Mueller J, Barbour A, Paulus W, Tyler WJ. Is sham cTBS real cTBS? The effect on EEG dynamics. *Front Hum Neurosci.* 2014;8:1043.

91. Conde V, Tomasevic L, Akopian I, Stanek K, Saturnino GB, Thielscher A, et al. The non-transcranial TMS-evoked potential is an inherent source of ambiguity in TMS-EEG studies. *NeuroImage.* 2019;185:300–312.

92. Fitzgerald PB, Maller JJ, Hoy K, Farzan F, Daskalakis ZJ. GABA and cortical inhibition in motor and non-motor regions using combined TMS-EEG: A time analysis. *Clinical Neurophysiol.* 2009;120(9):1706–1710.

93. Premoli I, Rivolta D, Espenhahn S, Castellanos N, Belardinelli P, Ziemann U, et al. Characterization of GABAB-receptor mediated neurotransmission in the human cortex by paired-pulse TMS-EEG. *NeuroImage.* 2014;103:152–162.

94. Rogasch NC, Daskalakis ZJ, Fitzgerald PB. Cortical inhibition of distinct mechanisms in the dorsolateral prefrontal cortex is related to working memory performance: A TMS-EEG study. *Cortex.* 2015;64:68–77.

95. Farzan F, Barr MS, Wong W, Chen R, Fitzgerald PB, Daskalakis ZJ. Suppression of gamma-oscillations in the dorsolateral prefrontal cortex following long interval cortical inhibition: A TMS-EEG study. *Neuropsychopharmacology.* 2009;34(6):1543–1551.

96. Ferreri F, Pasqualetti P, Maatta S, Ponzo D, Ferrarelli F, Tononi G, et al. Human brain connectivity during single and paired pulse transcranial magnetic stimulation. *NeuroImage.* 2011;54(1):90–102.

97. Noda Y, Zomorrodi R, Cash RF, Barr MS, Farzan F, Rajji TK, et al. Characterization of the influence of age on GABAA and glutamatergic mediated functions in the dorsolateral prefrontal cortex using paired-pulse TMS-EEG. *Aging (Albany NY).* 2017;9(2):556–572.

98. Rogasch NC, Daskalakis ZJ, Fitzgerald PB. Mechanisms underlying long-interval cortical inhibition in the human motor cortex: A TMS-EEG study. *J Neurophysiol.* 2013;109(1):89–98.

99. Opie GM, Rogasch NC, Goldsworthy MR, Ridding MC, Semmler JG. Investigating TMS-EEG indices of long-interval intracortical inhibition at different interstimulus intervals. *Brain Stimul.* 2017;10(1):65–74.

100. Stefan K, Kunesch E, Cohen LG, Benecke R, Classen J. Induction of plasticity in the human motor cortex by paired associative stimulation. *Brain.* 2000;123 Pt 3:572–584.

101. Carson RG, Kennedy NC. Modulation of human corticospinal excitability by paired associative stimulation. *Front Hum Neurosci.* 2013;7:823.

102. Huber R, Maatta S, Esser SK, Sarasso S, Ferrarelli F, Watson A, et al. Measures of cortical plasticity after transcranial paired associative stimulation predict changes in electroencephalogram slow-wave activity during subsequent sleep. *J Neurosci.* 2008;28(31):7911–7918.

103. Veniero D, Ponzo V, Koch G. Paired associative stimulation enforces the communication between interconnected areas. *J Neurosci.* 2013;33(34):13773–13783.

104. Casula EP, Pellicciari MC, Picazio S, Caltagirone C, Koch G. Spike-timing-dependent plasticity in the human dorso-lateral prefrontal cortex. *NeuroImage.* 2016;143:204–213.

105. Ziemann U, Paulus W, Nitsche MA, Pascual-Leone A, Byblow WD, Berardelli A, et al. Consensus: Motor cortex plasticity protocols. *Brain Stimul.* 2008;1(3):164–182.

106. Van Der Werf YD, Paus T. The neural response to transcranial magnetic stimulation of the human motor cortex. I. Intracortical and cortico-cortical contributions. *Exp Brain Res.* 2006;175(2):231–245.

107. Huang YZ, Edwards MJ, Rounis E, Bhatia KP, Rothwell JC. Theta burst stimulation of the human motor cortex. *Neuron.* 2005;45(2):201–206.

108. Vernet M, Bashir S, Yoo WK, Perez JM, Najib U, Pascual-Leone A. Insights on the neural basis of motor plasticity induced by theta burst stimulation from TMS-EEG. *Eur J Neurosci.* 2013;37(4):598–606.

109. Rocchi L, Ibanez J, Benussi A, Hannah R, Rawji V, Casula E, et al. Variability and predictors of response to continuous theta burst stimulation: A TMS-EEG study. *Front Neurosci.* 2018;12:400.

110. Chung SW, Lewis BP, Rogasch NC, Saeki T, Thomson RH, Hoy KE, et al. Demonstration of short-term plasticity in the dorsolateral prefrontal cortex with theta burst stimulation: A TMS-EEG study. *Clin Neurophysiol.* 2017;128(7):1117–1126.

111. Chung SW, Rogasch NC, Hoy KE, Fitzgerald PB. The effect of single and repeated prefrontal intermittent theta burst stimulation on cortical reactivity and working memory. *Brain Stimul.* 2018;11(3):566–574.

112. Darmani G, Zipser CM, Bohmer GM, Deschet K, Muller-Dahlhaus F, Belardinelli P, et al. Effects of the selective alpha5-GABAAR antagonist S44819 on excitability in the human brain: A TMS-EMG and TMS-EEG phase I study. *J Neurosci.* 2016;36(49):12312–12320.

8 reason

113. Premoli I, Castellanos N, Rivolta D, Belardinelli P, Bajo R, Zipser C, et al. TMS-EEG signatures of GABAergic neurotransmission in the human cortex. *J Neurosci.* 2014;34(16):5603–5612.
114. Premoli I, Bergmann TO, Fecchio M, Rosanova M, Biondi A, Belardinelli P, et al. The impact of GABAergic drugs on TMS-induced brain oscillations in human motor cortex. *NeuroImage.* 2017;163:1–12.
115. Salavati B, Rajji TK, Zomorrodi R, Blumberger DM, Chen R, Pollock BG, et al. Pharmacological manipulation of cortical inhibition in the dorsolateral prefrontal cortex. *Neuropsychopharmacology.* 2018;43(2):354–361.
116. Premoli I, Kiraly J, Muller-Dahlhaus F, Zipser CM, Rossini P, Zrenner C, et al. Short-interval and long-interval intracortical inhibition of TMS-evoked EEG potentials. *Brain Stimul.* 2018;11(4):818–827.
117. Farzan F, Barr MS, Levinson AJ, Chen R, Wong W, Fitzgerald PB, et al. Evidence for gamma inhibition deficits in the dorsolateral prefrontal cortex of patients with schizophrenia. *Brain.* 2010;133(Pt 5):1505–1514.
118. Radhu N, Garcia Dominguez L, Farzan F, Richter MA, Semeralul MO, Chen R, et al. Evidence for inhibitory deficits in the prefrontal cortex in schizophrenia. *Brain.* 2015;138(Pt 2):483–497.
119. Frantseva M, Cui J, Farzan F, Chinta LV, Perez Velazquez JL, Daskalakis ZJ. Disrupted cortical conductivity in schizophrenia: TMS-EEG study. *Cerebral Cortex.* 2014;24(1):211–221.
120. Naim-Feil J, Bradshaw JL, Rogasch NC, Daskalakis ZJ, Sheppard DM, Lubman DI, et al. Cortical inhibition within motor and frontal regions in alcohol dependence post-detoxification: A pilot TMS-EEG study. *World J Biol Psychiatry.* 2016;17(7):547–556.
121. Kahkonen S. MEG and TMS combined with EEG for mapping alcohol effects. *Alcohol.* 2005;37(3):129–133.
122. Noda Y, Barr MS, Zomorrodi R, Cash RFH, Rajji TK, Farzan F, et al. Reduced short-latency afferent inhibition in prefrontal but not motor cortex and its association with executive function in schizophrenia: A combined TMS-EEG Study. *Schizophrenia Bull.* 2018;44(1):193–202.
123. Canali P, Sarasso S, Rosanova M, Casarotto S, Sferrazza-Papa G, Gosseries O, et al. Shared reduction of oscillatory natural frequencies in bipolar disorder, major depressive disorder and schizophrenia. *J Affect Dis.* 2015;184:111–115.
124. Julkunen P, Jauhiainen AM, Westeren-Punnonen S, Pirinen E, Soininen H, Kononen M, et al. Navigated TMS combined with EEG in mild cognitive impairment and Alzheimer's disease: A pilot study. *J Neurosci Methods.* 2008;172(2):270–276.
125. Ferreri F, Vecchio F, Vollero L, Guerra A, Petrichella S, Ponzo D, et al. Sensorimotor cortex excitability and connectivity in Alzheimer's disease: A TMS-EEG Co-registration study. *Hum Brain Mapp.* 2016;37(6):2083–2096.
126. Casula EP, Mayer IMS, Desikan M, Tabrizi SJ, Rothwell JC, Orth M. Motor cortex synchronization influences the rhythm of motor performance in premanifest huntington's disease. *Move Dis.* 2018;33(3):440–448.
127. Sarasso S, Rosanova M, Casali AG, Casarotto S, Fecchio M, Boly M, et al. Quantifying cortical EEG responses to TMS in (un)consciousness. *Clin EEG Neurosci.* 2014;45(1):40–49.
128. Julkunen P, Jauhiainen AM, Kononen M, Paakkonen A, Karhu J, Soininen H. Combining transcranial magnetic stimulation and electroencephalography may contribute to assess the severity of Alzheimer's disease. *Int J Alzheimers Dis.* 2011;2011:654794.
129. Bagattini C, Mutanen TP, Fracassi C, Manenti R, Cotelli M, Ilmoniemi RJ, et al. Predicting Alzheimer's disease severity by means of TMS-EEG coregistration. *Neurobiol Aging.* 2019;80:38–45.
130. Manganotti P, Acler M, Masiero S, Del Felice A. TMS-evoked N100 responses as a prognostic factor in acute stroke. *Funct Neurol.* 2015;30(2):125–130.
131. Sun Y, Farzan F, Mulsant BH, Rajji TK, Fitzgerald PB, Barr MS, et al. Indicators for remission of suicidal ideation following magnetic seizure therapy in patients with treatment-resistant depression. *JAMA Psychiatry.* 2016;73(4):337–345.
132. Premoli I, Biondi A, Carlesso S, Rivolta D, Richardson MP. Lamotrigine and levetiracetam exert a similar modulation of TMS-evoked EEG potentials. *Epilepsia.* 2017;58(1):42–50.

133. Pellicciari MC, Ponzo V, Caltagirone C, Koch G. Restored asymmetry of prefrontal cortical oscillatory activity after bilateral theta burst stimulation treatment in a patient with major depressive disorder: A TMS-EEG study. *Brain Stimul.* 2017;10(1):147–149.

134. Casarotto S, Canali P, Rosanova M, Pigorini A, Fecchio M, Mariotti M, et al. Assessing the effects of electroconvulsive therapy on cortical excitability by means of transcranial magnetic stimulation and electroencephalography. *Brain Topogr.* 2013;26(2):326–337.

135. Thut G, Bergmann TO, Frohlich F, Soekadar SR, Brittain JS, Valero-Cabre A, et al. Guiding transcranial brain stimulation by EEG/MEG to interact with ongoing brain activity and associated functions: A position paper. *Clin Neurophysiol.* 2017;128(5):843–857.

136. Zrenner C, Belardinelli P, Muller-Dahlhaus F, Ziemann U. Closed-loop neuroscience and non-invasive brain stimulation: A tale of two loops. *Front Cell Neurosci.* 2016;10:92.

137. Rotenberg A. Prospects for clinical applications of transcranial magnetic stimulation and real-time EEG in epilepsy. *Brain Topogr.* 2010;22(4):257–266.

138. Kraus D, Naros G, Bauer R, Leao MT, Ziemann U, Gharabaghi A. Brain-robot interface driven plasticity: Distributed modulation of corticospinal excitability. *NeuroImage.* 2016;125:522–532.

Combining TMS with Neuroimaging

8.1 INTRODUCTION

A variety of neuroimaging techniques have been used over the past 20 years to markedly enhance our understanding of normal and abnormal brain function. Although no neuroimaging techniques are able to provide a perfect representation of brain structure and function, the techniques used in modern neuroscience are increasingly sophisticated and able to provide critical information about how the brain works and how it is affected in various illness states. Because of the considerable value of information that can be derived from neuroimaging studies, it is not surprising that a variety of researchers have turned to neuroimaging tools to better understand how stimulation techniques like transcranial magnetic stimulation (TMS) affect brain activity. Studies of this type have used positron emission tomography (PET)-, single photon emission computed tomography (SPECT)-, and magnetic resonance imaging (MRI)-based techniques. Studies have investigated the immediate impact of single sessions of brain stimulation on a variety of aspects of brain activity. Studies have also been conducted to investigate the types of changes induced with longer periods of stimulation, as in the context of the treatment of a disorder like depression, with these neuroimaging tools.

These types of studies, where scans are conducted before and after a period of brain stimulation, are usually referred to as "offline" studies. In contrast, a smaller set of studies has directly combined TMS and neuroimaging in so-called online protocols (Figure 8.1). These studies aim to directly capture or study what happens in the brain immediately during brain stimulation. For example, single TMS pulses can be applied in an MRI scanner and the immediate response to these pulses studied. This type of approach can

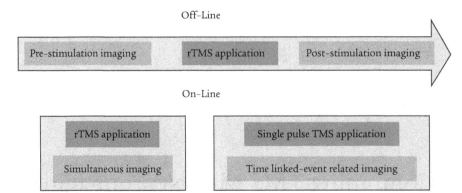

FIGURE 8.1 *Online and offline study designs.*

be used to better understand the effects of TMS but also as a mechanism to understand brain networks and the connections between brain regions. This chapter describes these types of neuroimaging studies and provides an overview of some of the more critical findings to emerge from them so far.

A number of issues must be considered in interpreting the results of both off- and online TMS neuroimaging studies. One of the most critical of these relates to the conclusions that can be drawn from these studies, especially those where stimulation is applied in an online manner. When provided at suprathreshold intensities, and even to some degree when provided at subthreshold intensities, TMS is a depolarizing form of brain stimulation. Unlike other techniques, such as transcranial direct current stimulation, TMS produces the direct firing of cortical neurons underneath the coil when applied at sufficient intensity. This allows us to study the pattern of activation that stimulation of a group of nerve cells from one cortical region produces.

However, it is important to remember that the firing of neurons under these circumstances cannot be considered physiological. In other words, the way in which neurons are activated by a TMS pulse is likely to be substantially different from the way these neurons become active during normal cognitive function. This is likely to be reflected in the size of a cortical region spontaneously or artificially activated and the degree to which neurons fire simultaneously. This might limit the conclusions that can be drawn about the outcomes of this type of stimulation.

As alluded to earlier, the issue of timing of brain imaging measurement in regards to TMS stimulation is also critical. What occurs during the provision of stimulation is likely to be quite different to what is seen once the period of stimulation ceases. For example, during low-frequency stimulation, it is likely that the cortex will be activated to a degree greater than seen at rest as neurons fire repeatedly in response to TMS pulses. However, this might lead to a down-regulation in cortical activity that is reflected in a very different pattern of activation once stimulation has ceased, quite possibly the opposite. As neuroimaging tools typically take a defined period of time to complete an image of the entire brain (e.g., a minimum of several seconds with MRI), it is unlikely that these tools are by necessity able to image all of the cortical evoked events produced with TMS stimulation. Therefore, in the design of neuroimaging experiments, it is critical to very clearly elucidate the desired outcomes and how these can be best achieved.

There is also a degree of complexity introduced by the nature of the TMS pulse and how this interacts with various types of neurons in the brain. It has been well documented that the processes of neurons that sit parallel to the surface of the brain, especially across the top of a gyrus, are more likely to be depolarized by a TMS pulse than the descending pyramidal neurons that project away from the cortex. It is possible to activate these projecting excitatory neurons at high enough stimulation intensities both directly and through the activation of excitatory imports onto these cells. At lower intensities, however, there is a preferential stimulation of inhibitory interneurons, potentially dampening down cortical activity as evidenced in basic physiological measures such as the cortical silent period and short-interval cortical inhibition (described in an earlier chapter).

When a significantly suprathreshold pulse is applied to the cortex, this will produce activation of excitatory pyramidal cells where the intensity of the magnetic pulse is at its peak. However, there will be an area surrounding this where the prime activation induced by the TMS pulse will be of inhibitory neurons. All of this complex activity ultimately adds up to a physiological and behavioral response, but we lack the sophistication in our imaging techniques to have any capacity to separate out these effects at the moment.

8.2 OFFLINE TMS-NEUROIMAGING STUDIES: STUDIES OF SINGLE STIMULATION SESSIONS

8.2.1 General Principles

Offline imaging techniques have been utilized for a number of important experimental purposes. Offline experiments can be conducted in several ways:

1. *When brain imaging is performed before TMS.* In these experiments, neuroimaging is most commonly used to identify a site for brain stimulation in an experimental or clinical context. In a cognitive study context, TMS is most commonly done to disrupt activity thought to be underpinned by a certain brain region: a scan is performed to identify areas of potential involvement in a task, and then one or more of these is the subject of stimulation to try to establish a causative relationship between the brain site and task performance. Brain imaging might also be used to individualize the site of stimulation within an experimental or clinical study context.

2. *Brain imaging performed after TMS.* These studies are typically done to understand the effects of repetitive transcranial magnetic stimulation (rTMS) on brain activity. Stimulation is applied, and then a recording is made to try to understand how brain activity is influenced by stimulation. This may be done with task-related imaging (mapping activity during a certain cognitive or emotional task) or with resting state scanning.

3. *Brain imaging performed both before and after stimulation,* most commonly with rTMS.

As alluded to earlier, neuroimaging before and after the provision of TMS allows us to make meaningful inferences about the nature of the effects of the type of TMS used on brain activity. This information can be gained about the local influences of TMS on the cortex underlying the coil as well as about impacts on more distal brain regions.

Perhaps more importantly, however, this type of experimental approach can also be used to study the role of specific brain regions and networks in the conduct of certain cognitive activities. One critical feature of the use of TMS is that it allows for greater causal inferences to be drawn about the role of brain regions in certain cognitive functions than can imaging alone. When traditional cognitive brain imaging studies are done, a pattern of activation may be seen in response to a certain cognitive task. However, it is difficult to draw an inference about whether specific regions are necessary for the performance of that task because activation of one or more regions may not be essential for task performance or may be an epiphenomena.

It has been increasingly recognized that TMS can be used to help deal with this experimental problem. If stimulation can be targeted to one or more of the sites identified in a neuroimaging experiment, and performance on that task enhanced or disrupted, this allows us to be more certain about the role of that brain region in underpinning past performance. This approach has been termed at times a "map and perturb" approach.

However, as the effects of TMS are not just local but propagate through multiple brain regions, this inference still cannot be drawn with complete confidence. It is possible that an experimenter could stimulate site X which is directly anatomically connected to site Y. Stimulation of site X could cause disruption of a task performance not because of the role of site X in that task but because trans-synaptic activation of site Y disrupted task performance.

However, if one combines studying the effect of stimulation on a behavioral variable (e.g., performance on the task being studied) with the simultaneous study of brain activation during that task before and after TMS stimulation, one can build a more sophisticated model and make greater causal inferences. For example, if TMS produces a transient impairment in performance on a certain task associated with a significant alteration in activity in the stimulated brain region but not necessarily other brain sites involved in the performance of that task, this will allow us to draw much stronger inferences about the role of the primary brain region in the task than might otherwise be possible.

The conduct of repeated imaging, pre- and post-stimulation, does introduce a potential confounding factor. A change in task performance and brain activation seen across the two imaging sessions may well arise directly from repeating task performance. The study participants might become conditioned to the task or improve performance through practice effects. Therefore, in conducting this type of experiment, it is critical to include at least one separate control testing session. In this separate session, pre- and post-task performance is assessed either side of stimulation being applied with a sham condition or to what is thought to be a control cortical site. The order of active and control sessions should be counterbalanced across participants and ideally sufficiently separated in time to ensure that there are no holdover effects from one session to the next. In practice, this is commonly done with a week-long break between sessions, although this degree of separation may not be always necessary.

The choice of sham or control stimulation in this type of design is critical. An ideal sham stimulation will produce a scalp sensation similar to that produced with true rTMS as well as a similar degree of sound. Sham stimulation systems have been developed for rTMS experiments, for example with a mechanism to induce scalp sensation using electrical stimulation. However, recent research into the brain effects of transcranial direct current stimulation and alternating current stimulation should make one cautious about the possibility that electrical stimulation of the scalp might produce some brain effects itself.

The choice of an active control stimulation site can also be problematic. Ideally, TMS would be provided to a different site on the scalp that has no functional relevance to the task or brain process being studied. However, as many cognitive tasks rely on the complex interplay between activation in complimentary brain regions (and possibly the deactivation of uninvolved circuitry), choosing an appropriate site that is truly neutral can be problematic.

8.2.2 PET and SPECT Imaging of Blood Flow and Metabolism

One of the first TMS neuroimaging approaches to be adopted involved studying cortical blood flow or metabolism before and after rTMS stimulation. Cortical metabolism may be assessed with SPECT and with a greater degree of anatomical resolution with PET imaging methods. As PET has considerably greater structural resolution, its use has mostly supplanted SPECT in this context. PET relies on the injection of a compound which has been tagged with a positron emitting isotope, for example carbon-11 or oxygen-15.

Most commonly glucose is used, which is taken up by metabolically active regions of the brain. This approach effectively assesses brain activity over a temporal scale of minutes as the glucose is taken up during a cognitive process. An alternative approach is to use an oxygen-15–based tracer to map cerebral blood flow. Water that incorporates the radioactive oxygen is typically used. Oxygen-based assessments allow one to study rapid changes in blood flow, usually with a subminute level degree of resolution.

SPECT imaging is somewhat more widely available because SPECT scanners do not require access to a closely located cyclotron as they tend to use isotopes with a longer half-life. Clearly both of these techniques involve the administration of tracers that involve exposure to radiation. This poses safety concerns which significantly limit the number of scans that a single participant can undertake. For example, it would not be possible to repeatedly scan somebody multiple times with PET during the therapeutic course of rTMS.

As the temporal resolution of PET and SPECT is somewhat limited, these techniques are primarily used to study the effects of trains of stimulation applied over minutes, rather than single- or paired-pulse TMS effects. These studies can be done in an online or offline manner. It is quite possible to apply rTMS stimulation within a PET scanner, and it is also possible to provide stimulation during the injection of a radiotracer such as [18]FDG-PET for measurement of metabolism. In this latter study design, stimulation is applied while the radiotracer is injected, and the participant is then transferred into the scanner for measurement of brain activity. PET scans are also ideal for studying brain activity before and after a course of rTMS treatment in a clinical context.

An early example of the type of study that can be done using PET simultaneously with rTMS explored the cerebral blood flow changes induced with high-frequency rTMS applied to the motor cortex. This study used $H_2{}^{15}O$-PET to assess changes produced by 10 Hz stimulation at a subthreshold intensity. Decreases in blood flow were seen in the stimulated as well as the contralateral motor cortical region.[1] A subsequent study investigated the effects of progressively increasing stimulation intensity (from 80% to 120% of the motor threshold) on regional blood flow produced with 1 Hz stimulation trains.[2] A local increase in blood flow was accompanied by increases and decreases across a wide range of brain regions including in auditory cortex, cerebellum, basal ganglia, insula, and the anterior cingulate and occipital cortex. This clearly demonstrates the widespread effects of rTMS stimulation. This approach can also be used to study the connectivity of nonmotor regions. For example, Paus et al. applied several forms of rTMS to the left mid-dorsolateral frontal cortex and demonstrated a complex relationship between frontal and anterior cingulate cortex activation.[3]

Studies have also been conducted to investigate the effects of rTMS in nonmotor regions in the context of investigating illness states and the response to treatment. For example, $H_2{}^{15}O$-PET was used to assess the response to high- and low-frequency rTMS given for 10 days to patients with major depression.[4] High-frequency stimulation produced increases in blood flow in prefrontal regions, the cingulate gyrus, the left amygdala, and a number of other brain regions. Low-frequency stimulation produced widespread decreases in blood flow although in areas less distributed than with high-frequency stimulation. In a more recent study, ^{18}FDG-PET was used to assess metabolic changes produced with 10 sessions of high-frequency rTMS in 21 depressed patients.[5] Successful treatment was related to changes in metabolism in several areas of the anterior cingulate cortex. Interestingly, higher baseline metabolism in the prefrontal region and anterior cingulate cortex was associated with improved clinical outcomes. A broader pattern of altered metabolism was seen in a second study exploring baseline metabolic activity in response to treatment.[6] In this report, responders to treatment had greater activity in left lateral orbitofrontal cortex and lower activity in the left amygdala and uncinate fasciculus.

8.2.3 Imaging the Effects of rTMS Treatment with MRI

Functional magnetic resonance imaging (fMRI) has also been used to study the impact over time of rTMS treatment, especially when applied in patients with depression. In one of the first of these studies, the effects of low-frequency right-sided rTMS was contrasted with the effects of high-frequency stimulation applied on the left.[7] Low-frequency stimulation produced a bilateral reduction in task-related activation in the middle frontal gyrus in treatment responders. In contrast, high-frequency stimulation produced increased task-related activation in responders in the left precuneus and several additional regions. This study demonstrated that these two different forms of rTMS produce substantially different changes in task-related activation across the brain regions, even when the degree of clinical response was similar. Activation during an emotional task was used in a study contrasting the effects of rTMS treatment and treatment with the antidepressant drug fluoxetine in a group of depressed patients with Parkinson's disease.[8] rTMS treatment was associated with increased task-related activity in the left prefrontal cortex and anterior cingulate gyrus as well as reductions in activity in several other brain regions. This pattern of response differed from that seen with fluoxetine.

Beyond imaging specific functional changes, fMRI has also been used to study the impact that rTMS stimulation has on activation patterns across brain networks. A recent review synthesized the results of 33 such studies where offline fMRI was used to investigate changes in resting state functional connectivity following rTMS stimulation[9] (see Figure 8.2). The review included studies with a diversity of stimulation targets and paradigms but came to some interesting conclusions. First, distal connectivity impacts of rTMS stimulation did not follow a simple low frequency → inhibition, high-frequency

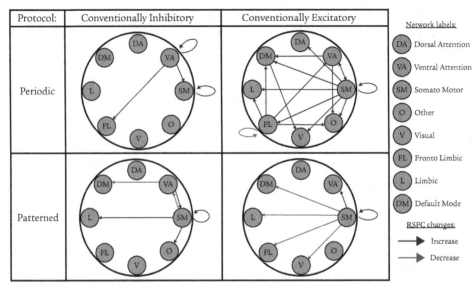

FIGURE 8.2 *Repetitive transcranial magnetic stimulation (rTMS)-induced changes in resting-state functional connectivity (RSFC) by resting-state functional networks for each type of stimulation protocol separated into conventional inhibitory/excitatory and periodic versus patterned pulse sequences (Periodic conventionally inhibitory: 1 Hz; periodic conventionally excitatory: 5, 10, and 20 Hz; patterned conventionally inhibitory: cTBS and iQPS; patterned conventionally excitatory: iTBS and eQPS). The starting point of each arrow indicates the stimulated network, and the head of each arrow represents a network where corresponding rTMS-induced changes were observed. The thickness of the arrow indicates the number of studies finding the same result (e.g., FL-DM is thicker because four studies were associated with changes between these networks). Blue arrows indicate increased RSFC after rTMS, and red arrows indicate decreased RSFC.*
From Beynel et al., Neuroimage. 2020;211:116596.

→ excitation type model. Second, substantial effects of stimulation were seen in networks other than the network targeted. The authors concluded that the effects of rTMS extended substantially across networks rather than being confined to local effects or even effects in the network being targeted.

Studies have also used MRI-based approaches to study patterns of brain activation that might predict response to treatment. For example, one study analyzed baseline task related activation and response to high-frequency left-sided stimulation or sham.[10] In the actively treated group, response was associated with larger task-related activation in the left ventral caudate-putamen and several regions of task-related deactivation.

Beyond functional imaging, a limited body of research has used structural imaging to investigate changes in regional brain volume before and after rTMS treatment. Furtado et al. measured regional brain volumes in depressed patients undergoing rTMS before treatment and at 3-month follow-up.[11] Response to treatment was associated with an increase in left amygdala volume in contrast to a small reduction in hippocampal volume seen over time in treatment nonresponders. A few studies have also used diffusion tensor imaging (DTI) measures of white matter integrity to study the effects of rTMS treatment as well as to correlate the effect of rTMS stimulation and DTI measures of connectivity. For example, a recent study correlated the effects of rTMS used in a disruptive paradigm on an aspect of movement with fractional anisotropy (FA) in the superior longitudinal fasciculus.[12] In depression, research has suggested that rTMS treatment of depression is associated with an increase in frontal FA[13] with similar findings in a second small study which did not quite reach significance.[14]

Studies have also begun to use magnetic resonance spectroscopy (MRS) to examine the effects of rTMS on cortical metabolites, also concentrated on the context of the treatment of depression. In the first study of this type, 17 patients with depression were studied with MRS before and after a course of high-frequency left prefrontal rTMS, with 6 patients responding to treatment.[15] Responders, compared to nonresponders, had lower baseline left prefrontal glutamate levels which increased with rTMS treatment, but no changes were at observed in the anterior cingulate cortex. Zheng et al. found a significant increase in N-acetylaspartate (NAA) in the anterior cingulate cortex following high-frequency left-sided rTMS treatment in depressed subjects.[16] NAA levels were reduced in patients pretreatment and returned to a level equivalent to healthy controls. A more recent study examined the effects of high-frequency left prefrontal rTMS treatment in depression by examining medial prefrontal cortex gamma-aminobutyric acid (GABA) and combined glutamate and glutamine (Glx) concentrations.[17] The study found a significant increase in GABA concentration but no change in Glx across all subjects who received rTMS treatment

8.3 ONLINE TMS-FMRI

The technique that appears to have the greatest potential for directly uncovering the effects of TMS stimulation on real-time activity in brain networks is concurrent TMS-fMRI when stimulation is provided directly during the process of image acquisition (see Figure 8.3 from Vink et al.[18]). This technique is not new: it was actually first demonstrated in the late 1990s but has only slowly been adopted as a method of studying the effects of brain stimulation, probably due to the complexity of establishing a successful experimental setup. The initial TMS-fMRI studies predominantly examined the effects of stimulation on primary motor cortical regions. These studies demonstrated that TMS pulses would activate local cerebral regions but also connected regions in remote sites. Studies have progressively attempted to deal with experimental confounds including the brain response to stimulation noise and the sensory responses to scalp stimulation as well as induced motor responses. As controlled conditions have developed to deal with some of these, more interest has grown in the use of TMS-fMRI to study the effects of stimulation

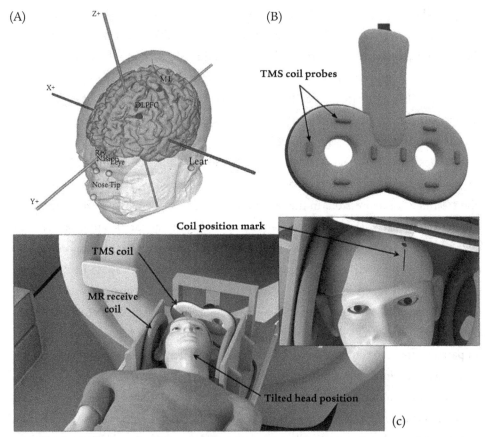

FIGURE 8.3 *Schematic showing concurrent functional magnetic resonance imaging (fMRI) and repetitive transcranial magnetic stimulation (rTMS). (A) Location of facial markers and TMS targets in the neural navigator (neuronavigation software). The statistical map of voluntarily induced motor activity is thresholded and shown in red. Facial markers: Tip of the nose; nasion, left and right inner eyelid; left and right upper and lower ear. TMS targets: Primary motor cortex (M1); dorsolateral prefrontal cortex (DLPFC). (B) TMS coil probes. The probes are visualized in a T2-weighted scan to determine their location with respect to the head. (C) Participant is lying on the MR bed with the head positioned in between two MR receiver coils and the TMS coil is located over the cranium.*

FROM VINK ET AL., *HUM BRAIN MAPP*. 2018;39:4580–4592.

in nonmotor regions. These studies have been almost exclusively done in a cognitive neuroscience context to understand the role of specific neural circuits underpinning aspects of cognition. For example, Ruff et al. was able to conduct a series of studies exploring how frontal and parietal brain activity modulates aspects of visual perception.[19–21] In another example, researchers studied the effects of parietal stimulation during spatial and nonspatial control tasks and were able to draw conclusions about the role of parietal and frontal interactions in task performance.[22]

Methods for application of TMS-fMRI continue to evolve with the development of new coil systems,[23,24] and methods of controlling for stimulation artifacts[25] are likely to

TABLE 8.1. Neuroimaging methods combined with transcranial magnetic stimulation (TMS): Features and challenges

Imaging type	Main applications	Comments
Single photon emission computed tomography (SPECT)	Pre-post therapy designs	Limited spatial resolution, inexpensive and widely available
Positron emission tomography (PET)	Pre-post therapy designs Online/during stimulation	Better spatial resolution, expensive Poor temporal resolution (better with O^{15} based imaging)
Functional magnetic resonance imaging (fMRI)	Pre-post therapy designs Online/during stimulation	Excellent spatial resolution, widely available Excellent spatial resolution, moderate temporal resolution, expensive, technically challenging

continue to expand the usability of these approaches. This will allow the approach to become a powerful tool for exploring causal brain–behavior relationships.[26]

8.4 CONCLUSION

TMS can be usefully combined with a variety of neuroimaging techniques to allow researchers and clinicians to better understand the effects of stimulation, address complex questions about the relationship between brain activity and cognitive functions, and increase our understanding of how therapeutic applications of rTMS produce their effects both locally in the brain and on distributed circuitry. It is likely that there will be increasing emphasis on combining TMS with MRI-based imaging approaches, with studies that potentially combine metabolic, structural, and functional approaches. In addition, recent research has suggested that measures of electrical activity may well be combined into a TMS and imaging framework to provide a broader multimodal understanding of the effects of stimulation (Table 8.1).[27]

REFERENCES

1. Paus T, Jech R, Thompson CJ, Comeau R, Peters T, Evans AC. Dose-dependent reduction of cerebral blood flow during rapid-rate transcranial magnetic stimulation of the human sensorimotor cortex. *J Neurophysiol*. 1998;79:1102–1107.
2. Speer AM, Willis MW, Herscovitch P, Daube-Witherspoon M, Shelton JR, Benson BE, et al. Intensity-dependent regional cerebral blood flow during 1-Hz repetitive transcranial magnetic stimulation (rTMS) in healthy volunteers studied with H215O positron emission tomography: I. Effects of primary motor cortex rTMS. *Biol Psychiatry*. 2003;54:818–825.

3. Paus T, Castro-Alamancos MA, Petrides M. Cortico-cortical connectivity of the human mid-dorsolateral frontal cortex and its modulation by repetitive transcranial magnetic stimulation. *Eur J Neurosci.* 2001;14:1405–1411.

4. Speer AM, Kimbrell TA, Wassermann EM, Rapella JD, Willis MW, Herscovitch P, et al. Opposite effects of high and low frequency rTMS on regional brain activity in depressed patients. *Biol Psychiatry.* 2000;48:1133–1141.

5. Baeken C, De Raedt R, Van Hove C, Clerinx P, De Mey J, Bossuyt A. HF-rTMS treatment in medication-resistant melancholic depression: Results from 18FDG-PET brain imaging. *CNS Spectr.* 2009;14:439–448.

6. Paillere Martinot ML, Martinot JL, Ringuenet D, Galinowski A, Gallarda T, Bellivier F, et al. Baseline brain metabolism in resistant depression and response to transcranial magnetic stimulation. *Neuropsychopharmacology.* 2011;36:2710–2719.

7. Fitzgerald PB, Sritharan A, Daskalakis ZJ, de Castella AR, Kulkarni J, Egan G. A functional magnetic resonance imaging study of the effects of low frequency right prefrontal transcranial magnetic stimulation in depression. *J Clin Psychopharmacol.* 2007;27:488–492.

8. Cardoso EF, Fregni F, Martins Maia F, Boggio PS, Luis Myczkowski M, Coracini K, et al. rTMS treatment for depression in Parkinson's disease increases BOLD responses in the left prefrontal cortex. *Int J Neuropsychopharmacol.* 2008;11:173–183.

9. Beynel L, Powers JP, Appelbaum LG. Effects of repetitive transcranial magnetic stimulation on resting-state connectivity: A systematic review. *Neuroimage.* 2020;211:116596.

10. Hernandez-Ribas R, Deus J, Pujol J, Segalas C, Vallejo J, Menchon JM, et al. Identifying brain imaging correlates of clinical response to repetitive transcranial magnetic stimulation (rTMS) in major depression. *Brain Stimul.* 2013;6:54–61.

11. Furtado CP, Hoy KE, Maller JJ, Savage G, Daskalakis ZJ, Fitzgerald PB. An investigation of medial temporal lobe changes and cognition following antidepressant response: A prospective rTMS study. *Brain Stimul.* 2013;6:346–354.

12. Rodriguez-Herreros B, Amengual JL, Gurtubay-Antolin A, Richter L, Jauer P, Erdmann C, et al. Microstructure of the superior longitudinal fasciculus predicts stimulation-induced interference with online motor control. *Neuroimage.* 2015;120:254–265.

13. Peng H, Zheng H, Li L, Liu J, Zhang Y, Shan B, et al. High-frequency rTMS treatment increases white matter FA in the left middle frontal gyrus in young patients with treatment-resistant depression. *J Affect Disord.* 2012;136:249–257.

14. Kozel FA, Johnson KA, Nahas Z, Nakonezny PA, Morgan PS, Anderson BS, et al. Fractional anisotropy changes after several weeks of daily left high-frequency repetitive transcranial magnetic stimulation of the prefrontal cortex to treat major depression. *J ECT.* 2011;27:5–10.

15. Luborzewski A, Schubert F, Seifert F, Danker-Hopfe H, Brakemeier EL, Schlattmann P, et al. Metabolic alterations in the dorsolateral prefrontal cortex after treatment with high-frequency repetitive transcranial magnetic stimulation in patients with unipolar major depression. *J Psychiatr Res.* 2007;41:606–615.

16. Zheng H, Jia F, Guo G, Quan D, Li G, Wu H, et al. Abnormal anterior cingulate n-acetylaspartate and executive functioning in treatment-resistant depression after rTMS therapy. *Int J Neuropsychopharmacol.* 2015;18:pyv059.

17. Dubin MJ, Mao X, Banerjee S, Goodman Z, Lapidus KA, Kang G, et al. Elevated prefrontal cortex GABA in patients with major depressive disorder after TMS treatment measured with proton magnetic resonance spectroscopy. *J Psychiatry Neurosci.* 2016;41:150223.

18. Vink JJT, Mandija S, Petrov PI, van den Berg CAT, Sommer IEC, Neggers SFW. A novel concurrent TMS-fMRI method to reveal propagation patterns of prefrontal magnetic brain stimulation. *Hum Brain Mapp.* 2018;39:4580–4592.

19. Ruff CC, Blankenburg F, Bjoertomt O, Bestmann S, Weiskopf N, Driver J. Hemispheric differences in frontal and parietal influences on human occipital cortex: direct confirmation with concurrent TMS-fMRI. *J Cogn Neurosci.* 2009;21:1146–1161.

20. Ruff CC, Blankenburg F, Bjoertomt O, Bestmann S, Freeman E, Haynes JD, et al. Concurrent TMS-fMRI and psychophysics reveal frontal influences on human retinotopic visual cortex. *Curr Biol.* 2006;16:1479–1488.

21. Ruff CC, Bestmann S, Blankenburg F, Bjoertomt O, Josephs O, Weiskopf N, et al. Distinct causal influences of parietal versus frontal areas on human visual cortex: evidence from concurrent TMS-fMRI. *Cereb Cortex.* 2008;18:817–827.

22. Sack AT, Kohler A, Bestmann S, Linden DE, Dechent P, Goebel R, et al. Imaging the brain activity changes underlying impaired visuospatial judgments: Simultaneous FMRI, TMS, and behavioral studies. *Cereb Cortex.* 2007;17:2841–52.

23. Navarro de Lara LI, Windischberger C, Kuehne A, Woletz M, Sieg J, Bestmann S, et al. A novel coil array for combined TMS/fMRI experiments at 3 T. *Magn Reson Med.* 2015;74:1492–1501.

24. de Weijer AD, Sommer IE, Bakker EJ, Bloemendaal M, Bakker CJ, Klomp DW, et al. A setup for administering TMS to medial and lateral cortical areas during whole-brain FMRI recording. *J Clin Neurophysiol.* 2014;31:474–487.

25. Bungert A, Chambers CD, Phillips M, Evans CJ. Reducing image artefacts in concurrent TMS/fMRI by passive shimming. *Neuroimage.* 2012;59:2167–2174.

26. Sliwinska MW, Vitello S, Devlin JT. Transcranial magnetic stimulation for investigating causal brain-behavioral relationships and their time course. *J Vis Exp.* 2014;18(89):51735.

27. Peters JC, Reithler J, Schuhmann T, de Graaf T, Uludag K, Goebel R, et al. On the feasibility of concurrent human TMS-EEG-fMRI measurements. *J Neurophysiol.* 2013;109:1214–1227.

RTMS AS TREATMENT OF NEUROLOGICAL AND PSYCHIATRIC DISORDERS

The Use of rTMS and Other Forms of Brain Stimulation in the Treatment of Neuropsychiatric Disorders

9.1 INTRODUCTION

Over the past 15 years, repetitive transcranial magnetic stimulation (rTMS) has progressed from an experimental technique to something that is now widely being used in clinical practice, with its range of applications progressively expanding and likely to continue to do so for some time. rTMS in many places has become a common and regular part of the treatment armamentarium for psychiatrists managing patients with significant mood disorders, and there are a range of other applications where rTMS is progressively moving toward or becoming part of clinical practice. There are an even greater number of clinical indications for which we already have preliminary data for the potential use of this treatment but at this stage lack the larger multisite trials required to facilitate transition to clinical practice.

One of the major challenges that has slowed the progression of rTMS treatment into clinical practice across most disorders has been the nature of many of the trials conducted to date. Beginning with the first therapeutic use of rTMS in the treatment of depression in the mid-1990s, the vast majority of rTMS trials across disorders have been investigator-initiated studies conducted at single sites on limited budgets. For this reason, the vast majority of studies across all applications have been relatively small and, in many cases, underpowered to provide sufficient evidence of clinical efficacy. There have been only a handful of larger multisite clinical trials, some independently and some industry funded.

The challenge that this proliferation of small, often underpowered studies has provided to the field has been significantly exacerbated by the large degree of variability evident in the methods that can be used in any individual clinical application.

In fact, the development of rTMS therapeutic paradigms is complicated by the existence of a very wide parameter space and the reality that, for many applications, individual investigative groups have adopted slightly or significantly diverging approaches which makes pooling data from multiple small studies highly problematic. In fact, an increasing number of meta-analyses of rTMS studies have been published which include studies applying treatment with markedly different paradigms even including multiple different brain regions. This clearly is problematic, and individual therapeutic paradigms utilizing specific frequencies of stimulation and stimulation targets should be regarded as different from one another.

The parameter space relevant to the development of clinical applications of rTMS includes the following issues.

9.2 THE SELECTION OF STIMULATION LOCATION

The selection of stimulation location for rTMS paradigms has typically used neuroimaging research to identify localized changes in brain function in a specific disorder at a region accessible to TMS stimulation on the cortical surface. For example, the application of rTMS to the dorsolateral prefrontal cortex (DLPFC) in the treatment of major depressive disorder was originally motivated by findings from resting positron emission tomography (PET) scanning (for example [1]). Initial studies using PET in depression identified reductions in blood flow or metabolism in lateral areas of the prefrontal cortex, a site that was accessible to TMS stimulation and hence a logical target for treatment development. In contrast, research had suggested dysfunctional activity of relevant brain processes in the region of the temporoparietal junction in individuals experiencing persistent auditory hallucinations,[2] again motivating a localized approach to treatment.[3] It is notable that, even in this early research, it was recognized that there might be a significant variation in the pathophysiology of brain processes underlying specific disorders or syndromes resulting in heterogeneity in response to rTMS therapy,[3] indicating the potential value of personalization of stimulation targeting.

Although this has generally been a fruitful method to drive the development of therapeutic applications of rTMS, an approach that seeks to identify localized changes in blood flow or metabolism may be insufficient to adequately identify targets that are more critical to the pathophysiology of most neuropsychiatric disorders. As is often the case, thinking about the pathophysiology of neuropsychiatric disorders has progressed with the evolution of the neuroscientific techniques that we are able to apply to understand these disorders. The initial use of structural imaging and metabolism and task-based functional magnetic resonance imaging (sMRI) generally identified specific regions in the brain that appeared to be abnormally active in individuals with specific disorders. This motivated theories around the role of individual brain regions and has certainly driven the development of a wide range of brain stimulation paradigms targeting specific localized brain changes.

However, our thinking about the pathophysiology of most neuropsychiatric disorders has progressed with the evolution of neuroscientific techniques. The use of diffusion tensor imaging to map white matter pathways and structural connectivity and the use of resting state fMRI scanning as well as other techniques being used to study functional connectivity has driven a major interest in understanding the role of distributed brain networks and increasing emphasis on trying to understand how dysfunction in these networks underpins disease. In this context, we are increasingly thinking of neuropsychiatric disorders as disorders of abnormal networks rather than of dysfunction in specific brain regions.[4]

9.2.1 Target Validation

A relevant aspect of the choice of stimulation location is the validation of whether the particular stimulation paradigm being utilized actually engages the target of relevance. This is relatively straightforward when rTMS is being applied to the motor cortex, where the evocation of a motor evoked potential is a clear demonstration of the activation of the relevant pathway. However, target validation is considerably more complicated for almost all other brain regions. However, prior to embarking on a substantive new therapeutic application with a brain stimulation technique like rTMS (but not limited to rTMS), it is a sensible first step to ensure that the stimulation parameters being adopted engage in a meaningful way the relevant target through which the proposed application is likely to work. This might involve the use of electrical field modeling or the conduct of preclinical studies demonstrating relevant changes with stimulation in some aspect of the function of the network being stimulated (e.g., demonstrating the change in a specific oscillation or basic cognitive function). Likewise, in interpreting the results of clinical trials of new brain stimulation techniques, it is important to understand whether or not the investigators have adequately established target validation. This is likely to become an increasingly critical part of justifying clinical trial design.

This has significant implications for how we conceptualize therapeutic targets for brain stimulation applications. If the intent is to modulate activity around a dysfunctional circuit, rather than changing local activity in a defined anatomical region, there are likely to be multiple targets to access this network either directly or indirectly. There are also likely to be nodes in these networks that are more critical. Some of these nodes may be

important because their stimulation allows us to have secondary effects around the network through the stimulation of neurons with projecting axons to other relevant regions.
Other nodes may be critical because they have specific properties such as "pacemaker
type" functions that drive the oscillatory frequencies relevant to specific network activity.
Therefore, the justification for a specific stimulation site should consider not just the local
anatomical properties and functional relevance of the targeted region but the specifics of
its connectivity and its role in broader network function. As such, we should consider
whether our primary target is in fact defined by local anatomy or whether the actual target
could be better defined as a specific structural or functional circuit of relevance to the disorder being targeted.

9.3 DETERMINATION OF A RELEVANT METHOD
TO ENSURE THAT STIMULATION IS APPLIED
ACCURATELY TO THE CHOSEN LOCATION

When rTMS was first used to stimulate the DLPFC, the target for an individual patient
was determined using the so-called *5 cm method*. This involved localizing the relevant
scalp motor area for activation of activity in a thumb or other hand muscle using single-
pulse stimulation around the motor cortex and then measuring 5 cm anterior to this along
the scalp surface. This produced an approximation of the localization of the DLPFC, but
the method was relatively quickly shown to be inaccurate, especially because it fails to
take into account any variation in head size and in general appears to fail to move the
coil sufficiently forward to ensure localization in the DLPFC in the majority of study
participants.[5]

A variety of alternative methods have been developed to address this limitation.
Simple modifications of the 5 cm rule have moved the coil further forward[6] and sometimes lateral (e.g., 6 cm forward and 1 cm lateral). A more significant divergence, which
does take head size into account, has been to adopt an approach based on measurements
of the location of electroencephalogram (EEG) electrodes, including the 10-20 EEG
system. Most commonly, the F3 EEG point has been used as an approximation of the
site of the relevant DLPFC. A specific algorithm has been developed and popularized
to allow for an estimation of the F3 EEG point without the requirement of complicated
scalp measurements (the *beam F3 method*).[7] This is an efficient method for localizing
an approximation of the F3 site, which is found to be systematically more anterior than
measurement 5 or 5.5 cm forward from the motor cortex.[5,8]

It is worth noting that the original research establishing the beam F3 method suggested that this produced localization consistent with that achieved by measuring up the
location of the F3 electrode using traditional 10-20 EEG methods. More recent research

has suggested that the beam F3 method results in a somewhat more anterior location to that produced with standard measurement. In fact, analysis of the brain location established across multiple studies using traditional 10-20 EEG measurements suggest that this method can produce quite variable location depending on the methods and the study approach adopted (see Figure 9.1).

The other significantly different technique that has evolved has used neuronavigational techniques to base scalp localization on individual MRI scan data (also see Chapter 2). Neuronavigational methods typically involve obtaining a relatively high-resolution T1 structural MRI scan and then using relevant hardware to co-register an individual participant's MRI scan to their head in 3D space. The neuronavigational equipment tracks the position of a probe or TMS coil in 3D space relevant to the participant's head and brain to allow the researcher to identify a specific region on the scalp that corresponds to a target on the brain as shown by the relevant software. Neuronavigational methods can simply show the coil and the projected magnetic field relevant to the target but can also include mapping of the e-field induced with the specific coil being utilized. Neuronavigational targeting can be based on simple brain anatomy or can use overlaid diffusion tensor imaging (DTI) or functional imaging data to allow the specific targeting of a pathway or functional region of interest. Targeting can also utilize normalized scans to allow consistent use of a specific target coordinate

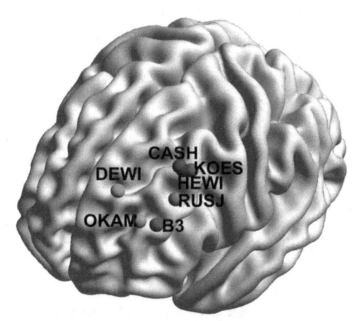

FIGURE 9.1 *Cortical representation of the site of stimulation produced with the Beam F3 method and standard 10-20 measurement across a series of published studies.*
From F3 sites: CASH = Cash et al.[9]; KOES = Koessler et al.[10]; HEWI = Herwig et al.[11]; DEWI = De Witte et al.[12]; RUSJ = Rusjan et al.[13]; OKAM = Okamoto et al.[14]

or use template brains to give an approximate location when individual MRI scans are not available.

A number of studies have compared the accuracy and fidelity of using different techniques to determine stimulation localization. These have clearly demonstrated that neuronavigational techniques are superior in ensuring accurate coil localization.[15] However, few studies have explored whether this degree of increased localization accuracy is associated with improved clinical outcomes. One clinical study showed that neuronavigationally localized stimulation produced superior outcomes in the treatment of depression compared to the 5 cm method, although this requires replication in a larger sample.[16] A more recent study failed to find differences in response to intermittent theta burst stimulation (iTBS) provided at the border between the anterior and middle third of the middle frontal gyrus using neuronavigation compared to localization to the F3 EEG site.[17] It is likely that there would have been a high degree of overlap between the treatment sites provided in the two arms in this study as the comparison condition, using treatment at the F3 EEG point, is likely to be more anterior to that found using the 5 cm method and would commonly overlap with the neuronavigationally targeted site.[18]

It is important to distinguish between the use of neuronavigational tools to determine stimulation location and the use of these tools in maximizing the fidelity of stimulation across multiple sessions of stimulation. In the former, neuronavigation is used to identify a particular scalp region corresponding to the desired brain target. Across multiple stimulation sessions, it may not be necessary to repeat the neuronavigational localization but to use other methods to ensure the coil is repeatedly placed in the same position. The use of neuronavigation to try to maximize fidelity of coil placement across multiple sessions requires repetition of the technique, which may have significant implications for treatment duration and cost. The value of these two elements should be evaluated separately.

A third element to consider is the use of this form of equipment to maximize fidelity *during* each treatment session. Neuronavigational tools can be used to ensure the coil has not moved off a target site during therapy and even be combined with robotic arms to automatically compensate when a patient moves their head.[19] There has not been any systematic evaluation of the implementation of tools of this sort.

Of note, it is also important not to automatically assume that improved fidelity or consistency of stimulation location will translate into improved outcomes. Although this seems like an obvious premise, if we are trying to stimulate a relatively large brain region, then some degree of variation in the stimulation location across time may actually enhance rather than undermine treatment efficacy. Determination of whether this is the case is likely to only be knowable through an optimal understanding of the methods through which the specific target can be engaged and then large-scale evaluation in clinical trials.

9.4 FREQUENCY OF STIMULATION

The choice of frequency of stimulation is a basic but critical element in developing and understanding rTMS treatment paradigms. Traditionally, rTMS paradigms are considered to be either low- or high-frequency, with stimulation frequencies around 1 Hz considered low-frequency and pretty much any frequency above this considered high although for practical purposes high-frequency protocols are usually between 5 and 20 Hz. One study found equivalent outcomes between 1 and 2 Hz stimulation applied to the right DLPFC in depressed patients, suggesting that there is not a clear frequency cutoff above 1 Hz.[20] Low-frequency stimulation has typically been regarded as inhibitory in nature or able to produce persistent reductions in cortical excitability.[21] In contrast, high-frequency stimulation is believed to induce increases in cortical excitability and local activation.

Although this distinction has been widely adopted, studies demonstrating these changes, predominately in motor cortex, do show a considerable degree of heterogeneity in responses across individual subjects.[21] In a similar way, more modern stimulation paradigms, including continuous and intermittent TBS (cTBS and iTBS, respectively) show similar but at times frustratingly inconsistent effects. cTBS has been shown to have effects similar to those induced with 1 Hz stimulation and iTBS to high-frequency stimulation, but, in individual participants, either paradigm can produce no change in cortical excitability or an opposite effect to that expected.[22] Thus, it remains somewhat unclear whether the effects of specific frequencies of rTMS utilized in therapeutic paradigms produce their effects in a frequency-dependent manner or whether the actual stimulation frequency is of relatively less importance than typically assumed.

Interpretation of these effects is also complicated by the investigative paradigms utilized. Generally speaking, most of our knowledge about the effects of individual frequencies of stimulation comes from single-session studies conducted in healthy control participants. In these studies, some measurement of cortical excitability (usually the size of motor evoked potentials produced by stimulation of the motor cortex or cortical evoked potentials measured with EEG outside the motor cortex) are assessed before and after a single session of stimulation. Clearly it is likely that differing effects on cortical excitability will be produced when stimulation sessions are repeated in therapeutic paradigms on a daily basis over multiple days. It also seems likely that the accumulative effect of stimulation will also significantly differ in patients with neuropsychiatric disorders who have abnormalities in cortical excitability compared to the effects we might see in healthy control individuals. There is clearly evidence that patients with disorders such as depression and schizophrenia display different neuroplastic responses to single trains of rTMS administered in experimental studies[23] but little research has explored the implications of this for therapy development.

9.5 TREATMENT SCHEDULING AND DOSE

How individual rTMS treatment sessions are structured and applied varies widely across clinical trials conducted to date and varies substantially even within one clinical application. The variables in this area include the number of rTMS trains applied in each stimulation session, the intertrain interval between stimulation trains, the number of treatment sessions applied, and the scheduling of these sessions across days and weeks. Although there is considerable variability in methods applied, some features of clinical protocol development (e.g., applying treatment once per day 5 days per week) have carried over from the very initial clinical rTMS trials and been little studied in a systematic way to establish optimal outcomes.

The majority of early clinical trials using TMS methods generally applied a relatively low number of stimulation trains (e.g., 10–20 trains of 10 Hz stimulation) for a relatively limited duration of often 5–10 days. Over time, there has been a progressive increase in most dose-related variables. Treatment paradigms have applied an increasingly large number of stimulation trains and have done so over increasingly longer courses of treatment. The pivotal rTMS trial that led to US approval in depression involved a 6-week treatment regime with an additional 2 weeks of tapering of therapy,[24] a substantial increase from the trials conducted prior to this, most of which ran for a maximum of 4 weeks. There certainly does appear to be indirect evidence that longer periods of treatment are associated with improved clinical outcomes because response and remission rates in depression seem to increase with longer periods of therapy.

Outside of the number of treatment days or duration of treatment, the majority of the other dose variables that are used to construct an rTMS treatment course have been subject to extremely limited or no systematic research whatsoever. For example, although the number of trains in an average rTMS treatment paradigm in depression has increased from around 20 to 75 per day across time, at this stage there are almost no published dose-finding studies exploring whether an increased number of trains is associated with improved clinical outcomes. A recent study found no clear and significant benefit of increasing the number of 10 Hz trains from 50 to 125 per day or increasing the duration of 1 Hz right-sided rTMS from 20 to 60 min per day.[25]

As alluded to earlier, there are also very few studies exploring the scheduling of rTMS treatment. The first conducted trials provided treatment on a daily basis 5 days per week, and this has really been mimicked in almost all therapeutic applications for more than 20 years. One clinical trial in depression has shown that applying treatment three times a week produces equivalent clinical benefits, although more slowly, then when treatment is applied in the standard 5 days.[26] The major innovation currently under way in this space is the exploration of so-called *accelerated* or *intensive treatment protocols*.[27–31] These have been developed with an intent to try to induce a more rapid antidepressant response through the provision of high doses of stimulation across a very limited number of days. There is evidence from these initial studies that accelerated or intensive TMS or TBS protocols produce similar efficacy to standard treatment approaches, but substantive trials have not yet established a more rapid onset of clinical benefits. Little research has explored these accelerated protocols in the treatment of other conditions beyond depression.

9.6 STIMULATION INTENSITY

The intensity of TMS pulses applied during rTMS therapy is typically determined in most applications as a proportion of an individual's resting motor threshold (RMT). This does provide a general estimation of cortical excitability for an individual participant although there are very limited grounds on which to assume that cortical excitability in nonmotor areas such as the DLPFC is going to closely reflect an individual's RMT. There is emerging research exploring whether electrical field modeling can be used as a better way of determining the intensity of stimulation required in an individual participant,[32] but this is not yet clinically applicable.

The overall intensity of stimulation in treatment paradigms has also increased progressively over time in the absence of a systematic demonstration that this has produced improved clinical outcomes. For example, early rTMS trials in depression applied stimulation at subthreshold intensities, often 80–90% of the RMT, whereas modern applications typically use stimulation intensities of around 120% of the RMT. The maximum stimulation intensity that can be used in any one application is limited due to safety concerns, but the field has progressively increased dose in most cases to the maximal limit without necessarily demonstrating the therapeutic benefit of this approach.

Of interest, studies have now demonstrated that there is a biphasic vascular response to increasing stimulation intensity. Stimulation applied to the DLPFC at sub-RMT levels typically produce a transient increase in blood flow consistent with a physiological vascular response to increased neuronal activity. In contrast, when stimulation intensity is increased in an individual participant to usually 110–120% of the RMT, a large reduction in oxygenation is seen on a nonphysiological scale suggesting the induction of some form of vasoconstrictor response.[33] No research has explored whether the pattern of better response to stimulation is associated with clinical or other neuroplastic physiological effects.

The change over time in stimulation intensity seen in rTMS studies has also been observed in the area of TBS research. TBS paradigms were initially developed using quite low intensities of stimulation, typically below the active motor threshold (which is again below the resting motor threshold). In fact, the neurophysiological effects of TBS have only really been seen at the subthreshold intensities. Initial clinical trials using TBS in depression adopted subthreshold stimulation, but, in more recent years, stimulation at 120% of the resting motor threshold has been widely adopted, including in the signifi-cant noninferiority trial that led to Food and Drug Administration approval of TBS in the United States.[34] There is some suggestion that the effects of TBS in prefrontal cortex may be bimodal, with a greater effects seen in healthy controls in single sessions at modest subthreshold intensities,[35] but how this translates to clinical outcomes remains com-pletely unclear.

9.7 COIL ORIENTATION

The orientation of the stimulation coil during the application of rTMS as a therapeutic tool is something that is almost universally ignored as a significant factor in the design of therapeutic applications. When single TMS pulses are applied to the motor cortex, it is well-established that a 45-degree angulation from the sagittal plane is usually optimal for the evocation of motor evoked potentials. When rTMS treatment was first proposed in the DLPFC, this coil angle was adopted by default. However, the orientation of gyri and superficial cortical neurons in the DLPFC differs substantially from that in the motor cortex, and it is unlikely that the optimal coil orientation for stimulation of the motor cortex will directly translate to the DLPFC or, for that matter, any other brain region. The limited research conducted addressing this issue supports this notion, demonstrating that the optimal coil angle for DLPFC stimulation varies substantially between individu-als[36] (also see Figure 9.2). Currently, however, we do not have a way to clinically utilize this information to optimize coil orientation during the treatment of individual patients, although approaches using electrical field modeling may prove useful.[32]

9.8 BRAIN ACTIVATION

Another factor that has been fairly systematically ignored until recently is consideration of the interaction between external brain stimulation and the state of the brain at the time of stimulation application. Studies using rTMS in depression have almost univer-sally done so when patients are at rest, although the vast majority of manuscripts do not describe the conditions for treatment or the instructions given to patients other than to indicate that they sat in a comfortable/reclining chair. There is considerable variability between clinics and how patients are managed during treatment: this can vary from patients falling asleep or watching television to being actively engaged in some sort of concurrent psychotherapy.

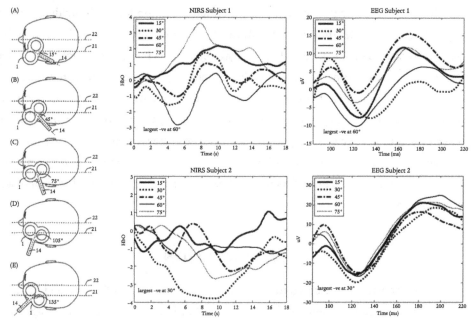

FIGURE 9.2 *Data from two individual participants showing differing patterns of physiological response assessed with near infrared spectroscopy (NIRS) and electroencephalography (EEG) to single transcranial magnetic stimulation (TMS) pulses applied to the left DLPFC at differing angles (15–75 degrees from the sagittal plane). In study participant 1, the greatest response is seen at an angle of 60 degrees, whereas the greatest effect in participant 2 is seen at 30 degrees.*

Despite this lack of research, there is a reasonably convincing number of studies emerging from cognitive neuroscience to suggest that the effects of exogenous brain stimulation are substantially influenced by underlying elements of brain activity. For example, the effects of single sessions of transcranial direct current stimulation (tDCS) on working memory are substantially greater if individuals engage in working memory tasks during stimulation.[37]

In addition, a small clinical study also demonstrated that the antidepressant effects of tDCS are significantly greater when patients engage in a cognitive activation task engaging the prefrontal cortex during exogenous stimulation of the same site.[38] More directly relevant, there is a slowly emerging literature to suggest that the effects of TMS are brain state–dependent in specific clinical applications. For example, the ability of rTMS to moderate symptoms of posttraumatic stress disorder (PTSD) was greater when patients were engaged in a process of recalling trauma stimuli prior to each rTMS treatment session compared to when rTMS was applied without any form of stimulus activation.[39] In addition, the protocol used in the recent development of deep TMS as a therapeutic option in obsessive-compulsive disorder (OCD) involves the induction of significant OCD symptoms prior to the provision of brain stimulation during each treatment session.[40]

Clearly, considering the optimal aspect of brain activation for any individual clinical application is a complex one and probably needs to be developed in consideration of the factors just discussed in regards to target engagement. The clinician must decide whether to activate a circuit or network that is dysfunctionally "overactive" with the intent to down-regulate or interrupt this overactivity with exogenous stimulation. In contrast, stimulation could be designed to help reinforce a healthy/functioning or underactive brain circuit, such as that underpinning positive affect. Regardless, an increased understanding of how exogenous stimulation such as rTMS interacts with ongoing symptom or non–symptom-related brain function will be critical to the future development of advanced protocols.

9.9 CONCLUSION

A series of important principles underpin the development and application of rTMS protocols regardless of the potential therapeutic application. Attempting to treat a mental health disorder or a specific symptom or subsyndrome of a disorder (e.g., auditory hallucinations in patients with schizophrenia) requires a careful consideration of the brain activity that underpins the relevant psychopathology and the development of a hypothesis about how this may be modified with brain stimulation alone or in combination with some form of activation paradigms. Once this target is established, the choice of stimulation parameters that may be utilized is extremely broad and should be strongly influenced by the development of methods to validate target engagement. We continue to require substantial systematic research to optimize stimulation parameters in all of the therapeutic areas of interest with rTMS, including in the most widely explored area, the use of this treatment in patients with depression.

REFERENCES

1. George MS, Ketter TA, Post RM. Prefrontal cortex dysfunction in clinical depression. *Depression.* 1994;2:59–72.
2. Silbersweig DA, Stern E, Frith C, Cahill C, Holmes A, Grootoonk S, et al. A functional neuroanatomy of hallucinations in schizophrenia. *Nature.* 1995;378:176–179.
3. Hoffman RE, Boutros NN, Berman RM, Roessler E, Belger A, Krystal JH, et al. Transcranial magnetic stimulation of left temporoparietal cortex in three patients reporting hallucinated "voices." *Biol Psychiatry.* 1999;46:130–132.
4. Downar J, Daskalakis ZJ. New targets for rTMS in depression: A review of convergent evidence. *Brain Stimul.* 2013;6:231–240.
5. Fitzgerald PB, Maller JJ, Hoy KE, Thomson R, Daskalakis ZJ. Exploring the optimal site for the localization of dorsolateral prefrontal cortex in brain stimulation experiments. *Brain Stimul.* 2009;2:234–237.
6. Johnson KA, Baig M, Ramsey D, Lisanby SH, Avery D, McDonald WM, et al. Prefrontal rTMS for treating depression: Location and intensity results from the OPT-TMS multi-site clinical trial. *Brain Stimul.* 2013;6:108–117.

7. Beam W, Borckardt JJ, Reeves ST, George MS. An efficient and accurate new method for locating the F3 position for prefrontal TMS applications. *Brain Stimul.* 2009;2:50–54.

8. Trapp NT, Bruss J, King Johnson M, Uitermarkt BD, Garrett L, Heinzerling A, et al. Reliability of targeting methods in TMS for depression: Beam F3 vs. 5.5 cm. *Brain Stimul.* 2020;13:578–581.

9. Cash RFH, Cocchi L, Lv J, Fitzgerald PB, Zalesky A. Functional magnetic resonance imaging–guided personalization of transcranial magnetic stimulation treatment for depression. *JAMA Psychiatry.* 2020;78(3):337–339.

10. Koessler L, Maillard L, Benhadid A, Vignal JP, Felblinger J, Vespignani H, et al. Automated cortical projection of EEG sensors: Anatomical correlation via the international 10-10 system. *Neuroimage.* 2009;46:64–72.

11. Herwig U, Satrapi P, Schonfeldt-Lecuona C. Using the international 10-20 EEG system for positioning of transcranial magnetic stimulation. *Brain Topogr.* 2003;16:95–99.

12. De Witte S, Klooster D, Dedoncker J, Duprat R, Remue J, Baeken C. Left prefrontal neuronavigated electrode localization in tDCS: 10-20 EEG system versus MRI-guided neuronavigation. *Psychiatry Res Neuroimaging.* 2018;274:1–6.

13. Rusjan PM, Barr MS, Farzan F, Arenovich T, Maller JJ, Fitzgerald PB, et al. Optimal transcranial magnetic stimulation coil placement for targeting the dorsolateral prefrontal cortex using novel magnetic resonance image-guided neuronavigation. *Hum Brain Mapp.* 2010;31(11):1643–1652.

14. Okamoto M, Dan H, Sakamoto K, Takeo K, Shimizu K, Kohno S, et al. Three-dimensional probabilistic anatomical cranio-cerebral correlation via the international 10-20 system oriented for transcranial functional brain mapping. *Neuroimage.* 2004;21:99–111.

15. Ahdab R, Ayache SS, Brugieres P, Goujon C, Lefaucheur JP. Comparison of "standard" and "navigated" procedures of TMS coil positioning over motor, premotor and prefrontal targets in patients with chronic pain and depression. *Neurophysiol Clin.* 2010;40:27–36.

16. Fitzgerald PB, Hoy K, McQueen S, Maller JJ, Herring S, Segrave R, et al. A randomized trial of rTMS targeted with MRI based neuro-navigation in treatment-resistant depression. *Neuropsychopharmacology.* 2009;34:1255–1262.

17. Hebel T, Gollnitz A, Schoisswohl S, Weber FC, Abdelnaim M, Wetter TC, et al. A direct comparison of neuronavigated and non-neuronavigated intermittent theta burst stimulation in the treatment of depression. *Brain Stimul.* 2021;14:335–343.

18. Fitzgerald PB. Targeting repetitive transcranial magnetic stimulation in depression: Do we really know what we are stimulating and how best to do it? *Brain Stimul.* 2021;14:730–736.

19. Goetz SM, Kozyrkov IC, Luber B, Lisanby SH, Murphy DLK, Grill WM, et al. Accuracy of robotic coil positioning during transcranial magnetic stimulation. *J Neural Eng.* 2019;16:054003.

20. Fitzgerald PB, Huntsman S, Gunewardene R, Kulkarni J, Daskalakis ZJ. A randomized trial of low-frequency right-prefrontal-cortex transcranial magnetic stimulation as augmentation in treatment-resistant major depression. *Int J Neuropsychopharmacol.* 2006;9:655–666.

21. Fitzgerald PB, Fountain S, Daskalakis ZJ. A comprehensive review of the effects of rTMS on motor cortical excitability and inhibition. *Clin Neurophysiol.* 2006;117:2584–2596.

22. Davidson JR, Meltzer-Brody SE. The underrecognition and undertreatment of depression: What is the breadth and depth of the problem? *J Clin Psychiatry.* 1999;60(Suppl 7):4–9;discussion 10–11.

23. Fitzgerald PB, Brown TL, Marston NA, Oxley T, De Castella A, Daskalakis ZJ, et al. Reduced plastic brain responses in schizophrenia: A transcranial magnetic stimulation study. *Schizophr Res.* 2004;71:17–26.

24. O'Reardon JP, Solvason HB, Janicak PG, Sampson S, Isenberg KE, Nahas Z, et al. Efficacy and safety of transcranial magnetic stimulation in the acute treatment of major depression: A multisite randomized controlled trial. *Biol Psychiatry.* 2007;62:1208–1216.

25. Fitzgerald PB, Hoy KE, Reynolds J, Singh A, Gunewardene R, Slack C, et al. A pragmatic randomized controlled trial exploring the relationship between pulse number and response to repetitive transcranial magnetic stimulation treatment in depression. *Brain Stimul.* 2020;13:145–152.

26. Galletly C, Gill S, Clarke P, Burton C, Fitzgerald PB. A randomized trial comparing repetitive transcranial magnetic stimulation given 3 days/week and 5 days/week for the treatment of major depression: Is efficacy related to the duration of treatment or the number of treatments? *Psychol Med.* 2011:1–8.

27. Baeken C, Marinazzo D, Wu GR, Van Schuerbeek P, De Mey J, Marchetti I, et al. Accelerated HF-rTMS in treatment-resistant unipolar depression: Insights from subgenual anterior cingulate functional connectivity. *World J Biol Psychiatry*. 2014;15:286–297.

28. Holtzheimer PE, 3rd, McDonald WM, Mufti M, Kelley ME, Quinn S, Corso G, et al. Accelerated repetitive transcranial magnetic stimulation for treatment-resistant depression. *Depress Anxiety*. 2010;27:960–963.

29. Fitzgerald PB, Chen L, Richardson K, Daskalakis ZJ, Hoy KE. A pilot investigation of an intensive theta burst stimulation protocol for patients with treatment resistant depression. *Brain Stimul*. 2020;13:137–144.

30. Fitzgerald PB, Hoy KE, Elliot D, Susan McQueen RN, Wambeek LE, Daskalakis ZJ. Accelerated repetitive transcranial magnetic stimulation in the treatment of depression. *Neuropsychopharmacology*. 2018;43:1565–1572.

31. Kaster TS, Chen L, Daskalakis ZJ, Hoy KE, Blumberger DM, Fitzgerald PB. Depressive symptom trajectories associated with standard and accelerated rTMS. *Brain Stimul*. 2020;13:850–857.

32. Gomez LJ, Dannhauer M, Koponen LM, Peterchev AV. Conditions for numerically accurate TMS electric field simulation. *Brain Stimul*. 2020;13:157–166.

33. Thomson RH, Rogasch NC, Maller JJ, Daskalakis ZJ, Fitzgerald PB. Intensity dependent repetitive transcranial magnetic stimulation modulation of blood oxygenation. *J Affect Disord*. 2012;136:1243–1246.

34. Blumberger DM, Vila-Rodriguez F, Thorpe KE, Feffer K, Noda Y, Giacobbe P, et al. Effectiveness of theta burst versus high-frequency repetitive transcranial magnetic stimulation in patients with depression (THREE-D): A randomised non-inferiority trial. *Lancet*. 2018;391:1683–1692.

35. Chung SW, Rogasch NC, Hoy KE, Sullivan CM, Cash RFH, Fitzgerald PB. Impact of different intensities of intermittent theta burst stimulation on the cortical properties during TMS-EEG and working memory performance. *Hum Brain Mapp*. 2018;39:783–802.

36. Thomson RH, Cleve TJ, Bailey NW, Rogasch NC, Maller JJ, Daskalakis ZJ, et al. Blood oxygenation changes modulated by coil orientation during prefrontal transcranial magnetic stimulation. *Brain Stimul*. 2013;6:576–581.

37. Andrews SC, Hoy KE, Enticott PG, Daskalakis ZJ, Fitzgerald PB. Improving working memory: The effect of combining cognitive activity and anodal transcranial direct current stimulation to the left dorsolateral prefrontal cortex. *Brain Stimul*. 2011;4:84–89.

38. Segrave RA, Arnold S, Hoy K, Fitzgerald PB. Concurrent cognitive control training augments the antidepressant efficacy of tDCS: A pilot study. *Brain Stimul*. 2014;7:325–331.

39. Isserles M, Shalev AY, Roth Y, Peri T, Kutz I, Zlotnick E, et al. Effectiveness of deep transcranial magnetic stimulation combined with a brief exposure procedure in post-traumatic stress disorder: A pilot study. *Brain Stimul*. 2013;6:377–383.

40. Carmi L, Tendler A, Bystritsky A, Hollander E, Blumberger DM, Daskalakis J, et al. Efficacy and safety of deep transcranial magnetic stimulation for obsessive-compulsive disorder: A prospective multicenter randomized double-blind placebo-controlled trial. *Am J Psychiatry*. 2019;176:931–938.

Clinical Applications of Transcranial Magnetic Stimulation in Stroke

10.1 INTRODUCTION

Single- and paired-transcranial magnetic stimulation (TMS), discussed in detail in Chapter 3, have been used in stroke as a prognostic tool, to understand the pathophysiology of stroke and the mechanisms of recovery. Different repetitive TMS (rTMS) protocols (discussed in Chapter 4), mainly low- and high-frequency rTMS and theta burst stimulation (TBS) protocols, are being tested as a treatment to modulate cortical excitability to promote beneficial plasticity.

10.2 ROLE OF TMS IN THE PROGNOSIS OF RECOVERY FROM STROKE

While the degree of early motor impairment is related to recovery of function in stroke patients, there is wide variation in recovery in patients with similar initial presentations.[1] The ability of TMS to evoke motor-evoked potentials (MEPs) in the upper limb is associated with greater potential for recovery.[2,3] A systematic review found that 14 out of 15 studies reported that TMS of the motor cortex eliciting MEPs within 2 weeks of stroke is a prognostic tool for recovery of upper limb function.[4] Stroke patients who had recordable MEP in their upper limbs can be expected to recover about 70% of their maximum potential recovery as measured with the Fugl-Meyer upper limb scale, known as the *proportional recovery rule*, whereas patients without recordable MEP had less recovery (Figure 10.1).[5,6] However, patients without recordable MEP may also achieve meaningful

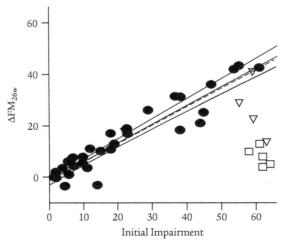

FIGURE 10.1 *Proportional resolution of impairment depends on corticomotor pathway integrity and initial impairment. The vertical axis represents change in Fugl-Meyer scale scores from 2 weeks to 26 weeks post-stroke after standardized upper limb therapy. The horizontal axis represents the initial impairment and the available improvement. Dashed line indicates the 70% rule prediction. Linear regression and 95% confidence intervals are plotted for those expected to conform to the rule (filled circles). Participants are coded by motor-evoked potential (MEP) status and fractional anisotropy asymmetric index (FAAI) in the posterior limb of the internal capsule. Circles: MEP+; open triangles: MEP– and FAAI <0.15 (no symmetry); open squares: MEP– and FAAI >0.15 (asymmetry). For MEP+ patients, recovery is proportional to the available improvement.*
FROM BYBLOW ET AL., *ANN NEUROL.* 2015;78(6):848–859, WITH PERMISSION.

improvement with neuromodulation paired with motor training.[7] Stroke patients with absence of MEP in the biceps muscle are more likely to have voluntary contraction of the muscle compared to those with absence of MEP in the first dorsal interosseous (FDI) muscle, suggesting that alternative pathways to the corticospinal tract are more likely to mediate volitional contraction of proximal than distal muscles.[8]

Algorithms that combine clinical assessment together with TMS and magnetic resonance imaging (MRI) to predict upper limb function have been developed.[9] An updated algorithm, the Predict Recovery Potential 2 (PREP2), uses clinical scores and presence or absence of MEP at 3–7 days post-stroke can make accurate prediction of upper limb function in 75% of patients (Figure 10.2).[10] Predictions made within days of stroke was accurate for 80% of patients at 2-year post-stroke,[11] but predictions made at 2 weeks post-stroke may be less accurate.[12] Thus, TMS is a useful measure to test the integrity of the corticospinal pathway to help predict recovery and direct rehabilitation therapies.

The presence of ipsilateral MEP in the paretic limb from M1 stimulation in the healthy hemisphere has been associated with poor recovery from stroke,[13,14] and this was also observed in children.[15] However, ipsilateral MEP in the paretic arm from premotor stimulation could be associated with good recovery.[16] A study showed that study participants with stroke had higher ipsilateral MEP amplitudes in the biceps muscle but lower ipsilateral MEP amplitude in the first dorsal interosseous (FDI) muscle compared

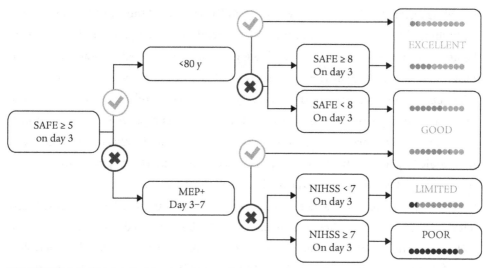

FIGURE 10.2 *The Predict Recovery Potential 2 (PREP2) algorithm predicts upper limb functional outcome at 3 months post-stroke. The four possible upper limb outcomes are color-coded. The colored dots depict the proportion of patients expected to achieve each color-coded outcome, depending on their pathway through the algorithm, based on the results of the classification and regression tree analysis. Patients who achieve a SAFE score (sum of Medical Research Council grades for shoulder abduction and finger extension for the paretic arm 3 days after stroke) of five or more within 72 h of stroke symptom onset and are younger than 80 years are most likely to have an Excellent upper limb outcome. Patients who achieve a SAFE score of five or more within 72 h of stroke symptom onset and are 80 years old or older are most likely to have an Excellent upper limb outcome provided their SAFE score is at least 8; otherwise, they are likely to have a Good upper limb outcome. Patients whose SAFE score is less than 5 at 72 h after stroke symptom onset need transcranial magnetic stimulation (TMS) to determine motor-evoked potential (MEP) status in the paretic upper limb, a key biomarker of corticospinal tract integrity. If a MEP can be elicited (MEP+) approximately 5 days post-stroke, then the patient is likely to have at least a Good upper limb outcome. If a MEP cannot be elicited, the National Institutes of Health Stroke Scale (NIHSS) score obtained 3 days post-stroke can be used to predict either a Limited outcome if the score is less than 7 or a Poor outcome if the score is 7 or more.*FROM STINEAR ET AL., ANN CLIN TRANSLAT NEUROL. 2017;4(11):811–820, WITH PERMISSION.

to normal individuals, suggesting that there is stronger corticoreticulospinal projections to proximal muscles after stroke.[17]

10.3 ROLE OF TMS IN UNDERSTANDING THE PATHOPHYSIOLOGY OF STROKE AND IN OUTCOME ASSESSMENT

The motor cortex plays a critical role in the motor deficits and recovery from stroke. The motor cortex is the primary contributor to corticospinal tract fibers and is particularly important for fine finger movements. In stroke, there are changes in cortical excitability such as motor threshold (MT), recruitment curve, and cortical inhibition, and these changes depend on lesion location.[18] As expected, a meta-analysis of TMS measures in adult stroke patients that included 112 studies reported that basic measures of M1 excitability including resting MT (RMT), active MT (AMT), MEP amplitude, and latency consistently showed lower excitability in the affected hemisphere compared to the unaffected hemisphere and healthy controls.[19] Following motor cortical rTMS, motor function improvement was associated with increased excitability of the affected motor cortex.[20-23] Silent period duration was longer in the early post-stroke period in the affected than the unaffected hemisphere but was shorter in the affected hemisphere in chronic stroke.[19] Short-interval intracortical inhibition (SICI) was reduced in the affected hemisphere in both adult[18,24] and pediatric stroke subjects.[15] In the unaffected hemisphere, SICI was initially decreased but may return to normal values with recovery of motor functions.[25] These results were consistent with a meta-analysis which reported that SICI was decreased early after stroke in the affected hemisphere compared to the unaffected hemisphere and controls but that there were no differences in chronic stroke patients compared to controls.[19]

TMS mapping studies showed that a shift in the TMS motor map correlated with grip strength in the affected hand, suggesting that cortical plasticity after subcortical stroke is associated with better motor function.[26] Moreover, enlargement of the hand area of the motor cortex assessed by TMS mapping correlates with better motor outcome after stroke[27,28] and with improvement after rehabilitation therapy.[29]

A meta-analysis found that measures of interhemispheric inhibition (IHI) including ipsilateral silent period and IHI measured by the double-coil method were not different between the affected and unaffected hemispheres. Moreover, no difference was found between the unaffected hemisphere and controls, but there were few studies with high heterogeneity and most studies had a small number of subjects.[19] A study examined changes in IHI at interstimulus interval of 10 ms (IHI10) in the reaction time (pre-movement) period, which in normal subject decreases close to the time of movement onset. Premovement IHI10 was normal the acute and subacute stages of stroke but became abnormal in chronic stroke, with excessive inhibition near the time of movement onset.[30] These findings raised questions regarding the interhemispheric balance model of stroke (see later discussion).

A meta-analysis found that central motor conduction time (CMCT) did not show overall difference between affected hemispheres and controls, but may be prolonged in patients with chronic stroke.[19] A study suggested that CMCT may be prolonged in the unaffected hemisphere and could be associated with poor recovery of upper limb functions.[31]

10.4 RTMS AS TREATMENT OF STROKE

Most rTMS treatment studies in stroke are based on the widely held model of disturbance of hemispheric balance in stroke. Cortical excitability is increased in the unaffected motor cortex compared to the affected motor cortex due to decreased transcallosal inhibition from the affected to the unaffected motor cortex and increased transcallosal inhibition from the unaffected to the affected motor cortex, resulting in hemispheric imbalance.[32–34] Thus, the lesioned cortex is considered underactive and the homologous contralateral region is considered overactive. However, some studies found normal IHI in stroke patients, suggesting that excessive IHI may not be the cause of poor motor recovery.[19,30] Nevertheless, this proposal led to the concept of treatment of stroke by increasing the excitability of the lesioned cortex or by decreasing the excitability of the contralateral, unaffected cortex. The intervention may change local cortical excitability and also affects connectivity.

10.4.1 Excitatory rTMS to the Affected Hemisphere

In patients with acute to subacute stroke, a study reported benefit with 3 and 10 Hz rTMS to the affected M1 for 5 days, which persisted at 1 year.[35] The beneficial effects in subcortical stroke may be more marked than in cortical stroke.[36] In an evidence-based guideline, ipsilesional high-frequency rTMS was given Level B evidence of probable efficacy in subacute (between 1 week and 6 months of stroke onset) stroke.[37] There are few studies of intermittent TBS (iTBS) of the ipsilesional motor cortex in subacute stroke but one study found that it led to stronger recovery of grip strength.[38]

A study in chronic stroke found that 10 Hz rTMS to the M1 in the affected hemisphere increased cortical excitability and enhanced motor performance compared to sham stimulation.[21] One study found that iTBS of the affected hemisphere did not augment the results of a rehabilitation program in chronic stroke,[39] but another study reported that iTBS improved hand motor function.[40] An evidence-based guideline concluded that there are too few studies to provide recommendation for ipsilesional high-frequency rTMS or iTBS in chronic stroke.[37]

10.4.2 Inhibitory rTMS to the Unaffected Hemisphere

An evidence-based guideline concluded that the number and quality of studies of low-frequency (1 Hz) rTMS to contralesional motor cortex for subacute stroke reached Level A evidence of definite efficacy for improvement in hand function.[37] Previous studies have used between 5 and 30 daily sessions of low-frequency rTMS. rTMS was often used as priming before 30–60 min of physical therapy, and the effects may persist up to 6 months.[37] This is similar to the finding of an earlier systematic review of low-frequency rTMS of the unaffected hemisphere in stroke patients that examined 67 articles.[41] Inhibitory rTMS was found to have beneficial effects in stroke patients with motor impairment, spasticity, aphasia, hemispatial neglect, and dysphagia. Multiple sessions of rTMS in combination with rehabilitation therapy may increase the therapeutic effect. The effects in patients treated early after stroke could be long-lasting.[41] Another meta-analysis also reached similar conclusions.[42] However, large, randomized controlled trials are still needed to confirm these findings.

In chronic stroke, five sessions of inhibitory 1 Hz rTMS to the unaffected M1 were found to improve motor functions of the affected hand for 2 weeks,[20] and several other studies reported similar results.[43] However, a large study with results from 169 participants at 3 to 12 months post-stroke found no effect of 1 Hz rTMS to the unaffected hemisphere compared to sham stimulation before motor rehabilitation.[44] An evidence-based guideline concluded that there is a Level C recommendation of probable efficacy for low-frequency rTMS for recovery of hand function in chronic stroke.[37] Two studies found no benefit of cTBS of the unaffected hemisphere in subacute or chronic stroke.[39,45]

10.4.3 Excitatory TMS to the Unaffected Hemisphere

In patients with severe hemiplegia from subacute stroke (2 weeks to 3 months earlier), 2 weeks of high-frequency (10 Hz) rTMS to the contralesional motor cortex produced significant improvement in motor function, whereas the results of low-frequency (1 Hz) rTMS was no different from sham stimulation.[46]

10.4.4 Comparison of rTMS to Affected Versus Unaffected Hemisphere

Some studies compared treatment that aimed to increase the excitability of the stroke hemisphere to those that aimed to decrease the excitability of the unaffected hemisphere. One study in acute stroke found that high-frequency rTMS to the lesioned hemisphere produced better recovery of motor function than low-frequency rTMS to the contralesional hemisphere, but there was no long-term follow-up.[47] Another acute stroke study reported that both high-frequency (10 Hz) rTMS to the affected hemisphere and low-frequency (1 Hz) rTMS to the unaffected hemisphere led to greater improvement than sham stimulation, with no significant difference between high- and low-frequency stimulation.[48] A study in acute stroke reported that ipsilesional iTBS improved movement of the affected limb whereas 1 Hz rTMS of the unaffected motor cortex reduced spasticity.[49] In contrast, another study reported that both 1 Hz rTMS to the unaffected hemisphere and 3 Hz rTMS to the affected hemisphere improved motor function in acute stroke, with greater improvement in arm function for 1 Hz rTMS at 3 months.[50] Thus, the relative efficacy of excitatory versus inhibitory rTMS protocols in different types of stroke has not been established.

10.4.5 Combining Excitatory rTMS to Affected Hemisphere and Inhibitory rTMS to Unaffected Hemisphere

Several studies applied excitatory rTMS to the affected hemisphere and inhibitory rTMS to the unaffected hemisphere in the same session. In a study in acute (within 2 weeks) stroke, 4 weeks of 10 Hz rTMS to the affected motor cortex followed by 1 Hz rTMS to the unaffected motor cortex produced greater motor improvement than 10 Hz or 1 Hz rTMS alone or sham stimulation.[51] In patients with subacute[52] or chronic stroke,[53] combined 1 Hz rTMS to the unaffected motor cortex and iTBS to the affected motor cortex resulted in greater improvement compared to 1 Hz rTMS or iTBS alone. Thus, combining excitatory stimulation to the affected hemisphere and inhibitory stimulation to the unaffected hemisphere is a promising approach, but more studies are needed.

10.4.6 Treatment of Aphasia and Hemineglect

In addition to treatment of motor deficit, rTMS has also been tested as treatment of aphasia and hemineglect from stroke. Most studies in post-stroke aphasia applied contralesional low-frequency 1 Hz rTMS to the right homologue of Broca's area in the inferior frontal gyrus. This approach may be more effective in nonfluent Broca's aphasia than in other forms of aphasia. An evidence-based guideline concluded that there is Level B evidence of probable efficacy for low-frequency rTMS to the right inferior gyrus for treatment of nonfluent aphasia, particularly when combined with speech therapy.[37] A meta-analysis also concluded that low-frequency rTMS can improve language performance in chronic stroke.[54]

Hemispatial neglect is typically caused by stroke in the right middle cerebral territory affecting the right posterior parietal and superior temporal areas. Most studies used inhibitory rTMS (e.g., 1 Hz[55] or cTBS[56]) to the left posterior parietal cortex. However, some studies used high-[57] or low-frequency[58] rTMS to the posterior parietal cortex in the lesioned right hemisphere and reported beneficial results. Based on several studies of cTBS to the contralesional left posterior parietal cortex,[56,59–61] an evidence-based guideline concluded that there was Level C evidence of possible efficacy for this treatment.[37] However, a study reported that cTBS to the intact left parietal cortex did not produce additional benefit when combined with prism adaptation.[62]

10.4.7 Treatment of Pediatric Stroke

Most rTMS studies in stroke are in the adult populations, and only a few studies examined pediatric stroke, even though the potential for brain plasticity may be higher in children. A study in children with cerebral palsy reported that 5 Hz but not 1 Hz rTMS or sham stimulation reduced spasticity.[63] Contralesional 1 Hz rTMS was found to improve hand functions in study of 10 pediatric patients with subcortical arterial ischemic stroke.[64] Another study observed an additive effect of contralesional 1 Hz rTMS and constraint-induced movement therapy in 45 children with perinatal stroke-induced hemiparesis (Figure 10.3).[65] rTMS is safe in children,[66] although syncope has been reported.[67]

10.4.8 Variability of Response to rTMS and Genetic Factors in Stroke

Similar to other neurological and psychiatric conditions, the responses to rTMS in stroke patients are variable and this is a barrier in developing TMS as a treatment. A study reported that stroke patients with the Val/Val genotype of brain-derived neurotrophic factor (BDNF) val66met polymorphism showed greater improvement with 10 Hz rTMS to the M1 in the ipsilesional hemisphere than participants with the Met allele.[68] The Val/Val group also showed greater increase in MEP amplitude with high-frequency, supra-threshold rTMS than Met carriers in another study.[69] However, more work is needed to determine how genetic variations influence the effects of rTMS and rehabilitation in stroke.

10.5 CONCLUSION AND FUTURE PERSPECTIVES

The effects of rTMS on stroke likely depend on many factors including the lesion location (i.e., cortical, subcortical), brainstem strokes, lesion size, and the time since stroke occurred. The effects in acute, subacute, and chronic stroke may differ. Most published studies examined upper limb functions in subacute or chronic stroke. There are relatively few studies in acute stroke[70] and in the lower limbs.

While rTMS is a promising treatment for stroke, there is currently insufficient evidence to recommend it as a standard treatment. Further large randomized controlled trials with adequate sham control are needed. While earlier studies mostly used rTMS as the only treatment, more recent studies have tested rTMS combined with rehabilitation therapies to harness their potentially synergistic effects on neuroplasticity.

A potentially important consideration is the role of the contralateral, unaffected hemisphere in recovery from stroke. In patients with intact or minimal damage to the corticospinal tract, descending drive from the unaffected ipsilateral reticulospinal tract may interfere with the function of the contralateral corticospinal pathway.[71] In these patients, inhibitory rTMS to the contralesional hemisphere may be a useful treatment. However, in patients with severely damaged corticospinal pathway, involvement of the unaffected, ipsilateral cortico-reticulo-propriospinal pathway may be beneficial.[71] In this situation,

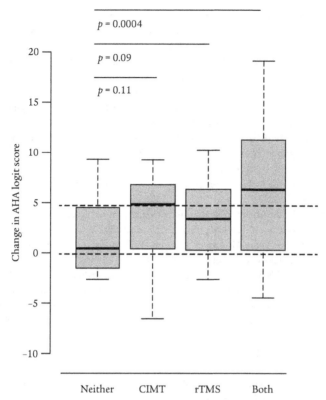

FIGURE 10.3 *Brain stimulation and constraint for perinatal stroke hemiparesis. Assisting Hand Assessment (AHA) scores across time and treatment. Largest changes at 6 months were observed with repetitive transcranial magnetic stimulation (rTMS) + constraint-induced movement therapy (CIMT). Top dashed line indicates clinically significant change of ≥5 logit units.*
From Kirton et al., Neurology. 2016;86(18):1659–1667, with permission.

excitatory rather than inhibitory stimulation of the contralesional hemisphere may be indicated.[46]

It will be crucial to understand factors that account for the variability in response to rTMS including corticospinal excitability; cortical inhibitory and facilitatory circuits; clinical measures; imaging findings such as lesion size and location; functional connectivity; and genetic factors. A combination of these factors may determine the optimal stimulation site and parameters and predict the response to rTMS. Future work may lead to a personalized approach to the treatment of stroke.

REFERENCES

1. Smith MC, Stinear CM. Transcranial magnetic stimulation (TMS) in stroke: Ready for clinical practice? *J Clin Neurosci Australasia.* 2016;31:10–14.
2. Heald A, Bates D, Cartlidge NE, French JM, Miller S. Longitudinal study of central motor conduction time following stroke. 1. Natural history of central motor conduction. *Brain.* 1993;116 (Pt 6):1355–1370.

3. Delvaux V, Alagona G, Gerard P, De Pasqua V, Pennisi G, Maertens de Noordhout A. Post-stroke reorganization of hand motor area: A 1-year prospective follow-up with focal transcranial magnetic stimulation. *Clin Neurophysiol.* 2003;114(7):1217–1225.

4. Bembenek JP, Kurczych K, Karli Nski M, Czlonkowska A. The prognostic value of motor-evoked potentials in motor recovery and functional outcome after stroke: A systematic review of the literature. *Funct Neurol.* 2012;27(2):79–84.

5. Byblow WD, Stinear CM, Barber PA, Petoe MA, Ackerley SJ. Proportional recovery after stroke depends on corticomotor integrity. *Ann Neurol.* 2015;78(6):848–859.

6. Stinear CM, Byblow WD, Ackerley SJ, Smith MC, Borges VM, Barber PA. Proportional Motor Recovery After Stroke: Implications for Trial Design. *Stroke.* 2017;48(3):795–798.

7. Powell ES, Westgate PM, Goldstein LB, Sawaki L. Absence of motor-evoked potentials does not predict poor recovery in patients with severe-moderate stroke: An exploratory analysis. *Arch Rehabil Res Clin Transl.* 2019;1(3-4):100023.

8. Schambra HM, Xu J, Branscheidt M, et al. Differential post-stroke motor recovery in an arm versus hand muscle in the absence of motor evoked potentials. *Neurorehabil Neural Repair.* 2019;33(7):568–580.

9. Stinear CM, Barber PA, Petoe M, Anwar S, Byblow WD. The PREP algorithm predicts potential for upper limb recovery after stroke. *Brain.* 2012;135(Pt 8):2527–2535.

10. Stinear CM, Byblow WD, Ackerley SJ, Smith MC, Borges VM, Barber PA. PREP2: A biomarker-based algorithm for predicting upper limb function after stroke. *Ann Clin Transl Neurol.* 2017;4(11):811–820.

11. Smith MC, Ackerley SJ, Barber PA, Byblow WD, Stinear CM. PREP2 algorithm predictions are correct at 2 years post-stroke for most patients. *Neurorehabil Neural Repair.* 2019;33(8):635–642.

12. Lundquist CB, Nielsen JF, Arguissain FG, Brunner IC. Accuracy of the upper limb prediction algorithm PREP2 applied 2 weeks post-stroke: A prospective longitudinal study. *Neurorehabil Neural Repair.* 2021;35(1):68–78.

13. Netz J, Lammers T, Homberg V. Reorganization of motor output in the non-affected hemisphere after stroke. *Brain.* 1997;120 (Pt 9):1579–1586.

14. Gerloff C, Bushara K, Sailer A, et al. Multimodal imaging of brain reorganization in motor areas of the contralesional hemisphere of well recovered patients after capsular stroke. *Brain.* 2006;129(Pt 3):791–808.

15. Zewdie E, Damji O, Ciechanski P, Seeger T, Kirton A. Contralesional corticomotor neurophysiology in hemiparetic children with perinatal stroke. *Neurorehabil Neural Repair.* 2017;31(3):261–271.

16. Caramia MD, Palmieri MG, Giacomini P, Iani C, Dally L, Silvestrini M. Ipsilateral activation of the unaffected motor cortex in patients with hemiparetic stroke. *Clin Neurophysiol.* 2000;111(11):1990–1996.

17. Taga M, Charalambous CC, Raju S, et al. Corticoreticulospinal tract neurophysiology in an arm and hand muscle in healthy and stroke subjects. *J Physiol.* 2021;599(16):3955–3971.

18. Liepert J, Restemeyer C, Kucinski T, Zittel S, Weiller C. Motor strokes: The lesion location determines motor excitability changes. *Stroke.* 2005;36(12):2648–2653.

19. McDonnell MN, Stinear CM. TMS measures of motor cortex function after stroke: A meta-analysis. *Brain Stimul.* 2017;10(4):721–734.

20. Fregni F, Boggio PS, Valle AC, et al. A sham-controlled trial of a 5-day course of repetitive transcranial magnetic stimulation of the unaffected hemisphere in stroke patients. *Stroke.* 2006;37(8):2115–2122.

21. Kim YH, You SH, Ko MH, et al. Repetitive transcranial magnetic stimulation-induced corticomotor excitability and associated motor skill acquisition in chronic stroke. *Stroke.* 2006;37(6):1471–1476.

22. Hummel F, Celnik P, Giraux P, et al. Effects of non-invasive cortical stimulation on skilled motor function in chronic stroke. *Brain.* 2005;128(Pt 3):490–499.

23. Khedr EM, Ahmed MA, Fathy N, Rothwell JC. Therapeutic trial of repetitive transcranial magnetic stimulation after acute ischemic stroke. *Neurology.* 2005;65(3):466–468.

24. Manganotti P, Patuzzo S, Cortese F, Palermo A, Smania N, Fiaschi A. Motor disinhibition in affected and unaffected hemisphere in the early period of recovery after stroke. *Clin Neurophysiol.* 2002;113(6):936–943.

25. Bütefisch CM, Wessling M, Netz J, Seitz RJ, Hömberg V. Relationship between interhemispheric inhibition and motor cortex excitability in subacute stroke patients. *Neurorehabil Neural Repair.* 2008;22(1):4–21.

26. Thickbroom GW, Byrnes ML, Archer SA, Mastaglia FL. Motor outcome after subcortical stroke correlates with the degree of cortical reorganization. *Clin Neurophysiol.* 2004;115(9):2144–2150.

27. Traversa R, Cicinelli P, Bassi A, Rossini PM, Bernardi G. Mapping of motor cortical reorganization after stroke. A brain stimulation study with focal magnetic pulses. *Stroke.* 1997;28:110–117.

28. Cicinelli P, Traversa R, Rossini PM. Post-stroke reorganization of brain motor output to the hand: A 2-4 month follow-up with focal magnetic transcranial magnetic stimulation. *Electroencephalogr Clin Neurophysiol.* 1997;105:438–450.

29. Liepert J, Bauder H, Wolfgang HR, Miltner WH, Taub E, Weiller C. Treatment-induced cortical reorganization after stroke in humans. *Stroke.* 2000;31(6):1210–1216.

30. Xu J, Branscheidt M, Schambra H, et al. Rethinking interhemispheric imbalance as a target for stroke neurorehabilitation. *Ann Neurol.* 2019;85(4):502–513.

31. Hoonhorst MHJ, Nijland RHM, Emmelot CH, Kollen BJ, Kwakkel G. TMS-induced central motor conduction time at the non-infarcted hemisphere is associated with spontaneous motor recovery of the paretic upper limb after severe stroke. *Brain Sci.* 2021;11(5):648.

32. Shimizu T, Hosaki A, Hino T, et al. Motor cortical disinhibition in the unaffected hemisphere after unilateral cortical stroke. *Brain.* 2002;125(Pt 8):1896–1907.

33. Murase N, Duque J, Mazzocchio R, Cohen LG. Influence of interhemispheric interactions on motor function in chronic stroke. *Ann Neurol.* 2004;55(3):400–409.

34. Fregni F, Pascual-Leone A. Technology insight: Noninvasive brain stimulation in neurology-perspectives on the therapeutic potential of rTMS and tDCS. *Nat Clin Pract Neurol.* 2007;3(7):383–393.

35. Khedr EM, Etraby AE, Hemeda M, Nasef AM, Razek AA. Long-term effect of repetitive transcranial magnetic stimulation on motor function recovery after acute ischemic stroke. *Acta Neurol Scand.* 2010;121(1):30–37.

36. Lefaucheur JP, André-Obadia N, Antal A, et al. Evidence-based guidelines on the therapeutic use of repetitive transcranial magnetic stimulation (rTMS). *Clin Neurophysiol.* 2014;125(11):2150–2206.

37. Lefaucheur JP, Aleman A, Baeken C, et al. Evidence-based guidelines on the therapeutic use of repetitive transcranial magnetic stimulation (rTMS): An update (2014-2018). *Clin Neurophysiol.* 2020;131(2):474–528.

38. Volz LJ, Rehme AK, Michely J, et al. Shaping early reorganization of neural networks promotes motor function after stroke. *Cerebral Cortex (New York, NY: 1991).* 2016;26(6):2882–2894.

39. Talelli P, Wallace A, Dileone M, et al. Theta burst stimulation in the rehabilitation of the upper limb: A semirandomized, placebo-controlled trial in chronic stroke patients. *Neurorehabil Neural Repair.* 2012;26(8):976–987.

40. Lai CJ, Wang CP, Tsai PY, et al. Corticospinal integrity and motor impairment predict outcomes after excitatory repetitive transcranial magnetic stimulation: A preliminary study. *Arch Phys Med Rehabil.* 2015;96(1):69–75.

41. Sebastianelli L, Versace V, Martignago S, et al. Low-frequency rTMS of the unaffected hemisphere in stroke patients: A systematic review. *Acta Neurol Scand.* 2017;136(6):585–605.

42. Zhang L, Xing G, Shuai S, et al. Low-frequency repetitive transcranial magnetic stimulation for stroke-induced upper limb motor deficit: A meta-analysis. *Neural Plasticity.* 2017;2017:2758097.

43. Bonin Pinto C, Morales-Quezada L, de Toledo Piza PV, et al. Combining fluoxetine and rTMS in post-stroke motor recovery: A placebo-controlled double-blind randomized phase 2 clinical trial. *Neurorehabil Neural Repair.* 2019;33(8):643–655.

44. Harvey RL, Edwards D, Dunning K, et al. Randomized sham-controlled trial of navigated repetitive transcranial magnetic stimulation for motor recovery in stroke. *Stroke.* 2018;49(9):2138–2146.

45. Nicolo P, Magnin C, Pedrazzini E, et al. Comparison of neuroplastic responses to cathodal transcranial direct current stimulation and continuous theta burst stimulation in subacute stroke. *Arch Phys Med Rehabil.* 2018;99(5):862–872.e861.

46. Wang Q, Zhang D, Zhao YY, Hai H, Ma YW. Effects of high-frequency repetitive transcranial magnetic stimulation over the contralesional motor cortex on motor recovery in severe hemiplegic stroke: A randomized clinical trial. *Brain Stimul.* 2020;13(4):979–986.

47. Sasaki N, Mizutani S, Kakuda W, Abo M. Comparison of the effects of high- and low-frequency repetitive transcranial magnetic stimulation on upper limb hemiparesis in the early phase of stroke. *J Stroke Cerebrovasc Dis.* 2013;22(4):413–418.

48. Du J, Yang F, Hu J, et al. Effects of high- and low-frequency repetitive transcranial magnetic stimulation on motor recovery in early stroke patients: Evidence from a randomized controlled trial with clinical, neurophysiological and functional imaging assessments. *Neuro Image Clin.* 2019;21:101620.

49. Watanabe K, Kudo Y, Sugawara E, et al. Comparative study of ipsilesional and contralesional repetitive transcranial magnetic stimulations for acute infarction. *J Neurol Sci.* 2018;384:10–14.

50. Khedr EM, Abdel-Fadeil MR, Farghali A, Qaid M. Role of 1 and 3 Hz repetitive transcranial magnetic stimulation on motor function recovery after acute ischaemic stroke. *Eur J Neurol.* 2009;16(12):1323–1330.

51. Chen Q, Shen D, Sun H, et al. Effects of coupling inhibitory and facilitatory repetitive transcranial magnetic stimulation on motor recovery in patients following acute cerebral infarction. *Neurorehabil.* 2021;48(1):83–96.

52. Meng Y, Zhang D, Hai H, Zhao YY, Ma YW. Efficacy of coupling intermittent theta-burst stimulation and 1 Hz repetitive transcranial magnetic stimulation to enhance upper limb motor recovery in subacute stroke patients: A randomized controlled trial. *Restor Neurol Neurosci.* 2020;38(1):109–118.

53. Sung WH, Wang CP, Chou CL, Chen YC, Chang YC, Tsai PY. Efficacy of coupling inhibitory and facilitatory repetitive transcranial magnetic stimulation to enhance motor recovery in hemiplegic stroke patients. *Stroke.* 2013;44(5):1375–1382.

54. Hong Z, Zheng H, Luo J, et al. Effects of low-frequency repetitive transcranial magnetic stimulation on language recovery in post-stroke survivors with aphasia: An updated meta-analysis. *Neurorehabil Neural Repair.* 2021;35(8):680–691.

55. Yang NY, Fong KN, Li-Tsang CW, Zhou D. Effects of repetitive transcranial magnetic stimulation combined with sensory cueing on unilateral neglect in subacute patients with right hemispheric stroke: A randomized controlled study. *Clin Rehabil.* 2017;31(9):1154–1163.

56. Koch G, Bonnì S, Giacobbe V, et al. θ-burst stimulation of the left hemisphere accelerates recovery of hemispatial neglect. *Neurology.* 2012;78(1):24–30.

57. Kim BR, Chun MH, Kim DY, Lee SJ. Effect of high- and low-frequency repetitive transcranial magnetic stimulation on visuospatial neglect in patients with acute stroke: A double-blind, sham-controlled trial. *Arch Phys Med Rehabil.* 2013;94(5):803–807.

58. Cha HG, Kim MK. Effects of repetitive transcranial magnetic stimulation on arm function and decreasing unilateral spatial neglect in subacute stroke: A randomized controlled trial. *Clin Rehabil.* 2016;30(7):649–656.

59. Cazzoli D, Müri RM, Schumacher R, et al. Theta burst stimulation reduces disability during the activities of daily living in spatial neglect. *Brain.* 2012;135(Pt 11):3426–3439.

60. Fu W, Song W, Zhang Y, et al. Long-term effects of continuous theta-burst stimulation in visuospatial neglect. *J Intl Med Res.* 2015;43(2):196–203.

61. Nyffeler T, Vanbellingen T, Kaufmann BC, et al. Theta burst stimulation in neglect after stroke: Functional outcome and response variability origins. *Brain.* 2019;142(4):992–1008.

62. Vatanparasti S, Kazemnejad A, Yoonessi A, Oveisgharan S. The effect of continuous theta-burst transcranial magnetic stimulation combined with prism adaptation on the neglect recovery in stroke patients. *J Stroke Cerebrovasc Dis.* 2019;28(11):104296.

63. Valle AC, Dionisio K, Pitskel NB, et al. Low and high frequency repetitive transcranial magnetic stimulation for the treatment of spasticity. *Develop Med Child Neurol.* 2007;49(7):534–538.

64. Kirton A, Chen R, Friefeld S, Gunraj C, Pontigon AM, Deveber G. Contralesional repetitive transcranial magnetic stimulation for chronic hemiparesis in subcortical paediatric stroke: A randomised trial. *Lancet Neurol.* 2008;7(6):507–513.

65. Kirton A, Andersen J, Herrero M, et al. Brain stimulation and constraint for perinatal stroke hemiparesis: The PLASTIC CHAMPS Trial. *Neurology.* 2016;86(18):1659–1667.

66. Zewdie E, Ciechanski P, Kuo HC, et al. Safety and tolerability of transcranial magnetic and direct current stimulation in children: Prospective single center evidence from 3.5 million stimulations. *Brain Stimul.* 2020;13(3):565–575.

67. Kirton A, Deveber G, Gunraj C, Chen R. Neurocardiogenic syncope complicating pediatric transcranial magnetic stimulation. *Pediatr Neurol.* 2008;39(3):196–197.

68. Chang WH, Bang OY, Shin YI, Lee A, Pascual-Leone A, Kim YH. BDNF polymorphism and differential rTMS effects on motor recovery of stroke patients. *Brain Stimul.* 2014;7(4):553–558.

69. Uhm KE, Kim YH, Yoon KJ, Hwang JM, Chang WH. BDNF genotype influence the efficacy of rTMS in stroke patients. *Neurosci Lett.* 2015;594:117–121.

70. Schambra HM. Repetitive transcranial magnetic stimulation for upper extremity motor recovery: Does it help? *Curr Neurol Neurosci Rep.* 2018;18(12):97.

71. Bradnam LV, Stinear CM, Byblow WD. Ipsilateral motor pathways after stroke: Implications for non-invasive brain stimulation. *Front Hum Neurosci.* 2013;7:184.

rTMS as Treatment for Movement Disorders

11.1 INTRODUCTION

Many studies have tested the effects of repetitive transcranial magnetic stimulation (rTMS) in movement disorders. The principles underlying different types of rTMS are discussed in Chapter 4. Most studies used high- or low-frequency regular rTMS and a few studies have used theta burst stimulation (TBS). This chapter discusses several of the more common movement disorders: Parkinson's disease (PD), dystonia, and functional movement disorders.

11.2 PARKINSON'S DISEASE

The effects on rTMS as treatment for PD have been evaluated in many studies. Most initial studies focused on the cardinal motor symptoms of bradykinesia, rigidity, and tremor, but other features of PD such as levodopa-induced dyskinesia, freezing of gait (FOG), depression, and cognitive impairment have also been examined.

11.2.1 PD Motor Symptoms

Many studies have used rTMS to treat PD motor symptoms. The results of several meta-analyses and larger randomized controlled trials are highlighted here. All studies have used the Unified Parkinson's Disease Rating Scale (UPDRS) as their main outcome measure. Earlier systematic reviews of randomized, controlled trials have concluded that rTMS at different cortical sites, particularly high-frequency rTMS (typically ≥5 Hz), leads to improvement in motor signs.[1,2] More recent meta-analyses confirmed that rTMS, particularly high-frequency rTMS to the primary motor cortex (M1), improved motor signs (Figure 11.1).[3–6] The improvement occurred with both short- and long-term follow-up.[5–7] A greater number of TMS pulses within the same session or across sessions were associated with greater improvement.[4,6,7]

A relatively large study that involved 61 PD patients used a realistic sham condition that combined the use of a sham coil with electrical scalp stimulation. Patients who received bilateral 10 Hz motor cortical stimulation for 10 daily sessions over 2 weeks showed improvement in PD motor signs compared to sham stimulation at 1 month but not at 3 months (Figure 11.2).[8] Since some studies suggested that higher frequencies of rTMS may be more efficacious, another study tested eight sessions of 50 Hz rTMS at 80% of active motor threshold (AMT) to bilateral motor cortices over 2 weeks in 26 PD patients. The intervention was safe but did not improve PD motor performance or functional status.[9] Thus, there is evidence that rTMS may improve motor symptoms in PD,[10] and an evidence-based guideline concluded that there was Level B (probable) evidence for bilateral high-frequency M1 rTMS for treatment of PD motor symptoms.[11]

While most studies have used high-frequency rTMS, several studies used low-frequency (≤1 Hz) rTMS, which likely reduced cortical excitability.[12] An initial systematic review found no evidence that low-frequency rTMS improved motor signs in PD.[2] However, more recent systematic reviews that included a greater number of studies suggested that low-frequency rTMS,[5,7,13] particularly when applied to frontal regions outside the M1,[4] also improved PD motor signs. The results are largely due to a relatively large study with 106 PD patients.[14] Following weekly rTMS treatment to the supplementary motor area (SMA) for 8 weeks, the 1 Hz group showed improvement at 20 weeks whereas the 10 Hz and sham groups showed only transient improvement. A more recent study in 33 PD patients also reported that 1 Hz rTMS to the right dorsolateral prefrontal cortex (DLPFC) for 10 days improved motor signs, nonmotor symptoms, depression, and sleep quality that persisted for at least 3 months.[15]

11.2.2 Levodopa-Induced Dyskinesias

Levodopa-induced dyskinesias (LID) is a disabling complication in PD patients, producing excessive, involuntary movements. Several studies used 1 Hz rTMS since it reduces cortical excitability. Low-frequency rTMS over the SMA was found to transiently reduce LID, but 5 days of treatment produced no additional benefit.[16] Another sham controlled study reported that 1 Hz rTMS to the SMA for 10 days decreased LID for 24 hours.[17] A cross-over study applied a single session of 1 Hz rTMS (1,800 pulses) to the pre-SMA, which resulted in increased time to onset of dyskinesia and reduction in severity of

(A)

Studyname	Design	Cohn's d	95% CI Lower limit	95% CI Upper limit	p-Value
Arias, et al., 2010	Parallel	0.211	−0.716	1.137	0.656
Gonzalez-Garcaia, et al., 2011	Parallel	0.729	−0.268	1.725	0.152
Benninger, et al., 2012	Parallel	0.138	−0.632	0.907	0.726
Bornke, et al., 2004	Crossover	0.248	−0.555	1.051	0.545
Khedr, et al., 2003	Parallel	1.069	0.369	1.768	0.003
Filipovic, et at., 2010	Crossover	0.038	−0.838	0.915	0.932
Lefaucheur, et al., 2004	Crossover	0.435	−0.374	1.245	0.292
Siebner, et al., 2000	Crossover	0.380	−0.504	1.264	0.400
Lomarev, et al., 2006	Parallel	−0.039	−0.963	0.885	0.934
Benninger, et al., 2011	Parallel	−0.130	−0.899	0.640	0.741
Okabe, et al., 2003	Parallel	0.046	−0.465	0.556	0.861
Overall		0.268	0.034	0.502	0.025

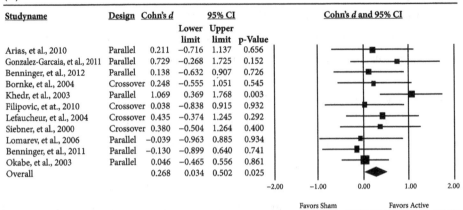

Favors Sham   Favors Active

(B)

Studyname	Design	Cohn's d	95% CI Lower limit	95% CI Upper limit	p-Value
Benninger, et al., 2012	Parallel	0.115	−0.654	0.885	0.769
Khedr, et al., 2003	Parallel	1.052	0.354	1.750	0.003
Lomarev, et al., 2006	Parallel	1.250	0.240	2.261	0.015
Benninger, et al., 2011	Parallel	0.004	−0.765	0.773	0.992
Okabe, et al., 2003	Parallel	−0.101	−0.611	0.410	0.699
Overall		0.312	−0.000	0.625	0.050

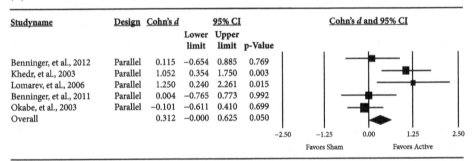

Favors Sham   Favors Active

(C)

Studyname	Design	Cohn's d	95% CI Lower limit	95% CI Upper limit	p-Value
Benninger, et al., 2012	Parallel	−0.036	−0.805	0.732	0.926
Khedr, et al., 2003	Parallel	−0.111	−0.766	0.544	0.740
Lomarev, et al., 2006	Parallel	1.346	0.323	2.369	0.010
Benninger, et al., 2011	Parallel	0.142	−0.627	0.912	0.717
Okabe, et al., 2003	Parallel	−0.164	−0.675	0.347	0.529
Overall		0.121	−0.309	0.550	0.582

Favors Sham   Favors Active

FIGURE 11.1 *Quantitative review of repetitive transcranial magnetic stimulation (rTMS) of the motor cortex in treatment of motor signs in Parkinson's disease. Effect sizes (Cohen's d) with corresponding 95% confidence intervals and P values for Unified Parkinson's Disease Rating Scale part III (UPDRS III) evaluations comparing active with sham rTMS groups are shown. (A) Baseline versus short-term (the same day or the day after the last stimulation session) follow-up assessment. (B) Baseline versus 1-month follow-up. (C) Short-term versus 1-month follow-up.*

FROM ZANJANI ET AL., *MOVEM DIS.* 2015;30(6):750–758, WITH PERMISSION.

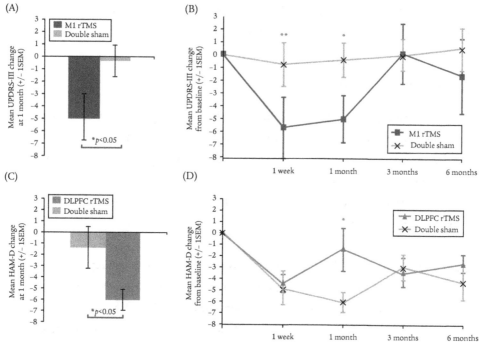

FIGURE 11.2 *Results from a study on multifocal repetitive transcranial magnetic stimulation (rTMS) for motor and mood symptoms of Parkinson's disease that randomized 61 patients. Unified Parkinson's Disease Rating Scale (UPDRS) part III scores at study time points in the M1 rTMS group compared to double-sham group, and Hamilton Depression Rating Scale (HAM-D) scores at study time points in dorsolateral prefrontal cortex (DLPFC) rTMS group compared to the double-sham group. (A,B) Improvement in motor symptoms after rTMS to primary motor cortex versus sham. There was a significant improvement in motor scores after M1 rTMS compared to double-sham at the primary endpoint (1 month after treatment) (A) that returned to baseline by 3 months (B). (C,D) Lack of improvement in mood symptoms after rTMS to DLPFC versus sham. rTMS to left DLPFC resulted in less antidepressant response at the primary 1-month endpoint than double-sham (C). This difference was specific to this single time point (D) and driven in part by a single outlier. *p, 0.05, **p, 0.001.*
FROM BRYS ET AL., *NEUROLOGY.* 2016;87(18):1907–1915, WITH PERMISSION.

dyskinesia following levodopa administration.[18] A different target for treatment of LID is the M1. In an open-label study with blinded assessment, 10 daily sessions of 1 Hz rTMS to the M1 showed decreased LID 1 day after treatment but not after 2 weeks.[19] A study of 1 Hz M1 rTMS over 4 days found a small but significant improvement in dyskinesia following real but not sham rTMS.[20] However, another study did not find effects of either a single session or five daily sessions of bilateral M1 rTMS on LID or motor function.[21] Another target for rTMS treatment of LID is the cerebellum. In a sham controlled study of 20 PD patients, 2 weeks of bilateral continuous TBS, which was designed to reduce cerebellar excitability, reduced LID in the real but not the sham treatment group for up to 4 weeks after the end of treatment.[22] The effects of cerebellar cTBS on LID may be related to brain-derived neurotrophic factor (BDNF) as the effects of single session was evident in study participants with the Val66Val genotype but not in those with Val66Met geno-type, and the treatment was associated with decrease in serum BDNF level.[23]

11.2.3 Gait Disturbance

Postural instability and FOG are common problems in PD and often respond poorly to dopaminergic medications. A study that stimulated bilateral M1 hand area and dorsal lateral prefrontal cortex with high-frequency rTMS for eight sessions found increased walking speed.[24] A small ($n = 10$) study reported that anodal transcranial direct current stimulation (tDCS) followed by 1 Hz rTMS to the hand area of M1 improved gait as measured with kinematics.[25]

Other studies that aimed to improve gait in PD targeted the leg area of M1. A study applied 5 Hz rTMS to both hand and leg areas of M1 for 10 days and reported increased walking speed for 1 month.[26] Application of 10 Hz rTMS to M1 leg area improved 10 m walking time.[27] Five Hz rTMS to leg M1 followed by treadmill training also improved walking speed.[28] A study that used 10 Hz rTMS to leg M1 with daily sessions for 5 days re-ported improvement in FOG in PD patients.[29] Another study with 51 PD patients found that 12 sessions of either 1 or 25 Hz rTMS to the leg motor cortex followed by treadmill training resulted in faster walking speed and improved PD motor signs that lasted for up to 3 months compared to sham stimulation.[30]

High-frequency (25 Hz) rTMS to SMA is also a promising approach for improving FOG in PD patients and may be a better target than the hand areas of M1.[31] In a study with 30 PD patients, a sessions of 10 Hz rTMS to SMA over 2 weeks improved FOG symptoms, gait parameters, and PD motor signs up to 4 weeks.[32] However, both contin-uous or intermittent TBS of the cerebellum were found to have no effect on FOG in PD.[33]

A meta-analysis of five studies in PD patients reported beneficial effects of rTMS on FOG.[34] Another meta-analysis of 14 studies found improved walking time but no sig-nificant change in FOG questionnaire and no long-term improvement in walking per-formance.[35] However, these meta-analyses combined studies that targeted hand and leg motor cortices and the frontal areas. Recent studies suggest that M1 leg area and the SMA[36] are promising targets for treating FOG in PD, particularly when combined with gait training.

11.2.4 Depression

Depression is a common symptom in PD and has been reported to occur in between 40% and 70% of PD patients. Chapter 13 contains more details on the use of rTMS in the treatment of depression.

High-frequency rTMS to the left DLFPC is an approved treatment for medication-resistant depression in many countries. Since pharmacological treatment may be ineffective or have intolerable side effects, nonpharmacological approaches, such as rTMS, may fill an unmet need in the treatment of PD patients. There are several randomized controlled trials of rTMS for the treatment of depression in PD. A meta-analysis reported that low-frequency rTMS of the right DLPFC was superior to sham stimulation, whereas high-frequency rTMS of the left DLPFC has been shown to have similar efficacy as antidepressant medications.[37] Two more recent meta-analyses came to the similar conclusion that rTMS of DLPFC improved depression in PD patients, similar to the effects of selective serotonin reuptake inhibitors.[7,38] A evidence-based guideline concluded that there was Level B evidence (probable efficacy) for high-frequency rTMS of the left DLPFC for treatment of depression in PD.[11] However, a relatively large study of 61 PD patients found no effect of 10 Hz rTMS to left DLPFC on depression.[8] This may be because the patients in this study had relatively mild depression and were therefore prone to spontaneous improvement or placebo effects (Figure 11.2).[8] While rTMS of DLPFC is a promising treatment of depression in PD patients, the subgroup that responds to this treatment requires further investigation. rTMS of M1 did not appear to have significant effect on mood symptoms in PD.[8,27]

11.2.5 Cognition

Cognitive impairment is common in PD, especially in more advanced stages. A meta-analysis examined 14 studies with 173 participants and reported that multiple sessions of high-frequency rTMS to the left DLPFC improved executive functions but not other cognitive domains.[39] However, another meta-analysis that examined 12 studies found no significant effect of rTMS on cognition in PD.[40]

Several studies used iTBS to the left DLPFC. A study with 28 PD patients applied left DLPFC iTBS twice a day for 3 days with 1–2 days between and reported overall improvement in cognition for up to 1 month, particularly in visuospatial ability.[41] However, a subsequent study by the same group in 41 PD patients with mild cognitive impairment found no significant effect of six session of left DLPFC iTBS after 1 week on cognition, although there was a trend for improved executive function.[42] Another study also found no significant effect of a single session of left DLPFC iTBS on executive function and working memory.[43] Thus, the use of rTMS for cognitive impairment in PD requires further study.

11.2.6 Other Nonmotor Symptoms

Other nonmotor symptoms, such as apathy and pain, are also major challenges in the treatment of PD. A few studies examined the effects of rTMS on these symptoms. A study with 106 PD patients reported that high- or low-frequency rTMS to the SMA did not change nonmotor symptoms.[14] A preliminary study found promising effect for low-frequency rTMS to the right DLPFC to reduce punding in 4 PD patients.[44]

11.2.7 Deep TMS

Several studies have tested the effects of the Hesed (H) coil, which is capable of reaching wider and deeper brain structures compared to conventional coils. An open-label study of high-frequency M1 and bilateral prefrontal cortex stimulation reported improvement in PD motor signs.[45] A subsequent sham-controlled study by the same group in 60 PD patients with 12 sessions over 4 weeks found improvement of PD motor signs with 10 Hz bilateral M1, with no additional effect of 10 Hz bilateral prefrontal cortex stimulation.[46] These findings are in keeping with the effects of high-frequency M1 rTMS with other types of coils in PD. However, a sham controlled study of low-frequency rTMS to M1 followed by high-frequency rTMS to the prefrontal cortex did not show significant benefit compared to sham stimulation.[47] A small pilot study suggested that medial prefrontal cortex stimulation may be further explored for treatment of FOG in PD.[48]

11.2.8 Safety of TMS in PD

A review of the safety of TMS in PD found that the incidence of adverse events was very low.[49] Transient headaches, tinnitus, scalp pain, nausea, increase in preexisting pain, and muscle jerks have been reported. Worsening of PD was reported in one rTMS study. No seizure has been reported in PD patients.

11.2.9 Summary of rTMS as Treatment for PD

High-frequency rTMS of the M1 and low-frequency rTMS to frontal areas outside of M1 are promising adjunctive treatment for PD. DLPFC stimulation may be effective for treatment of depression in PD. rTMS of the leg motor area and the SMA may be useful for improving gait disturbance. However, the results of meta-analyses are limited by the heterogeneity of the studies in terms of rTMS protocol, duration of treatment, patients studied, and methods of assessment. Further large, randomized controlled trials with realistic sham stimulation are needed to establish the therapeutic efficacy of rTMS in PD. rTMS as treatment of LID, cognitive impairment, and nonmotor symptoms also requires further study.

11.3 DYSTONIA

Dystonia is characterized by excessive muscle contractions, frequently leading to twisted postures. The pathophysiological findings in dystonia include loss of inhibition at multiple levels of the nervous system, excessive plasticity, and abnormal sensorimotor integration.

Most rTMS studies in dystonia used inhibitory paradigms. In patients with writer's cramp, an early study found that a single session of 1 Hz rTMS to M1 reduced writing pressure and restored deficient short-interval intracortical inhibition (SICI) and silent period.[50] Another study showed that 0.2 Hz rTMS to the premotor cortex improved writing in writer's cramp patients.[51] Pervious studies reported conflicting results of repeated administration of 1 Hz rTMS to the premotor cortex, and this may be related to heterogeneity of patient selection (writer's cramp vs. musician's cramp) and interindividual variability.[52-54] A study reported no clinical improvement with five sessions of cTBS of the premotor cortex in writer's cramp patients although there was increased cortical inhibition.[55] Improvement in handwriting was observed following five sessions of 1 Hz rTMS to the primary somatosensory cortex (S1) in writer's cramp patients.[56]

While most studies tested focal hand dystonia, some studies examined other types of dystonia. In patients with cervical dystonia, one study tested a single session of 0.2 Hz rTMS to several cortical locations and reported that dorsal premotor cortex and motor cortex stimulation led to the greatest reduction in dystonia (Figure 11.3).[57] However, an open-label study of five daily sessions of 1 Hz rTMS to the left dorsal premotor cortex in five cervical dystonia patients showed no benefit.[58] Ten sessions of bilateral cerebellar cTBS over 2 weeks was found to reduce the severity of cervical dystonia compared to sham stimulation,[59] while a single session of unilateral cerebellar cTBS did not change the clinical scores in focal hand dystonia or cervical dystonia patients.[60] A study using an opposite protocol of 10 sessions of iTBS in 16 patients with cervical dystonia showed a slight improvement compared to sham stimulation.[61] For blepharospasm, a study reported that a single session of 0.2 Hz rTMS over the anterior cingulate cortex with either a circular coil or an H-coil improved clinical outcome.[62] A 2-week course of daily 0.2 Hz rTMS over the anterior cingulate cortex delivered by a double-cone coil initiated 1 month after botulinum toxin injection was found to improve symptoms of blepharospasm compared to sham stimulation.[63]

In summary, inhibitory rTMS to the premotor cortex, motor cortex, and cerebellum are potential treatments for focal hand and cervical dystonia, while the anterior cingulate cortex is a promising site for the treatment of blepharospasm. However, large, randomized controlled trials are needed, particularly in combination with other treatments such as botulinum toxin injections or physical therapy.

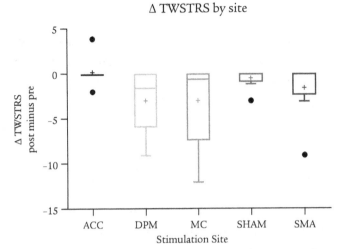

FIGURE 11.3 *Results of single sessions of 0.2 Hz repetitive transcranial magnetic stimulation to different cortical sites in cervical dystonia. Boxplots of changes in Toronto Western Spasmodic Torticollis Rating Scale (TWSTRS) severity scores by stimulation site showing greatest improvement over the dorsal premotor cortex (dPM) and motor cortex (MC). A box in the boxplot represents first to third quartile, with the median as the centerline. The outliers are represented by circles and the mean value as a cross. Note that the anterior cingulate cortex (ACC) boxplot is collapsed since the first quartile is equal to the third quartile. SMA, supplementary motor area.*
FROM PIRIO RICHARDSON ET AL., *PLOS ONE*. 2015;10(4):E0124937, WITH PERMISSION.

11.4 FUNCTIONAL MOVEMENT DISORDERS

In functional neurological disorders, patients have neurological symptoms that cannot be explained by observable brain lesions, neurological disease, or other medical conditions. These patients frequently have severe disabilities, and there are no effective treatments. In functional movement disorders (FMD), the symptoms manifest as abnormal movements.

Several studies tested rTMS as treatment for FMD. In a single case of functional myoclonus of the right leg, 1 Hz rTMS of the left premotor cortex 5 times a week for 6 weeks led to symptomatic benefit.[64] Another case of functional movement disorder associated with posttraumatic stress disorder improved after 36 sessions of 1 Hz rTMS targeting the cingulate gyrus, premotor cortex, and SMA.[65] An open label study with 24 patients reported improvement after a single session of 0.25 Hz rTMS with approximately 20 stimuli to the contralateral motor cortex.[66] A subsequent study by the same group found that spinal root magnetic stimulation was as effective as motor cortical rTMS, suggesting that the benefits were due to cognitive-behavioral effects rather than cortical neuromodulation.[67] This is consistent with a report that peripheral electrical stimulation was associated with improvement in functional neurological disorder.[68] An open-label study of 0.33 Hz rTMS to the motor or dorsal premotor cortex in six FMD patients did not show benefit, which may be related to the long-standing symptoms in this group of patients.[69] Interestingly, a parallel group, sham-controlled study in 18 patients with functional tremor reported greater improvement in those patients treated with five consecutive days of real 1 Hz motor cortical rTMS compared to the sham group.[70] Thus, rTMS, possibly combined with suggestion and behavioral therapy, is worth further investigation as a treatment for FMDs.

11.5 CONCLUSION

Studies have consistently showed that high-frequency rTMS to M1 and frontal motor area leads to improvement in motor symptoms in PD, although further large, randomized controlled trials are needed. rTMS also showed promise in treatment of levodopa-induced dyskinesia and FOG in PD. For dystonia, inhibitory rTMS to premotor cortex, motor cortex, and cerebellum may be further investigated as potential treatment. Low-frequency rTMS to M1 together with suggestion or cognitive behavioral therapy can be tested as possible treatments in functional movement disorders.

REFERENCES

1. Fregni F, Simon DK, Wu A, Pascual-Leone A. Non-invasive brain stimulation for Parkinson's disease: A systematic review and meta-analysis of the literature. *J Neurol Neurosurg Psychiatry.* 2005;76(12):1614–1623.
2. Elahi B, Elahi B, Chen R. Effect of transcranial magnetic stimulation on Parkinson motor function: Systematic review of controlled clinical trials. *Movem Dis.* 2009;24(3):357–363.
3. Zanjani A, Zakzanis KK, Daskalakis ZJ, Chen R. Repetitive transcranial magnetic stimulation of the primary motor cortex in the treatment of motor signs in Parkinson's disease: A quantitative review of the literature. *Movem Dis.* 2015;30(6):750–758.
4. Chou YH, Hickey PT, Sundman M, Song AW, Chen NK. Effects of repetitive transcranial magnetic stimulation on motor symptoms in Parkinson disease: A systematic review and meta-analysis. *JAMA Neurol.* 2015;72(4):432–440.
5. Wagle Shukla A, Shuster JJ, Chung JW, et al. Repetitive transcranial magnetic stimulation (rTMS) therapy in Parkinson disease: A meta-analysis. *PM&R.* 2016;8(4):356–366.
6. Chung CL, Mak MK. Effect of repetitive transcranial magnetic stimulation on physical function and motor signs in Parkinson's Disease: A systematic review and meta-analysis. *Brain Stimul.* 2016;9(4):475–487.
7. Li S, Jiao R, Zhou X, Chen S. Motor recovery and antidepressant effects of repetitive transcranial magnetic stimulation on Parkinson disease: A PRISMA-compliant meta-analysis. *Medicine (Baltimore).* 2020;99(18):e19642.
8. Brys M, Fox MD, Agarwal S, et al. Multifocal repetitive TMS for motor and mood symptoms of Parkinson disease: A randomized trial. *Neurology.* 2016;87(18):1907–1915.
9. Benninger DH, Iseki K, Kranick S, Luckenbaugh DA, Houdayer E, Hallett M. Controlled study of 50-Hz repetitive transcranial magnetic stimulation for the treatment of Parkinson disease. *Neurorehabil Neural Repair.* 2012;26(9):1096–1105.
10. Latorre A, Rocchi L, Berardelli A, Bhatia KP, Rothwell JC. The use of transcranial magnetic stimulation as a treatment for movement disorders: A critical review. *Movem Dis.* 2019;34(6):769–782.

11. Lefaucheur JP, Aleman A, Baeken C, et al. Evidence-based guidelines on the therapeutic use of re-petitive transcranial magnetic stimulation (rTMS): An update (2014-2018). *Clin Neurophysiol.* 2020;131(2):474–528.

12. Chen R, Classen J, Gerloff C, et al. Depression of motor cortex excitability by low-frequency transcranial magnetic stimulation. *Neurology.* 1997;48(5):1398–1403.

13. Zhu H, Lu Z, Jin Y, Duan X, Teng J, Duan D. Low-frequency repetitive transcranial magnetic stimulation on Parkinson motor function: A meta-analysis of randomised controlled trials. *Acta Neuropsychiatrica.* 2015;27(2):82–89.

14. Shirota Y, Ohtsu H, Hamada M, Enomoto H, Ugawa Y. Supplementary motor area stimulation for Parkinson disease: A randomized controlled study. *Neurology.* 2013;80(15):1400–1405.

15. Zhuang S, Wang FY, Gu X, et al. Low-frequency repetitive transcranial magnetic stimulation over right dorsolateral prefrontal cortex in Parkinson's disease. *Parkinson Dis* 2020;2020:7295414.

16. Brusa L, Versace V, Koch G, et al. Low frequency rTMS of the SMA transiently ameliorates peak-dose LID in Parkinson's disease. *Clin Neurophysiol.* 2006;117(9):1917–1921.

17. Sayın S, Cakmur R, Yener GG, Yaka E, Uğurel B, Uzunel F. Low-frequency repetitive transcranial mag-netic stimulation for dyskinesia and motor performance in Parkinson's disease. *J Clin Neurosci Australasia.* 2014;21(8):1373–1376.

18. Lohse A, Meder D, Nielsen S, et al. Low-frequency transcranial stimulation of pre-supplementary motor area alleviates levodopa-induced dyskinesia in Parkinson's disease: A randomized cross-over trial. *Brain Comm.* 2020;2(2):fcaa147.

19. Wagle-Shukla A, Angel MJ, Zadikoff C, et al. Low-frequency repetitive transcranial magnetic stimulation for treatment of levodopa-induced dyskinesias. *Neurology.* 2007;68(9):704–705.

20. Filipović SR, Rothwell JC, van de Warrenburg BP, Bhatia K. Repetitive transcranial magnetic stimula-tion for levodopa-induced dyskinesias in Parkinson's disease. *Movem Dis.* 2009;24(2):246–253.

21. Flamez A, Cordenier A, De Raedt S, et al. Bilateral low frequency rTMS of the primary motor cortex may not be a suitable treatment for levodopa-induced dyskinesias in late stage Parkinson's disease. *Parkinsonism Related Dis.* 2016;22:54–61.

22. Koch G, Brusa L, Carrillo F, et al. Cerebellar magnetic stimulation decreases levodopa-induced dyskine-sias in Parkinson disease. *Neurology.* 2009;73(2):113–119.

23. Sanna A, Follesa P, Puligheddu M, et al. Cerebellar continuous theta burst stimulation reduces levodopa-induced dyskinesias and decreases serum BDNF levels. *Neurosci Lett.* 2020;716:134653.

24. Lomarev MP, Kanchana S, Bara-Jimenez W, Iyer M, Wassermann EM, Hallett M. Placebo-controlled study of rTMS for the treatment of Parkinson's disease. *Movem Dis.* 2006;21(3):325–331.

25. von Papen M, Fisse M, Sarfeld AS, Fink GR, Nowak DA. The effects of 1 Hz rTMS preconditioned by tDCS on gait kinematics in Parkinson's disease. *J Neural Transmission (Vienna, Austria: 1996).* 2014;121(7):743–754.

26. Khedr EM, Farweez HM, Islam H. Therapeutic effect of repetitive transcranial magnetic stimulation on motor function in Parkinson's disease patients. *Eur J Neurol.* 2003;10(5):567–572.

27. Maruo T, Hosomi K, Shimokawa T, et al. High-frequency repetitive transcranial magnetic stimulation over the primary foot motor area in Parkinson's disease. *Brain Stimul.* 2013;6(6):884–891.

28. Yang YR, Tseng CY, Chiou SY, et al. Combination of rTMS and treadmill training modulates corticomo-tor inhibition and improves walking in Parkinson disease: A randomized trial. *Neurorehabil neural Repair.* 2013;27(1):79–86.

29. Kim MS, Chang WH, Cho JW, et al. Efficacy of cumulative high-frequency rTMS on freezing of gait in Parkinson's disease. *Restor Neurol Neurosci.* 2015;33(4):521–530.

30. Chung CL, Mak MK, Hallett M. Transcranial magnetic stimulation promotes gait training in Parkinson Disease. *Ann Neurol.* 2020;88(5):933–945.

31. Kim SJ, Paeng SH, Kang SY. Stimulation in supplementary motor area versus motor cortex for freezing of gait in Parkinson's Disease. *J Clin Neurol (Seoul, Korea).* 2018;14(3):320–326.

32. Mi TM, Garg S, Ba F, et al. High-frequency rTMS over the supplementary motor area improves freezing of gait in Parkinson's disease: A randomized controlled trial. *Parkinsonism Related Dis* 2019;68:85–90.

33. Janssen AM, Munneke MAM, Nonnekes J, et al. Cerebellar theta burst stimulation does not improve freezing of gait in patients with Parkinson's disease. *J Neurol*. 2017;264(5):963–972.

34. Kim YW, Shin IS, Moon HI, Lee SC, Yoon SY. Effects of non-invasive brain stimulation on freezing of gait in parkinsonism: A systematic review with meta-analysis. *Parkinsonism Related Dis*. 2019;64:82–89.

35. Xie YJ, Gao Q, He CQ, Bian R. Effect of repetitive transcranial magnetic stimulation on gait and freezing of gait in Parkinson Disease: A systematic review and meta-analysis. *Arch Phys Med Rehabil*. 2020;101(1):130–140.

36. Nardone R, Versace V, Brigo F, et al. Transcranial magnetic stimulation and gait disturbances in Parkinson's disease: A systematic review. *Neurophysiologie clinique/Clin neurophysiol*. 2020;50(3):213–225.

37. Xie CL, Chen J, Wang XD, et al. Repetitive transcranial magnetic stimulation (rTMS) for the treatment of depression in Parkinson disease: A meta-analysis of randomized controlled clinical trials. *Neurologic Sci*. 2015;36(10):1751–1761.

38. Hai-Jiao W, Ge T, Li-Na Z, et al. The efficacy of repetitive transcranial magnetic stimulation for Parkinson disease patients with depression. *Intl J Neurosci*. 2020;130(1):19–27.

39. Jiang Y, Guo Z, McClure MA, He L, Mu Q. Effect of rTMS on Parkinson's cognitive function: A systematic review and meta-analysis. *BMC Neurol*. 2020;20(1):377.

40. He PK, Wang LM, Chen JN, et al. Repetitive transcranial magnetic stimulation (rTMS) fails to improve cognition in patients with Parkinson's disease: A meta-analysis of randomized controlled trials. *Intl J Neurosci*. 2020:1–14.

41. Trung J, Hanganu A, Jobert S, et al. Transcranial magnetic stimulation improves cognition over time in Parkinson's disease. *Parkinsonism Related Dis*. 2019;66:3–8.

42. Lang S, Gan LS, Yoon EJ, et al. Theta-burst stimulation for cognitive enhancement in Parkinson's disease with mild cognitive impairment: A randomized, double-blind, sham-controlled trial. *Front Neurol*. 2020;11:584374.

43. Hill AT, McModie S, Fung W, Hoy KE, Chung SW, Bertram KL. Impact of prefrontal intermittent theta-burst stimulation on working memory and executive function in Parkinson's disease: A double-blind sham-controlled pilot study. *Brain Res*. 2020;1726:146506.

44. Nardone R, De Blasi P, Höller Y, et al. Repetitive transcranial magnetic stimulation transiently reduces punding in Parkinson's disease: A preliminary study. *J Neural Transmission (Vienna, Austria: 1996)*. 2014;121(3):267–274.

45. Spagnolo F, Volonté MA, Fichera M, et al. Excitatory deep repetitive transcranial magnetic stimulation with H-coil as add-on treatment of motor symptoms in Parkinson's disease: An open label, pilot study. *Brain Stimul*. 2014;7(2):297–300.

46. Spagnolo F, Fichera M, Chieffo R, et al. Bilateral repetitive transcranial magnetic stimulation with the H-coil in Parkinson's disease: A randomized, sham-controlled study. *Front Neurol*. 2020;11:584713.

47. Cohen OS, Rigbi A, Yahalom G, et al. Repetitive deep TMS for Parkinson disease: A 3-month double-blind, randomized sham-controlled study. *J Clin Neurophysiol*. 2018;35(2):159–165.

48. Dagan M, Herman T, Mirelman A, Giladi N, Hausdorff JM. The role of the prefrontal cortex in freezing of gait in Parkinson's disease: Insights from a deep repetitive transcranial magnetic stimulation exploratory study. *Exp Brain Res*. 2017;235(8):2463–2472.

49. Vonloh M, Chen R, Kluger B. Safety of transcranial magnetic stimulation in Parkinson's disease: A review of the literature. *Parkinsonism Related Dis*. 2013;19(6):573–585.

50. Siebner HR, Tormos JM, Ceballos-Baumann AO, et al. Low-frequency repetitive transcranial magnetic stimulation of the motor cortex in writer's cramp. *Neurology*. 1999;52(3):529–537.

51. Murase N, Rothwell JC, Kaji R, et al. Subthreshold low-frequency repetitive transcranial magnetic stimulation over the premotor cortex modulates writer's cramp. *Brain*. 2005;128(Pt 1):104–115.

52. Kimberley TJ, Borich MR, Arora S, Siebner HR. Multiple sessions of low-frequency repetitive transcranial magnetic stimulation in focal hand dystonia: Clinical and physiological effects. *Restor Neurol Neurosci*. 2013;31(5):533–542.

53. Borich M, Arora S, Kimberley TJ. Lasting effects of repeated rTMS application in focal hand dystonia. *Restor Neurol Neurosci*. 2009;27(1):55–65.

54. Kimberley TJ, Schmidt RL, Chen M, Dykstra DD, Buetefisch CM. Mixed effectiveness of rTMS and retraining in the treatment of focal hand dystonia. *Front Hum Neurosci.* 2015;9:385.

55. Huang YZ, Lu CS, Rothwell JC, et al. Modulation of the disturbed motor network in dystonia by multi-session suppression of premotor cortex. *PloS One.* 2012;7(10):e47574.

56. Havrankova P, Jech R, Walker ND, et al. Repetitive TMS of the somatosensory cortex improves writer's cramp and enhances cortical activity. *Neuro Endocrinol Lett.* 2010;31(1):73–86.

57. Pirio Richardson S, Tinaz S, Chen R. Repetitive transcranial magnetic stimulation in cervical dystonia: Effect of site and repetition in a randomized pilot trial. *PloS One.* 2015;10(4):e0124937.

58. Shin HW, Hallett M. Low-frequency transcranial magnetic stimulation of the left dorsal premotor cortex in patients with cervical dystonia. *Parkinsonism Related Dis.* 2020;76:13–15.

59. Koch G, Porcacchia P, Ponzo V, et al. Effects of two weeks of cerebellar theta burst stimulation in cervical dystonia patients. *Brain Stimul.* 2014;7(4):564–572.

60. Bologna M, Paparella G, Fabbrini A, et al. Effects of cerebellar theta-burst stimulation on arm and neck movement kinematics in patients with focal dystonia. *Clin Neurophysiol.* 2016;127(11):3472–3479.

61. Bradnam LV, McDonnell MN, Ridding MC. Cerebellar intermittent theta-burst stimulation and motor control training in individuals with cervical dystonia. *Brain Sci.* 2016;6(4).

62. Kranz G, Shamim EA, Lin PT, Kranz GS, Hallett M. Transcranial magnetic brain stimulation modulates blepharospasm: A randomized controlled study. *Neurology.* 2010;75(16):1465–1471.

63. Wagle Shukla A, Hu W, Legacy J, Deeb W, Hallett M. Combined effects of rTMS and botulinum toxin therapy in benign essential blepharospasm. *Brain Stimul.* 2018;11(3):645–647.

64. Naro A, Pignolo L, Billeri L, et al. A case of psychogenic myoclonus responding to a novel transcranial magnetic stimulation approach: Rationale, feasibility, and possible neurophysiological basis. *Front Hum Neurosci.* 2020;14:292.

65. Blades R, Jordan S, Becerra S, et al. Treating dissociative post-traumatic stress disorder presenting as a functional movement disorder with transcranial magnetic stimulation targeting the cingulate gyrus. *Neurologic Sci Italian.* 2020;41(8):2275–2280.

66. Garcin B, Roze E, Mesrati F, et al. Transcranial magnetic stimulation as an efficient treatment for psychogenic movement disorders. *J Neurol Neurosurg Psychiatry.* 2013;84(9):1043–1046.

67. Garcin B, Mesrati F, Hubsch C, et al. Impact of transcranial magnetic stimulation on functional movement disorders: Cortical modulation or a behavioral effect? *Front Neurol.* 2017;8:338.

68. Burke MJ, Isayama R, Jegatheeswaran G, et al. Neurostimulation for functional neurological disorder: Evaluating longitudinal neurophysiology. *Movem Dis Clin Pract.* 2018;5(5):561–563.

69. Shah BB, Chen R, Zurowski M, Kalia LV, Gunraj C, Lang AE. Repetitive transcranial magnetic stimulation plus standardized suggestion of benefit for functional movement disorders: An open label case series. *Parkinsonism related Dis.* 2015;21(4):407–412.

70. Taib S, Ory-Magne F, Brefel-Courbon C, et al. Repetitive transcranial magnetic stimulation for functional tremor: A randomized, double-blind, controlled study. *Movem Dis.* 2019;34(8):1210–1219.

rTMS as Treatment for Other Neurological Disorders

12.1 INTRODUCTION

This chapter covers the use of transcranial magnetic stimulation (TMS) and repetitive TMS (rTMS) in the treatment of several other neurological disorders. The principles and the use of different rTMS techniques to induce brain plasticity are discussed in Chapter 4. The disorders discussed include epilepsy, pain, multiple sclerosis (MS), and tinnitus, in which multiple studies have been conducted. While most studies used regular rTMS, some have used theta burst stimulation (TBS), while single and paired TMS have been used in the treatment of migraine.

12.2 EPILEPSY

12.2.1 Inhibitory rTMS as Treatment for Epilepsy

Since epilepsy is generally considered related to abnormally increased cortical excitability, most studies of rTMS in epilepsy have used low-frequency stimulation to decrease cortical excitability. The first report is an open label study of nine patients with refractory epilepsy treated with 0.33 Hz rTMS for 5 consecutive days using a circular coil, which led to reduced seizure frequencies for up to 4 weeks after treatment.[1] This is followed by several case reports and a small case series with varying results. In randomized controlled trials that used a focal figure-of-eight coil to target the epileptic focus with low-frequency (0.5–1 Hz) rTMS, two studies showed reduction in seizure frequency[2,3] but two studies were negative.[4,5] In randomized controlled studies that used low-frequency rTMS and a non-focal circular coil, one reported positive results[6] but two studies were negative.[5,7] All the published studies involved a relatively small number of participants (up to 60). Although all studies used low-frequency (0.3–1 Hz) rTMS, there are considerable variations in the stimulation parameters used, types of coils and regions stimulated (including the use of a nonfocal circular coil over the vertex or a focal figure-of-eight coil over the epileptic focus), and in the patient population studied (e.g., severity of epilepsy and location of epileptic focus). Patients with a neocortical epileptic focus on the convexity, particularly focal cortical dysplasia, may respond better than patients with mesial temporal lobe epilepsy.[8] An evidence-based guideline has Level C recommendation of "possible efficacy" of focal low-frequency rTMS delivered to the epileptic focus.[9] A meta-analysis that examined seven randomized controlled trials and found that low-frequency rTMS treatment decreased seizure frequency and interictal epileptiform discharges, but the effects decreased with the duration of follow-up, suggesting that the effects were short-lasting.[10] However, there are no large randomized controlled trials. Further studies are needed before low-frequency rTMS can be recommended for routine clinical use for treatment of epilepsy.

12.2.2 Treatment of Status Epilepticus

There are case reports and small series suggesting that low-frequency rTMS may be used in treating status epilepticus.[11,12] In five patients on multiple anti-epileptic drugs reported in four studies, low-frequency (0.5 to 1 Hz) rTMS aborted status epilepticus in all patients, with no adverse effect.[13]

12.2.3 Identification of Seizure Focus

Another potential use of rTMS is to induce seizures to help localize the epileptic focus and reduce the length of stay in an epilepsy monitoring unit. However, a study of seven patients with refractory epilepsy in an epilepsy monitoring unit found that intermittent or continuous TBS at the highest possible intensities applied to the presumed epileptic focus did not induce seizures or epileptic discharges.[14] Thus, the procedure appeared to be safe but did not help to localize the epileptic region.

12.3 MULTIPLE SCLEROSIS

MS is a demyelinating, autoimmune disorder of the central nervous system that also involves axonal degeneration and cortical atrophy. It is a major cause of disability in young individuals.

12.3.1 rTMS as Treatment for Spasticity

Lower limb spasticity is common in MS patients, and therefore several sham-controlled studies targeted the leg motor cortex as treatment for spasticity. The first study found that daily sessions of 5 Hz but not 1 Hz or sham rTMS to leg motor cortex over 2 weeks improved spasticity for at least 7 days.[15] Two subsequent studies reported that in 20 patients with relapsing-remitting MS, 10 sessions of iTBS over 2 weeks to the leg motor cortex contralateral to the more affected leg improved leg spasticity compared to sham stimulation, with better results when combined with exercise therapy.[16,17] Another study in 17 MS patients reported similar findings, although the reduction in spasticity lasted less than 2 weeks.[18] A study tested bilateral leg area iTBS using 20 Hz rTMS or sham stimulation for 10 daily sessions over 2 weeks in 34 secondary progressive MS patients.[19] Both iTBS and 20 Hz rTMS reduced spasticity. iTBS had longer lasting effects, but the 20 Hz rTMS group had reduction of pain and fatigue. Based on these studies, an evidence-based guideline concluded that there is Level B evidence (probable efficacy) for iTBS or high-frequency rTMS to the leg motor cortex for treatment of spasticity in MS.[9] A narrative review also arrived at similar conclusions.[20]

12.3.2 Stimulation of Hand Motor Cortical Area

A single session of 5 Hz rTMS but not sham stimulation to the hand area of the motor cortex in eight MS patients with cerebellar dysfunction led to transient improvement in hand dexterity.[21] Another study applied iTBS to the left motor cortex hand area with 10 daily sessions over 2 weeks in 36 relapsing-remitting MS patients. iTBS resulted in improvement in manual dexterity compared to sham stimulation.[22]

12.3.3 Fatigue

Fatigue is a common symptom in MS. A study used the two different Hesed (H)-coils with 18 Hz rTMS over left prefrontal cortex, 5 Hz rTMS for the bilateral motor cortex stimulation, and sham stimulation with 18 rTMS sessions over 6 weeks in 28 MS patients. Reduction in fatigue was observed in the group with motor cortex stimulation.[23] Reduction in pain and fatigue was observed with 20 Hz rTMS but not iTBS to leg M1 in another study.[19]

12.3.4 Gait and Balance

A study evaluated the effects of 10 sessions over 2 weeks of bilateral cerebellar iTBS followed by vestibular rehabilitation in 20 MS patients.[24] iTBS treatment led to greater improvement in gait and balance compared to sham stimulation.

In summary, there is evidence that excitatory rTMS to the leg motor cortex can improve spasticity in MS patients. Excitatory rTMS to the hand motor cortex may improve hand dexterity, while high-frequency M1 rTMS may reduce fatigue, and cerebellar iTBS has the potential to improve gait and balance. However, large sham-controlled trials are needed to conclusively demonstrate the efficacy of rTMS in MS.

12.4 PAIN

There is a large literature on the use of TMS as treatment for chronic pain. Here we focus on the treatment of neuropathic pain and primary headache disorders as these are the most common pain syndrome and have the largest number of studies to date.

12.4.1 Neuropathic Pain

Neuropathic pain refers to pain caused by disease or lesions of the central or peripheral somatosensory nervous system. It is major issue: the condition is prevalent (estimated to affect ~10% of the global population) and the current treatments, including pharmacological and surgical therapies, are of limited efficacy.

The most common protocol to treat neuropathic pain is rTMS to the primary motor cortex (M1). This is related to the initial reports of the efficacy of epidural motor cortex stimulation for medication-resistant neuropathic pain.[25] The initial studies of M1 rTMS for treatment of neuropathic pain was designed to select candidates who would respond to invasive motor cortex stimulation.[26]

12.4.1.1 *Motor Cortex Stimulation for Neuropathic Pain*

Most studies used high-frequency (5–20 Hz) rTMS to the M1, whereas low-frequency (0.5–1 Hz) is likely ineffective.[9] In a synthesis of 511 patients with chronic neuropathic pain, an evidence-based guideline provided Level A recommendation for high-frequency M1 rTMS contralateral to the pain side as treatment for neuropathic pain.[9] This is consistent with the conclusion of other systematic reviews,[27,28] although large variations and heterogeneity among studies were also noted. The efficacy of M1 rTMS may depend on the location of the pain. A systematic review suggested that the effects may be greater for trigeminal neuralgia, post-stroke pain, and spinal cord pain compared to peripheral nerve pain (Figure 12.1).[27] An expert consensus panel concluded that the level of evidence was high for M1 rTMS as treatment of neuropathic pain of supraspinal origin, moderate for phantom limb pain, and low for spinal cord and peripheral nerve pain.[29] While the effects of a single session of rTMS may persist for a few days, it may be increased and prolonged with repeated sessions.[9] For patients with neuropathic pain without severe depression, a

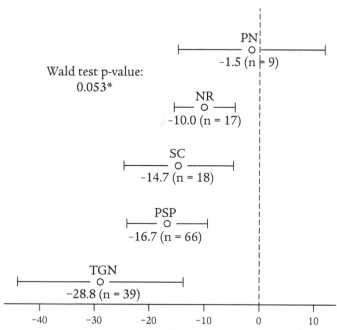

FIGURE 12.1 *Repetitive transcranial magnetic stimulation (rTMS) for suppressing neuropathic pain; a meta-analysis of diagnosis and treatment effect. Mean difference (95% confidence interval) in percent of pain visual analog scale (VAS) score change. *P value is from Wald test for the interaction effect of diagnosis and treatment on the percent decrease in VAS score. This P value increases to 0.140 when the Khedr study was excluded. The treatment effect was greater for trigeminal neuralgia, post-stroke pain and spinal cord pain compared to peripheral nerve pain. NR, nerve root; PN, peripheral nerve; PSP, post-stroke supraspinal related pain; TGN, trigeminal nerve or ganglion.*

From Leung et al., J Pain. 2009;10(12):1205–1216, with permission.

consensus panel recommended 5–10 sessions at 10–20 Hz and 2,000–3,000 pulses per session at 80–90% resting motor threshold for M1 contralateral to the pain.[29] A figure-of-eight coil with induced current in the anterior-posterior or posterior-anterior directions, as well as magnetic resonance imaging (MRI)-based neuronavigation are also recommended.[9,29]

High-frequency M1 rTMS is also considered useful to predict the response to epidural motor cortex stimulation, with a specificity of 60–100% and a positive predictive value of 75–100%.[28]

12.4.1.2 Other Cortical Targets for Neuropathic Pain

Dorsolateral prefrontal cortex (DLPFC) stimulation has also attracted interest because the symptoms of pain and depression frequently coexist, although the number of studies that have used DLPFC stimulation for neuropathic pain is much lower than that for M1 stimulation. A European evidence-based guideline did not provide recommendation for DLPFC stimulation as treatment for pain.[9] However, a consensus panel suggested that high-frequency left DLPFC rTMS can be used for diffuse neuropathic pain and for patients with neuropathic pain and severe comorbid depression.[29]

12.4.2 Primary Headache Disorders

Primary headache disorders are common and include migraine, tension-type headache, and cluster headache. Migraine is considered the third leading cause of disability for adults younger than 50. As migraine attacks are often episodic, treatment of migraine can be divided into treatment of acute migraine and prophylaxis or prevention.

12.4.2.1 Single-Pulse TMS as Treatment of Migraine

For acute treatment of migraine, a handheld device that delivers single-pulse TMS has been studied. The patient positions the device over the occiput and delivers a single pulse of TMS at the onset of headache or aura. Occipital TMS is hypothesized to disrupt spreading depression in migraine. The TMS pulse has a rise time of 180 μs and duration of less than 1 ms, with a strength of 1 Tesla measured 1 cm from the device.[30,31] If necessary, one or two additional pulses can be administered after the first pulse. A large, randomized controlled trial of 267 patients with migraine with aura showed that single-pulse TMS increased freedom from pain after 2 hours and the effect was sustained up to 48 hours (Figure 12.2).[30] The findings were confirmed in a 3-month post-marketing survey in the United Kingdom in 190 patients, which showed that the device was effective in treating migraine pain with no serious adverse effect.[31] This single-pulse TMS device was approved by the US Food and Drug Administration (FDA) for treatment of migraine with aura. A consensus guideline concluded that there was a moderate level of evidence and recommended offering this service based on professional judgment and patient preference.[29]

The post-marketing survey found reduction in headaches in patients with episodic or chronic migraine, suggesting that single-pulse TMS might be able to prevent migraine.[31] Another open-label post-marketing study involving 132 patients with migraine tested preventative treatment with four pulses twice daily and found a mean reduction of 2.75 headache days per month and a 45% responder rate.[32] The results were superior to a statistically derived placebo estimate. The FDA approved the device for migraine prevention based on this study. A small, open-label study testing migraine prevention reported promising results, but there were difficulties in adolescents following the treatment protocol.[33] An expert consensus panel indicated a moderate level of evidence and recommended the use of single-pulse TMS for migraine prevention based on professional judgment and patient preference.[29]

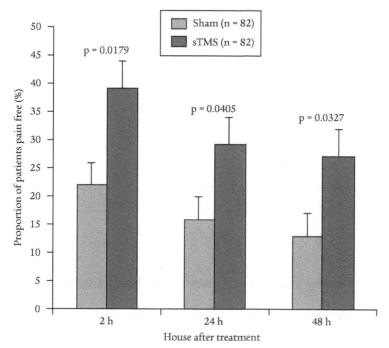

FIGURE 12.2 *Results of single-pulse transcranial magnetic stimulation (sTMS) for acute treatment of migraine with aura: a randomized, double-blind, parallel-group, sham-controlled trial. Proportion of patients pain-free at 2 hours, 24 hours, and 48 hours on active and sham treatment. Error bars =SE.* FROM LIPTON ET AL., *LANCET NEUROL.* 2010;9(4):373–380, WITH PERMISSION.

12.4.2.2 *Repetitive TMS for Migraine Prevention*

A small randomized controlled trial and an open-label study reported that high-frequency rTMS to the left DLPFC decreased migraine attack frequency,[34,35] but another small randomized controlled trial showed no benefit compared to sham stimulation.[36] Thus, there is only low-level evidence for left DLPFC rTMS for migraine prevention.

High-frequency M1 rTMS used to treat neuropathic pain has also been tested for migraine prevention. Several studies, including a randomized, controlled trial without a realistic sham control using 10 Hz rTMS to left M1, 600 pulses, 3 sessions on alternate days[37,38]; a nonrandomized study with sham stimulation[39]; and two open-label studies,[40] reported reduction in headache frequency with high-frequency M1 rTMS. Another study reported similar efficacy for M1 rTMS and botulinum toxin injection for migraine prevention.[41] An expert consensus group concluded that there was moderate level evidence and suggested implementation of high-frequency M1 rTMS for migraine prevention.[29]

An open-label study reported decreased number of headache days with 20 session of continuous TBS to right M1.[42] A randomized, unblinded study used the H1 deep TMS coil for bilateral DLPFC stimulation with 10 Hz, in 12 sessions of 600 pulses in 1 month, reported decreased pain intensity and number of attacks in seven patients.[43] However, there is not enough evidence to recommend these protocols for migraine prophylaxis.

For the treatment of cluster headache, one open-label study used 12 sessions of 10 Hz rTMS to the facial area of M1 over 3 weeks and reported a reduction in pain at 15 and 180 days after treatment initiation.[44]

12.5 TINNITUS

Tinnitus refers to abnormal auditory perception in the absence of auditory stimulus, usually the sensation of ringing in the ears. It is a common condition that leads to considerable distress and poor quality of life. There is no effective treatment. Therefore, many studies have investigated the use of rTMS as treatment for tinnitus. Several rTMS approaches have been used; the more common ones are discussed here.

12.5.1 Low-Frequency rTMS to Temporal Auditory Cortex

The most common approach is low-frequency rTMS (usually 1 Hz) to the left temporal auditory cortex or to the side contralateral to tinnitus in patients with unilateral tinnitus, with the rationale of downregulating the hyperactive auditory cortex.[45] A randomized controlled trial (64 participants) of 1 Hz rTMS with 2,000 pulses per session for 10 days showed a greater percentage of responders with real compared to sham stimulation.[46] However, a large trial (163 patients) found no difference between real and sham 1 Hz rTMS to the temporal cortex.[47] Two meta-analyses of 29 randomized studies concluded that rTMS is effective for chronic tinnitus with a moderate effect size,[48,49] although another meta-analysis of 10 randomized controlled trials reported no significant effect of rTMS for tinnitus.[50] An evidence-based guideline concluded that there was Level C (possible efficacy) evidence for repeated sessions of low-frequency rTMS to the left temporal cortex or contralateral to the tinnitus side for treatment of chronic tinnitus.[9]

12.5.2 High-Frequency rTMS to Dorsolateral Prefrontal Cortex or Dorsal Medial Prefrontal Cortex

Another approach is high-frequency rTMS to the left DLPFC. However, a study found no effect of 4 days of 3,000 pulses of rTMS to the left DLPFC alone.[51] A single blinded study in 29 patients showed greater benefit of 20 sessions of 10 Hz bilateral dorsal medial prefrontal cortex (DMPFC) rTMS compared to sham stimulation.[52]

12.5.3 Combination Studies

The combination of high-frequency rTMS to left DLPFC and low-frequency rTMS to the auditory cortex has been investigated. In a study with 32 patients, 10-day treatment with high-frequency rTMS to the left DLPFC followed by low-frequency rTMS to the left temporal cortex produced similar a reduction in tinnitus as left temporal cortex stimulation alone at the end of the treatment period, but the combined stimulation had greater effects at 3 months.[53] A similar study reported that 4 days of combined treatment showed improvement in tinnitus at 4, 8, and 12 weeks, but left temporal stimulation alone had no effect.[54] A study with 56 patients showed a nonsignificant trend for better outcome in the group treated with low-frequency rTMS to the right DLPFC followed by low-frequency rTMS to the left temporal cortex compared to left temporal stimulation alone.[55] Another study with 192 tinnitus patients showed no difference in treatment efficacy for combined high-frequency left DLPFC and low-frequency left temporal cortex stimulation compared to left temporal stimulation alone.[56]

Two studies from the same group examined triple-site stimulation with left DLPFC high-frequency rTMS and bilateral temporoparietal low-frequency rTMS versus left temporoparietal low-frequency rTMS alone and found reduction in tinnitus for both protocols without significant superiority of the triple-site compared to the single-site protocol.[57,58] However, another study reported that this triple stimulation approach did not produce significant benefit.[59] The benefits of combination stimulation with multiple sites over a single-site stimulation have not been convincingly demonstrated.

12.5.4 Theta Burst Stimulation for Tinnitus

Several studies used TBS as treatment of tinnitus. The most common procedure is continuous TBS to the left temporal auditory cortex in an attempt to downregulate the excitability of this area. However, a metanalysis of seven randomized controlled trials found no significant effect of TBS on the severity of tinnitus.[60]

12.5.5 Role of Neuronavigation

Two studies compared the efficacy of MRI-guided neuronavigation versus stimulation location based on the 10-20 EEG system (posterior to T3–C3 line) and found no advantage for neuronavigation.[61,62] Another approach is to stimulate the left temporal auditory cortex according to the tonotopic location of the pitch of the tinnitus, but no significant benefit was found for this approach, possibility related to a large placebo effect and high interindividual variation.[63]

12.5.6 Other Approaches

A personalized approach to the treatment of tinnitus has produced interesting results. In an open-label study, patients received different rTMS protocols of 1–20 Hz rTMS and continuous TBS to the right and left temporo-parietal cortices and DLPFC in the first session. The patients then received nine treatment sessions with the most effective temporo-parietal and frontal protocol. About half the patients responded to the test session. In these patients, the treatment benefit was sustained for 10 weeks.[64]

The mechanisms of rTMS treatment for tinnitus is not fully understood. While it is often presumed that it is related to downregulation of the left temporal auditory cortex, a modeling study suggested that this type of rTMS produced the strongest electric field in the insula.[49]

In summary, low-frequency rTMS to the left temporal auditory cortex is a promising approach for treatment of tinnitus, but there is considerable interindividual variability. Further, large, randomized controlled trials are needed. There is no good evidence for continuous TBS, and multisite stimulation does not appear to be superior to left temporal stimulation alone. Neuronavigation does not appear to produce added benefit.

REFERENCES

1. Tergau F, Naumann U, Paulus W, Steinhoff BJ. Low-frequency repetitive transcranial magnetic stimulation improves intractable epilepsy. *Lancet.* 1999;353(9171):2209.

2. Fregni F, Otachi PT, Do Valle A, et al. A randomized clinical trial of repetitive transcranial magnetic stimulation in patients with refractory epilepsy. *Ann Neurol.* 2006;60(4):447–455.

3. Sun W, Mao W, Meng X, et al. Low-frequency repetitive transcranial magnetic stimulation for the treatment of refractory partial epilepsy: A controlled clinical study. *Epilepsia.* 2012;53(10):1782–1789.

4. Theodore WH, Hunter K, Chen R, et al. Transcranial magnetic stimulation for the treatment of seizures: A controlled study. *Neurology.* 2002;59(4):560–562.

5. Seynaeve L, Devroye A, Dupont P, Van Paesschen W. Randomized crossover sham-controlled clinical trial of targeted low-frequency transcranial magnetic stimulation comparing a figure-8 and a round coil to treat refractory neocortical epilepsy. *Epilepsia.* 2016;57(1):141–150.

6. Tergau F, Neumann D, Rosenow F, Nitsche MA, Paulus W, Steinhoff B. Can epilepsies be improved by repetitive transcranial magnetic stimulation?: Interim analysis of a controlled study. *Suppl Clin Neurophysiol.* 2003;56:400–405.

7. Cantello R, Rossi S, Varrasi C, et al. Slow repetitive TMS for drug-resistant epilepsy: Clinical and EEG findings of a placebo-controlled trial. *Epilepsia.* 2007;48(2):366–374.

8. Hsu WY, Cheng CH, Lin MW, Shih YH, Liao KK, Lin YY. Antiepileptic effects of low frequency repetitive transcranial magnetic stimulation: A meta-analysis. *Epilepsy Res.* 2011;96(3):231–240.

9. Lefaucheur JP, Aleman A, Baeken C, et al. Evidence-based guidelines on the therapeutic use of repetitive transcranial magnetic stimulation (rTMS): An update (2014-2018). *Clin Neurophysiol.* 2020;131(2):474–528.

10. Mishra A, Maiti R, Mishra BR, Jena M, Srinivasan A. Effect of repetitive transcranial magnetic stimulation on seizure frequency and epileptiform discharges in drug-resistant epilepsy: A meta-analysis. *J Clin Neurol(Seoul, Korea).* 2020;16(1):9–18.

11. Zeiler FA, Matuszczak M, Teitelbaum J, Gillman LM, Kazina CJ. Transcranial magnetic stimulation for status epilepticus. *Epilepsy Res Treat.* 2015;2015:678074.

12. Liu A, Pang T, Herman S, Pascual-Leone A, Rotenberg A. Transcranial magnetic stimulation for refractory focal status epilepticus in the intensive care unit. *Seizure.* 2013;22(10):893–896.

13. San-Juan D, Dávila-Rodríguez DO, Jiménez CR, et al. Neuromodulation techniques for status epilepticus: A review. *Brain Stimul.* 2019;12(4):835–844.

14. Udupa K, Tai P, Saha U, et al. Theta burst transcranial magnetic stimulation to induce seizures in an epilepsy monitoring unit. *Brain Stimul.* 2020;13(6):1800–1802.

15. Centonze D, Koch G, Versace V, et al. Repetitive transcranial magnetic stimulation of the motor cortex ameliorates spasticity in multiple sclerosis. *Neurology.* 2007;68(13):1045–1050.

16. Mori F, Codecà C, Kusayanagi H, et al. Effects of intermittent theta burst stimulation on spasticity in patients with multiple sclerosis. *Eur J Neurol.* 2010;17(2):295–300.

17. Mori F, Ljoka C, Magni E, et al. Transcranial magnetic stimulation primes the effects of exercise therapy in multiple sclerosis. *J Neurol.* 2011;258(7):1281–1287.

18. Boutière C, Rey C, Zaaraoui W, et al. Improvement of spasticity following intermittent theta burst stimulation in multiple sclerosis is associated with modulation of resting-state functional connectivity of the primary motor cortices. *Multiple sclerosis (Houndmills, Basingstoke, England).* 2017;23(6):855–863.

19. Korzhova J, Bakulin I, Sinitsyn D, et al. High-frequency repetitive transcranial magnetic stimulation and intermittent theta-burst stimulation for spasticity management in secondary progressive multiple sclerosis. *Eur J Neurol.* 2019;26(4):680–e644.

20. Aloizou AM, Pateraki G, Anargyros K, et al. Transcranial magnetic stimulation (TMS) and repetitive TMS in multiple sclerosis. *Rev Neurosci.* 2021.

21. Koch G, Rossi S, Prosperetti C, et al. Improvement of hand dexterity following motor cortex rTMS in multiple sclerosis patients with cerebellar impairment. *Multiple sclerosis (Houndmills, Basingstoke, England).* 2008;14(7):995–998.

22. Azin M, Zangiabadi N, Iranmanesh F, Baneshi MR, Banihashem S. Effects of intermittent theta burst stimulation on manual dexterity and motor imagery in patients with multiple sclerosis: A quasi-experimental controlled study. *Iranian Red Crescent Med J.* 2016;18(10):e27056.

23. Gaede G, Tiede M, Lorenz I, et al. Safety and preliminary efficacy of deep transcranial magnetic stimulation in MS-related fatigue. *Neurol Neuroimmunol Neuroinflamm.* 2018;5(1):e423.

24. Tramontano M, Grasso MG, Soldi S, et al. Cerebellar intermittent theta-burst stimulation combined with vestibular rehabilitation improves gait and balance in patients with multiple sclerosis: A preliminary double-blind randomized controlled trial. *Cerebellum (London, England).* 2020;19(6):897–901.

25. Tsubokawa T, Katayama Y, Yamamoto T, Hirayama T, Koyama S. Chronic motor cortex stimulation for the treatment of central pain. *Acta Neurochirur Suppl.* 1991;52:137–139.

26. Lefaucheur JP. The use of repetitive transcranial magnetic stimulation (rTMS) in chronic neuropathic pain. *Neurophysiologie clinique/Clin Neurophysiol.* 2006;36(3):117–124.

27. Leung A, Donohue M, Xu R, et al. rTMS for suppressing neuropathic pain: A meta-analysis. *J Pain.* 2009;10(12):1205–1216.

28. Gatzinsky K, Bergh C, Liljegren A, et al. Repetitive transcranial magnetic stimulation of the primary motor cortex in management of chronic neuropathic pain: A systematic review. *Scand J Pain.* 2021;21(1):8–21.

29. Leung A, Shirvalkar P, Chen R, et al. Transcranial magnetic stimulation for pain, headache, and comorbid depression: INS-NANS expert consensus panel review and recommendation. *Neuromodulation.* 2020;23(3):267–290.

30. Lipton RB, Dodick DW, Silberstein SD, et al. Single-pulse transcranial magnetic stimulation for acute treatment of migraine with aura: A randomised, double-blind, parallel-group, sham-controlled trial. *Lancet Neurol.* 2010;9(4):373–380.

31. Bhola R, Kinsella E, Giffin N, et al. Single-pulse transcranial magnetic stimulation (sTMS) for the acute treatment of migraine: Evaluation of outcome data for the UK post market pilot program. *J Headache Pain.* 2015;16:535.

32. Starling AJ, Tepper SJ, Marmura MJ, et al. A multicenter, prospective, single arm, open label, observational study of sTMS for migraine prevention (ESPOUSE Study). *Cephalalgia.* 2018;38(6):1038–1048.

33. Irwin SL, Qubty W, Allen IE, Patniyot I, Goadsby PJ, Gelfand AA. Transcranial magnetic stimulation for migraine prevention in adolescents: A pilot open-label study. *Headache.* 2018;58(5):724–731.

34. Brighina F, Piazza A, Vitello G, et al. rTMS of the prefrontal cortex in the treatment of chronic migraine: A pilot study. *J Neurol Sci.* 2004;227(1):67–71.

35. O'Reardon JP, Fontecha JF, Cristancho MA, Newman S. Unexpected reduction in migraine and psychogenic headaches following rTMS treatment for major depression: A report of two cases. *CNS Spectrums.* 2007;12(12):921–925.

36. Conforto AB, Amaro E, Jr., Gonçalves AL, et al. Randomized, proof-of-principle clinical trial of active transcranial magnetic stimulation in chronic migraine. *Cephalalgia.* 2014;34(6):464–472.

37. Misra UK, Kalita J, Bhoi SK. High-rate repetitive transcranial magnetic stimulation in migraine prophylaxis: A randomized, placebo-controlled study. *J Neurol.* 2013;260(11):2793–2801.

38. Zardouz S, Shi L, Leung A. A feasible repetitive transcranial magnetic stimulation clinical protocol in migraine prevention. *SAGE Open Medical Case Reports.* 2016;4:2050313x16675257.

39. Misra UK, Kalita J, Tripathi G, Bhoi SK. Role of β endorphin in pain relief following high rate repetitive transcranial magnetic stimulation in migraine. *Brain Stimul.* 2017;10(3):618–623.

40. Misra UK, Kalita J, Bhoi SK. High frequency repetitive transcranial magnetic stimulation (rTMS) is effective in migraine prophylaxis: An open labeled study. *Neurol Res.* 2012;34(6):547–551.

41. Shehata HS, Esmail EH, Abdelalim A, et al. Repetitive transcranial magnetic stimulation versus botulinum toxin injection in chronic migraine prophylaxis: A pilot randomized trial. *J Pain Res.* 2016;9:771–777.

42. Chen PR, Lai KL, Fuh JL, et al. Efficacy of continuous theta burst stimulation of the primary motor cortex in reducing migraine frequency: A preliminary open-label study. *J Chinese Med Assoc.* 2016;79(6):304–308.

43. Rapinesi C, Del Casale A, Scatena P, et al. Add-on deep transcranial magnetic stimulation (dTMS) for the treatment of chronic migraine: A preliminary study. *Neurosci Lett.* 2016;623:7–12.

44. Hodaj H, Alibeu JP, Payen JF, Lefaucheur JP. Treatment of chronic facial pain including cluster headache by repetitive transcranial magnetic stimulation of the motor cortex with maintenance sessions: A naturalistic study. *Brain Stimul.* 2015;8(4):801–807.

45. Chen R, Classen J, Gerloff C, et al. Depression of motor cortex excitability by low-frequency transcranial magnetic stimulation. *Neurology.* 1997;48:1389–1403.

46. Folmer RL, Theodoroff SM, Casiana L, Shi Y, Griest S, Vachhani J. Repetitive transcranial magnetic stimulation treatment for chronic tinnitus: A randomized clinical trial. *JAMA Otolaryngol Head Neck Surg.* 2015;141(8):716–722.

47. Landgrebe M, Hajak G, Wolf S, et al. 1-Hz rTMS in the treatment of tinnitus: A sham-controlled, randomized multicenter trial. *Brain Stimul.* 2017;10(6):1112–1120.

48. Liang Z, Yang H, Cheng G, Huang L, Zhang T, Jia H. Repetitive transcranial magnetic stimulation on chronic tinnitus: A systematic review and meta-analysis. *BMC Psychiatry.* 2020;20(1):547.

49. Lefebvre-Demers M, Doyon N, Fecteau S. Non-invasive neuromodulation for tinnitus: A meta-analysis and modeling studies. *Brain Stimul.* 2021;14(1):113–128.

50. Dong C, Chen C, Wang T, et al. Low-frequency repetitive transcranial magnetic stimulation for the treatment of chronic tinnitus: A systematic review and meta-analysis of randomized controlled trials. *BioMed Res Intl.* 2020;2020:3141278.

51. Noh TS, Kyong JS, Chang MY, et al. Comparison of treatment outcomes following either prefrontal cortical-only or dual-site repetitive transcranial magnetic stimulation in chronic tinnitus patients: A double-blind randomized study. *Otol Neurotol.* 2017;38(2):296–303.

52. Ciminelli P, Machado S, Palmeira M, Coutinho ESF, Sender D, Nardi AE. Dorsomedial prefrontal cortex repetitive transcranial magnetic stimulation for tinnitus: Promising results of a blinded, randomized, sham-controlled study. *Ear Hearing.* 2020;42(1):12–19.

53. Kleinjung T, Eichhammer P, Landgrebe M, et al. Combined temporal and prefrontal transcranial magnetic stimulation for tinnitus treatment: A pilot study. *Otolaryngol Head Neck Surg.* 2008;138(4):497–501.

54. Noh TS, Kyong JS, Park MK, Lee JH, Oh SH, Suh MW. Dual-site rTMS is more effective than single-site rTMS in tinnitus patients: A blinded randomized controlled trial. *Brain Topogr.* 2020;33(6):767–775.

55. Kreuzer PM, Landgrebe M, Schecklmann M, et al. Can temporal repetitive transcranial magnetic stimulation be enhanced by targeting affective components of tinnitus with frontal rTMS? A randomized controlled pilot trial. *Front Syst Neurosci.* 2011;5:88.

56. Langguth B, Landgrebe M, Frank E, et al. Efficacy of different protocols of transcranial magnetic stimulation for the treatment of tinnitus: Pooled analysis of two randomized controlled studies. *World J Biol Psychiatry.* 2014;15(4):276–285.

57. Lehner A, Schecklmann M, Poeppl TB, et al. Multisite rTMS for the treatment of chronic tinnitus: Stimulation of the cortical tinnitus network--a pilot study. *Brain Topogr.* 2013;26(3):501–510.

58. Lehner A, Schecklmann M, Greenlee MW, Rupprecht R, Langguth B. Triple-site rTMS for the treatment of chronic tinnitus: A randomized controlled trial. *Sci Rep.* 2016;6:22302.

59. Formánek M, Migaľová P, Krulová P, et al. Combined transcranial magnetic stimulation in the treatment of chronic tinnitus. *Ann Clin Translat Neurol.* 2018;5(7):857–864.

60. Schwippel T, Schroeder PA, Fallgatter AJ, Plewnia C. Clinical review: The therapeutic use of theta-burst stimulation in mental disorders and tinnitus. *Prog Neuro-Psychopharmacol Biol Psychiatry.* 2019;92:285–300.

61. Noh TS, Rah YC, Kyong JS, et al. Comparison of treatment outcomes between 10 and 20 EEG electrode location system-guided and neuronavigation-guided repetitive transcranial magnetic stimulation in chronic tinnitus patients and target localization in the Asian brain. *Acta Oto-Laryngologica.* 2017;137(9):945–951.

62. Sahlsten H, Holm A, Rauhala E, et al. Neuronavigated versus non-navigated repetitive transcranial magnetic stimulation for chronic tinnitus: A randomized study. *Trends Hearing.* 2019;23:2331216518822198.

63. Sahlsten H, Virtanen J, Joutsa J, et al. Electric field-navigated transcranial magnetic stimulation for chronic tinnitus: A randomized, placebo-controlled study. *Intl J Audiol.* 2017;56(9):692–700.

64. Kreuzer PM, Poeppl TB, Rupprecht R, et al. Individualized repetitive transcranial magnetic stimulation treatment in chronic tinnitus? *Front Neurol.* 2017;8:126.

rTMS for the Treatment of Depression

13.1 INTRODUCTION

Major depressive disorder (MDD) is a highly prevalent and disabling disorder. The significant social, health, and economic burden associated with depression is related, in part, to the limited effectiveness of current treatment options. One-third of treated patients fail to respond to antidepressant medications and are considered treatment-resistant.[1] Similarly, treatment with psychotherapy, even intensive programs targeting treatment resistant depression (TRD), achieve remission in only 22% of cases.[2] While electroconvulsive therapy (ECT) is a mainstay for TRD, its use is often hindered by fear of cognitive adverse effects,[3–5] persistent stigma in the general public,[6] and the need for anesthesia and associated lack of broad access, limiting its uptake to fewer than 1% of TRD cases.[7] Thus, there is an urgent need for safe, well-tolerated, and effective antidepressant treatments. This chapter reviews evidence for the use of rTMS in adults with MDD and other populations with depression. This chapter also discusses novel treatment approaches, current clinical challenges, and future directions.

13.1.1 A Brief History of rTMS to Treat Depression

The ability of rTMS to affect mood was first noted in healthy controls in the late 1980s. Seminal work by Pascual-Leone and colleagues in the 1990s, demonstrating that the cortical effects of rTMS could outlast stimulation,[8] led to a growth of studies focusing on the therapeutic application of rTMS. Several early proof-of-concept studies investigated the antidepressant effects of rTMS in patients with drug-resistant depression.[9–11] One of the pilot study found that all patients who received active stimulation showed improvements in depressive symptoms.[9] These early studies highlighted the therapeutic possibilities of this novel treatment. Over the next two decades, the field of rTMS continued to evolve, leading to the approval of rTMS for the on-label treatment of depression by regulatory agencies across a number of countries including Canada, Israel, Brazil, and Australia. In 2008, rTMS obtained approval from the US Food and Drug Administration (FDA) for the treatment of medication-refractory depression (FDA approval K061053). While these early studies uncovered the therapeutic potential of rTMS, they also led to a number of questions regarding ethical and safety considerations as well as the clinical applications of this novel intervention.

13.2 THERAPEUTIC EFFECTS OF RTMS IN DEPRESSION

While the exact mechanisms underlying the clinical effects of rTMS in depression remain elusive, researchers have proposed several mechanistic models, including the activation of different neurotransmitter systems, hippocampal neurogenesis, and synaptic plasticity, as well as the alteration of molecular pathways and, importantly, neural circuits. rTMS is thought to directly target underlying neurobiological impairments observed in patients with depression. For example, studies have observed asymmetrical cortical excitability in depressed patients[12,13] with lower left dorsolateral prefrontal cortex (DLPFC) and higher right DLPFC activity compared to healthy individuals.[14,15] As such, high-frequency rTMS (stimulation at frequency >5Hz) has been shown to increase cortical excitability, enhance glucose metabolism and cerebral blood flow, modulate neurotransmission, and alter network connectivity.[16,17] In contrast, low-frequency rTMS (stimulation at frequency of 1 Hz) is thought to inhibit cortical activity[18] via enhanced gamma aminobutyric acid (GABA)-mediated inhibitory neurotransmission. In line with this, studies have found that GABAergic neurotransmission is disrupted in MDD[19] and enhanced through ECT and treatment with antidepressant and mood-stabilizing treatments (Table 13.1).[20,21]

13.2.1 High-Frequency Stimulation

Early rTMS studies applied at high frequencies (10–20 Hz) over the left DLPFC demonstrated efficacy in depression, even among those with treatment-refractory depression[10] and in medication-resistant depressed patients with psychotic features.[11] While these early studies provided promising evidence for the use of rTMS, the antidepressant effects were typically modest. As such, more recent research employing longer treatment durations, beyond the typical 2-week time frame reported in early studies, have consistently demonstrated better clinical efficacy.[23–25] One of the largest and earliest multicenter trials evaluating the efficacy of high-frequency rTMS involved a randomized trial in 301

TABLE 13.1 Standard treatment parameters for commonly used repetitive transcranial magnetic stimulation (rTMS) protocols

Approach	Frequency (Hz)	Coil	Train details
High-frequency left DLPFC	10	Figure of 8	75 trains
			4 s duration 15–26 s ITI
			120% RMT
Low-frequency right DLPFC	1	Figure of 8	1single train
Sequential bilateral	10 on left	Figure of 8	Left most commonly 50 trains of 4 s duration Right – one train of 20 min duration Both – 120 % RMT
Deep TMS	18	HCoil	2 s trains
			20s ITI
			55 trains
iTBS	50/5	Figure of 8	50 Hz triplets repeated at 5 Hz for 2 s in one train
			20 trains
			8 s intertrain interval
			70–120% RMT

DLPFC, Dorsolateral prefrontal cortex; ITI, intertrain interval; RMT, resting motor threshold; iTBS, intermittent theta burst stimulation.

From Fitzgerald.[22]

medication-free patients who had failed to respond to a prior antidepressant treatment.[26] Findings from this study demonstrated that, compared to sham stimulation, active rTMS significantly improved depressive symptoms following 4–6 weeks of treatment and led to greater response and remission rates. Importantly, this study also further substantiated the safety and tolerability of rTMS.[26] The results from this trial were subsequently replicated in multisite trial conducted in 199 unmedicated patients with TRD.[27]

Of note, there are rTMS trials in depression which have shown a lack of clinical efficacy or mixed results.[28–30] Several explanations may account for the discrepant findings, including heterogeneity within patient populations, such as patients with TRD and those with other psychiatric or medical comorbidities. Additionally, stimulation parameters including frequency, intensity, duration, and localization methods have varied from study to study, precluding the proper determination of these parameters to optimize therapeutic response. Finally, the concomitant use of medications makes it difficult to conclude whether improvements were related to rTMS alone, the medication, or the combination of both.

One approach to evaluating the strength and reliability of the therapeutic efficacy of high-frequency rTMS in depression has been through the use of meta-analyses.[31–33] The majority of these meta-analyses report positive findings, yet with varying effect sizes and typically modest clinical meaningfulness. Of note, one study, however, failed to find a significant difference between active rTMS (i.e., >1 Hz) and sham stimulation in depression. However, this report included only six studies with 91 participants and, as such, likely had less power than the more recent meta-analyses.[34] In sum, meta-analyses evaluating high-frequency stimulation suggest that rTMS demonstrates clear separation from placebo when delivered for the treatment of depression, though the magnitude of the effect is modest and consistent with the magnitude of clinical effects of other treatments for depression such as pharmacotherapy and psychotherapy.

13.2.2 Low-Frequency Stimulation

Several studies have also demonstrated that low-frequency rTMS over the right DLPFC is an effective treatment for MDD.[23,35,36] Studies directly comparing the clinical efficacy of high-frequency left versus low-frequency right DLPFC stimulation in patients with depression suggest that low-frequency may be equivalent to high-frequency stimulation, and this is supported by a recent pooled analysis of the head to head trials.[37] The clinical efficacy and equivalence of low-frequency rTMS has also been established in several meta-analyses and network meta-analyses.[33,38–40] In addition to its efficacy, low-frequency stimulation may be associated with a lower risk of seizure induction and a better tolerability profile compared to high-frequency rTMS.[41] In addition, the energy requirements required to deliver 1 Hz treatment are lower. Taken together, the safety and good tolerability as well as the lower energy requirements may one day lead to an at-home rTMS device.

13.2.3 Bilateral Sequential Stimulation

The use of bilateral rTMS was initiated, in part, as a result of evidence that bilateral ECT is superior to unilateral ECT at similar stimulus parameters.[42] However, an initial attempt at applying *simultaneous* bilateral high-frequency rTMS was proved unsuccessful.[43] As such, a sequential pattern of stimulation, whereby low-frequency right-sided rTMS was applied followed by high-frequency left-sided rTMS was employed and has become the convention when delivering bilateral rTMS to the DLPFC.

Current evidence regarding the benefit of bilateral over sham stimulation has yielded positive results.[44,45] In contrast, several studies comparing the efficacy of bilateral versus unilateral stimulation have failed to find significant differences between the two protocols.[46–48] This finding has been confirmed in two large-scale meta-analyses demonstrating that bilateral rTMS displays comparable, but not better, efficacy to unilateral rTMS.[49,50] In the absence of clear evidence demonstrating the superiority of bilateral stimulation, there does not appear to be support for the use of one protocol over the other as a first-line treatment option (Table 13.2).

13.3 IMPROVING EFFICACY AND EFFICIENCY

13.3.1 Alternative Protocols

13.3.1.1 Theta Burst Stimulation

As described in previous chapters, theta burst stimulation (TBS) delivers a patterned stimulation of triplet bursts at a gamma frequency (most commonly 50 Hz) that are repeated at a theta frequency (most commonly 5 Hz) via a continuous (i.e., cTBS) or intermittent (iTBS) pattern.[51] Similar to standard rTMS, iTBS is commonly applied to the left DLPFC, while cTBS is applied to the right DLPFC, or both protocols are combined using a sequential bilateral approach. In addition to reducing the amount of time required for each treatment from 19–37.5 min for standard rTMS to around 3 min, TBS has the potential to improve treatment capacity and reduce the cost per session.[52]

Studies investigating the use of TBS for the treatment of depression have recently become more common. One meta-analysis including 221 participants from five randomized controlled trials using various TBS protocols demonstrated a significant difference between active and sham TBS, favoring active stimulation. Furthermore, their results suggested that bilateral TBS and iTBS may have a greater therapeutic efficacy than cTBS alone.[53] A recent large randomized noninferiority trial including 414 patients with depression compared the efficacy, safety, and tolerability of 4–6 weeks of 3-min iTBS with standard 37.5-min 10 Hz rTMS (Figure 13.1). Results from this trial demonstrated that iTBS was noninferior to standard 10 Hz rTMS in reducing depressive symptoms as well as in response and remission rates. While self-rated intensity of pain was greater in the iTBS group, the dropout rates, and overall safety and tolerability profiles associated with the two protocols were similar.[54] Following this trial, iTBS was approved by the FDA for the treatment of MDD. Taken together, these findings suggest that TBS represents a potential time- and cost-effective alternative to standard rTMS for the treatment of depression.

13.3.2 Deep TMS

The use of deep TMS (dTMS) to target broader DLPFC and subcortical regions has recently been studied in the context of depression. Device clearance for dTMS use in

TABLE 13.2 Outcome measures across larger clinical studies investigating the use of several repetitive transcranial magnetic stimulation (rTMS) protocols for the treatment of treatment-resistant depression (TRD)

Type of study	rTMS	Sample	Response rate (%)	Remission rate (%)	Comments
Randomized blind trial, medication free (O'Reardon et al., 2007)	75 trains per day of 10 Hz stimulation	301 patients with TRD	23.9 vs. 15.1	17.4 vs. 8.2	Rate at 6 weeks
Randomized blind trial, medication free (George et al., 2010)	75 trains per day of 10 Hz stimulation	190 patients with TRD	15 vs. 5	14.1 vs. 5.1	Rates at 3 weeks
Randomized blinded 3-arm study: RTMS, venlafaxine (up to 225 mg/day) or combination (Brunelin et al., 2014)	Six trains per day of 60 s of 1 Hz (360 pulses)	155 patients with TRD	rTMS: 59 / venlafaxine: 60 combination: 54	rTMS: 40.7 / Venlafaxine: 43.1% Combination: 28%	Up to 6 weeks of treatment, rTMS and medication response were equivalent
Randomized double-blind trial, concomitant medication allowed (Yesvage et al., 2018)	100 trains per day of 10 Hz stimulation (4,000 pulses)	164 veterans with TRD, ~50% with posttraumatic stress disorder (PTSD), ~50% with substance use disorder		40.7vs. 37.4	Up to 6 weeks
Randomized double-blind trial, medication free (Levkovitz et al., 2015)	55 trains of 20 Hz stimulation daily (1,980 pulses), deep TMS coil	212 patients TRD, 181 patients in per protocol (PP) analysis	38.4vs. 21.4	32.6vs. 14.5	Response and remission rates at 5 weeks for PP analysis
Pooled outcome data from 11 clinical trials (Fitzgerald et al., 2016a)	Multiple protocols, left, right and bilateral rTMS	1,132 patients in multiple trials	46.8	31.4	Assessment based on end of acute treatment
Randomized 4 group trial (2 doses × 2 conditions – left and right) (Fitzgerald et al., 2020)	125or 50 10 Hz Trains per day or 20 min or 60 min of 1 Hz stimulation	300patients with TRD	47.3–52.5	18.6–31.9	Rates at 4 weeks across 4 groups
Randomized controlled comparative trial, on medication (Blumberger et al., 2018)	rTMS: 75 trains per day of 10 Hz stimulation (3,000 pulses) iTBS: 600 pulses over 189 s	385patients with TRD	47(rTMS) vs. 49 (iTBS)	27(rTMS) vs. 32 (iTBS)	Rates at 4 weeks

DLPFC, dorsolateral prefrontal cortex; ITI, intertrain interval; RMT, resting motor threshold; iTBS, intermittent theta burst stimulation.

From Fitzgerald.[22]

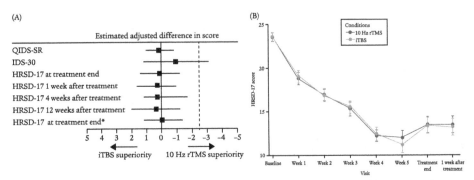

FIGURE 13.1 *Results from the THREE-D study. (A) Estimated adjusted differences in depression scores on several clinical scales, from baseline to the end of treatment, comparing standard 10 Hz repetitive transcranial magnetic stimulation (rTMS) and intermittent theta burst stimulation (iTBS). The dotted line indicates the non-inferiority margin (2·25 points). QIDS-SR, 16-item Quick Inventory of Depressive Symptomatology; IDS-30, 30-item Inventory of Depressive Symptomatology; HRSD-17, 17-item Hamilton Rating Scale for Depression. (B) The change in HRSD-17 scores over time, demonstrating the non-inferiority of iTBS compared to standard 10 Hz rTMS in treating depression.*
From Blumberger et al., *Lancet.* 2018;391(10131):1683–1692.

depression was granted based on a large, randomized control trial in 212 patients with depression. In this study, patients received either active or sham dTMS daily for 4 weeks, followed by biweekly stimulation for 12 weeks. Results demonstrated clinical efficacy of active dTMS compared to sham stimulation, which remained stable over the maintenance phase.[55]

Following this initial trial, studies have reported positive results in the treatment of bipolar depression (BD) at endpoint but not follow-up,[56] and in late-life depression.[57] One recent study aimed to directly compare dTMS, standard rTMS, and medication alone in 228 patients with depression. Both dTMS and standard rTMS were associated with better remission rates than medication alone. Additionally, moderate effects were observed in reduction of depressive symptoms and response rates in the dTMS group; however, the two rTMS treatment groups did not significantly differ in terms of remission rates.[58] Of note, among these studies, cases of increased application site pain[55,57] and serious adverse events associated with two seizures were reported.[55,59] In all, current evidence provides support for the use of dTMS as an efficacious treatment for depression, but data do not suggest that there is a benefit of dTMS over standard rTMS at this time.

13.3.3 Priming rTMS

Similar to the concept of priming in TMS cognition studies (reviewed in Chapter 6), priming rTMS (pTMS) suggests that a brief duration of high-frequency stimulation delivered immediately prior to low-frequency stimulation may act to enhance the neurophysiological response of the low-frequency stimulation.[60] Using 20 trains of 6 Hz stimulation preceding 15 min of low-frequency right prefrontal cortex stimulation, one study demonstrated greater therapeutic response compared to sham priming stimulation (i.e., a single train of 1 Hz rTMS) after 2 and 4 weeks of treatment.[61] When comparing sequential bilateral rTMS to this priming protocol, both groups demonstrated similar substantial remission and response rates.[48] A recent study investigated the effects of active (4–8 Hz stimulation, 400 pulses) versus sham pTMS, followed by low-frequency right stimulation and found a modest yet significantly greater antidepressant effect with active priming.[62] Given the small number of priming studies conducted to date, the use of pTMS in clinical practice for the treatment of depression has not occurred.

13.3.4 Novel Targets

In addition to the DLPFC, neuroimaging studies have identified several other brain regions and networks underlying the pathophysiology of depression.[63,64] For example, a chart view invetigating the efficacy of high-frequency rTMS and iTBS delivered to the dorsomedial prefrontal cortex (DMPFC) in 185 patients, found clinically meaningful response and remission rates that were comparable across the two protocols.[65] Importantly, DMPFC stimulation appears to be safe[65] and does not result in significant cognitive side effects.[66]

The anterior cingulate cortex (ACC) represents another potential target for rTMS given evidence demonstrating abnormal ACC activity in patients with depression.[67] Using a double-cone coil, it is possible to stimulate the deeper cortical structure of the ACC; one pilot trial demonstrated the feasibility and tolerability of this approach as a potential add-on treatment for depression.[68] Finally, preliminary evidence suggests that the orbitofrontal cortex (OFC), primarily the right lateral OFC, may represent an important treatment target in depression.[69] One key consideration when stimulating these deeper regions is the potential for more discomfort and pain. However, these preliminary results are promising and warrant further investigation with larger sham-controlled studies.

13.4 SCHEDULING AND MAINTENANCE APPROACHES

13.4.1 Standard Versus Accelerated Protocols

A typical therapeutic course of rTMS includes 20–30 sessions delivered daily for 4–6 weeks, which requires a large time commitment from patients. Recently, researchers and clinicians have begun to investigate accelerated protocols involving multiple rTMS sessions per day. This is made possible in part by the clinical success of shorter TBS

protocols. This novel approach to treatment scheduling not only has the potential to reduce the daily burden on patients, but it may also accelerate clinical improvements.

Using this approach, few studies have demonstrated the overall safety and efficacy
of twice-daily rTMS compared to sham stimulation[70] or once-daily stimulation.[71] One
important consideration when directly comparing once- and twice-daily rTMS is the
fact that patients in the twice-daily group receive a higher dose of treatment,[22] likely
contributing to the overall efficacy. In contrast, a recent retrospective analysis comparing once- and twice-daily rTMS reported similar rates of response and remission among
the two protocols; however, these rates were achieved faster in the twice-daily group. In
this study, the total number of pulses per day were equivalent among the two treatment
groups, which therefore suggests that the cumulative number of sessions rather than the
number of pulses impacts response.[72] Additional studies,[73] including one study in older
individuals,[74] provide further support for the safety, feasibility, and efficacy of twice-daily
rTMS to treat depression.

Fewer studies have investigated applying more than two treatment sessions per day of
high-frequency rTMS.[75,76] The first study administered 15 rTMS sessions over 2 days and
observed a decrease in symptoms of depression and anxiety, with comparable response
rates to that of the standard 4–6 weeks of treatment. Importantly, response remained fairly
stable at 36% during the 3- and 6-week follow-up assessments, with few side effects.[77] The
feasibility and efficacy of shorter rTMS sessions through the use of TBS has allowed for
further investigation of accelerated rTMS. Using a cross-over design, one study found
that while symptoms of depression[78,79] and suicidal ideation decreased[77] following accelerated iTBS, there was no difference between active and sham stimulation. More recently, an open-label study administered 10 daily sessions of iTBS for 5 consecutive days,
which resulted in a very high remission rate of greater than 90% and a 100% remission on
measures of suicidal ideation.[80] Taken together, accelerated rTMS protocols appear to be
promising, especially in terms of reducing the length of the treatment course; however,
continued investigation using appropriate sham-controlled study designs are needed before implementing this approach in clinical practice.

13.4.2 Treating and Preventing Relapse

The majority of previous rTMS research has focused on the acute effects of treatment;
however, it is well established that a relapse of symptoms following rTMS treatment is
common. For example, a meta-analysis estimated that only 53% of patients maintained
response 6 months after treatment[81] whereas a naturalistic study reported a relapse rate
of 77% after 6 months.[82] Overall, the clinical benefits of rTMS following an acute course
have been shown to last anywhere from 3[83] to 12 months.[84]

One common approach to addressing relapse involves restimulation using the same protocol that was used in the initial treatment course. In general, this approach appears to be successful in treating subsequent episodes[85,86] and may require a shorter duration of treatment.[84,87] For example, one study reported that of the 38 patients who reported symptom worsening and received restimulation at the 24-month follow-up, 32 of these patients (84.2%) showed symptom improvement.[86] While these initial findings are promising, identifying a method to successfully prevent relapse rather than initiating treatment following the onset of relapse is of great importance.

At present, there is limited evidence regarding the optimal approach to prevent relapse after a successful course of rTMS. However, several potential strategies have been identified and are currently under investigation. The first approach, which involves administering single sessions of rTMS either weekly or monthly following an acute course of rTMS, has demonstrated mixed results. For example, one study failed to find a significant benefit in prolonging clinical response with monthly rTMS maintenance treatments compared to observation (i.e., reintroduce rTMS if depressive symptoms worsen).[87] Similarly, similar relapse rates were reported in patients treated with either rTMS, venlafaxine, or a combination of the two when maintenance was tapered from twice weekly to once every 2 weeks.[88] In contrast, weekly maintenance rTMS, but not less frequent stimulation, appeared to be associated with a moderate clinical benefit when compared to sham stimulation.[89] Furthermore, twice-weekly dTMS was also associated with a sustained therapeutic effect for up to 16 weeks.[55]

An alternative to this approach, a "clustered" maintenance strategy that typically involves the monthly administration of two daily treatments, has shown success in maintaining response or remission.[90] In a large, randomized control trial in 281 patients who initially responded to medication, clustered rTMS (i.e., 5–10 sessions over 3–5-days) and combined rTMS plus antidepressants were associated with lower relapse rates compared to antidepressants alone.[91] Despite these data, currently there is insufficient information to guide the frequency and duration of maintenance rTMS. However, it is recommended that, in addition to rTMS, alternative evidence-based maintenance strategies, including medication, psychotherapy, or a combination of approaches, be considered following an acute course of rTMS.[92]

13.5 RTMS FOR SPECIAL POPULATIONS WITH DEPRESSION

13.5.1 Bipolar Depression

Several early studies investigating the efficacy of rTMS included patients with either unipolar or bipolar depression; therefore, the majority of what we know regarding the use of rTMS in this population is drawn from these mixed sample studies. Numerous rTMS protocols and target areas have been investigated in patients with BD; however, most studies employed high-frequency DLPFC stimulation followed by low-frequency and sequential bilateral protocols.[93] In general, these studies primarily demonstrated greater clinical efficacy of active compared to sham stimulation.[93,94] Additionally, mixed sample studies reported similar response rates among those with unipolar and bipolar depression,[95,96] suggesting that rTMS may be as effective in BD as it is in unipolar depression. However, one recent meta-analysis reported that of the nine sham-controlled randomized controlled trials included in their analysis, only three reported a benefits of active over sham stimulation.[93]

Similarly, the limited number of studies including samples with only BD patients provide conflicting results. For example, active dTMS was associated with a greater reduction in depression rating scores at end point but not at the follow-up visit. Furthermore, no differences were found between active or sham stimulation in response or remission rates.[56] Additional small-scale studies have failed to find clinical benefits of active sequential bilateral rTMS[97] or of active high- or low-frequency stimulation when administered in combination with quetiapine.[98] One important consideration noted in treating patients with BD is the risk of treatment-emergent affective switching. While a few cases of manic switching have been reported with sequential rTMS[99] and iTBS,[100] the risk associated with active rTMS appears to be relatively low.[93,101] A recent trial of iTBS to the left DLPFC was halted due to poor recruitment and lack of efficacy; conclusions from this trial are limited due to the small sample size.[102] In all, current evidence provides some support for the use of rTMS in the treatment of BD though the optimal parameters and target sites for stimulation warrant further investigation.

13.5.2 Depression in the Elderly

Depression in the elderly and aging population in general is associated with neurophysiological and anatomical changes, cognitive and functional impairments, and polypharmacy. All of these factors likely impact the overall efficacy of rTMS. As such, initial rTMS studies suggested that increased age may be associated with lower levels of treatment response.[103–106] This was in part, due to under-dosing of stimulus intensity associated with frontal cortical atrophy. To address this, some early studies investigated the use of modified rTMS parameters and reported some benefit in increasing the stimulus intensity to 120% as well as increasing the number of pulses in elderly patients.[107–109] In this context, more recent studies suggest that age may be a positive predictor of response,[110] while other studies have failed to find an association between age and treatment outcome.[111,112]

While few clinical trials specifically focusing on rTMS use in the elderly currently exist, available studies have revealed positive results using a number of rTMS protocols. For example, a double-blind, sham-controlled trial demonstrated significantly greater remission rates in patients with late-life depression who were treated with dTMS compared to sham stimulation.[57] Greater response rates were also observed in elderly patients treated with twice-daily rTMS.[74] Similarly, compared to sham stimulation, studies have shown that bilateral[113] and high-frequency left DLPFC[109] stimulation are superior and safe in elderly patients with late-life depression and vascular depression, respectively. While studies indicate that ensuring adequate stimulus intensity should be considered in treating depression in elderly populations, current findings provide support for the use of sequential bilateral rTMS when treating older depressed adults in clinical practice and for the ongoing inclusion of elderly patients in novel rTMS trials.[108]

13.5.3 Depression in Adolescents

In contrast to other clinical applications of rTMS, research on the antidepressant efficacy of rTMS in adolescents is fairly limited. Drawing primarily from case reports and small-scale open-label studies employing high-frequency stimulation, a recent meta-analysis including 10 studies and 112 patients found that rTMS represents a potentially effective, safe, and well-tolerated treatment for depression in adolescents.[114]

Of these studies, several rTMS protocols, along with varying rates of response, have been reported. For example, an early study employing high-frequency left stimulation at 80% intensity found clinical response in 3 out of 9 teenaged patients.[115] More recent studies, including an open-label trial in 32 patients with treatment-resistant MDD, found a response rate of 56% with high-frequency stimulation at 120% intensity. Importantly, the authors reported a high retention rate and no serious adverse effects.[116] High-frequency stimulation was also associated with a reduction in suicidal ideation in adolescents; however, this effect was accounted for by changes in depressive symptoms.[117] Compared to adults, higher response rates for symptoms of depression and anxiety were reported with high-frequency stimulation in a naturalistic study.[118] A recent multicenter trial in 103 adolescents aged 12–21 using high-frequency stimulation did not find differences in reduction of symptoms, response, or remission rates.[119] This trial highlighted the prominent placebo response that can be seen with antidepressant treatments in this population. In addition, low-frequency right and bilateral stimulation has shown some antidepressant efficacy, with a response rate of 40% reported in one retrospective analysis in 15 patients.[120] While evidence supporting the use of rTMS in adolescents is limited, these studies highlight its potential role, but also the challenge of demonstrating the efficacy of novel interventions in this population.

13.5.4 Pregnancy and Postpartum Depression

Postpartum depression is reported to affect between 10% and 15% of women; however, many women do not seek treatment or discontinue treatment during pregnancy.[121–123] rTMS is thought to pose minimal risk to the fetus, with one computational modeling study demonstrating that the exposure to the fetus is significantly below the exposure limits deemed to be potentially harmful.[124] Thus, rTMS offers a promising noninvasive approach to the treatment of peripartum and postpartum depression.

The majority of what is known about the efficacy and safety of rTMS treatment during pregnancy comes from case reports and series,[125–127] including one successful case report of iTBS use in the third trimester of pregnancy.[128] A recent RCT in 22 pregnant women found that low-frequency right DLPFC stimulation was safe and clinically beneficial compared to sham stimulation.[129] Importantly, follow-up studies have not reported abnormalities among the children born to mothers who were treated with rTMS,[130] although one study reported some language developmental delays at a rate similar to children born to mothers with untreated depression.[131] A systematic review of available evidence, including 87 pregnant women who received rTMS for depression, found that in addition to effectively reducing symptoms of depression, no serious adverse events were reported. Additionally, rates of side effects were similar to those reported in nonpregnant populations and patients receiving sham stimulation.[132] Similarly, available case series and small studies in women with postpartum depression provide evidence of reduced symptoms of depression[133] and improved infant bonding following rTMS treatment.[134] In all, these studies demonstrate clear support for the effectiveness, safety, and tolerability of rTMS in peripartum and postpartum depression. Large-scale randomized controlled trials are unlikely to occur, and alternative strategies to gather outcome and safety data in this population are needed.

13.6 CURRENT CHALLENGES AND FUTURE DIRECTIONS

While it is clear that previous research has demonstrated the clinical efficacy of rTMS in the treatment of depression, numerous clinical challenges and questions still remain. One key consideration and the focus of ongoing investigation lies in identifying strategies to optimize treatment outcomes. This includes not only rTMS-related factors, but also individualized patient-related factors.

13.6.1 rTMS Factors

Elucidating the dose-response relationship with regards to the optimal stimulation intensity, number of pulses, and overall treatment length remains a current topic of debate.

While it may be reasonable to assume that a greater rTMS dose would result in a greater antidepressant response, this is not necessarily supported in the research.[22,135] Similarly, available research regarding the optimal length of a treatment course suggests that an average of 4–6 weeks is needed to achieve clinical improvement; however, given the high relapse rate following an acute course of rTMS, it follows that longer treatment courses could be more beneficial. As such, studies have demonstrated that longer treatment courses are generally associated with higher response and remission rates,[136,137] but this must be weighed against the cost-effectiveness and capacity of clinics. One proposed strategy may be to extend treatment if patients have partially but not yet fully responded to a standard 4–6 week course.[22,137,138]

An alternative strategy to consider in treating patients who have not responded to an initial course of rTMS is to switch to a different protocol. Few studies have investigated this method, including switching from low-frequency to high-frequency stimulation[139] and vice versa,[137] as well as switching from high-frequency to sequential bilateral stimulation.[140] Finally, one study also assessed the efficacy of switching to low-frequency stimulation to the right orbitofrontal cortex in those who did not respond to dorsomedial stimulation.[69] Taken together these studies have found some support for the use of a second rTMS protocol in initial nonresponders. However, increasing the length of the treatment course, regardless of switching protocols, may account for some of the therapeutic benefits found in these studies.[22] Efforts to establish optimal stimulation parameters require further studies focusing specifically on the dose-response relationships in depression.

13.6.2 Patient Factors

In addition to optimizing response based on stimulation parameters, research efforts have sought to identify clinical predictors of response. Examples of interindividual variables that may alter the stimulation effects include anatomic features (e.g., skull-to-brain distance, skull thickness, tissue heterogeneity), age, sex, brain state, pharmacological interventions, and genetics.[141–143]

Research has revealed several clinical, sociodemographic, and environmental variables that are associated with rTMS response. For example, degree of treatment resistance, comorbid psychotic symptoms, and the presence of significant anxiety have previously been reported to predict poorer treatment response[110,112,144]; however, these variables do not appear to be reliable predictors of outcome. As such, researchers have begun to explore potential electrophysiological and neuroimaging-based predictive features using machine learning approaches.[145,146] Recent work suggests that coil location relative to the site within the DLPFC most anticorrelated with the subgenual cingulate may be highly predictive of treatment outcome.[147,148] Similarly coil location and the stimulation site within the DLPFC may also mediate symptom-specific response.[149] Understanding the impact of such interindividual variables on the neurophysiologic and circuit effects of rTMS may help identify and refine novel predictive markers. Importantly, prospective clinical trials are needed to test these promising functional magnetic resonance imaging (fMRI) predictors.

13.7 CONCLUSION

Research conducted over the past 25 years has clearly demonstrated the safety and efficacy of rTMS as a treatment for depression. Some have raised concerns about the efficacy of rTMS, questioning the entire field. These attempts are tantamount to questioning the efficacy of antidepressants in general. There is clear multicenter data that has established the efficacy of high-frequency rTMS delivered to the left DLPFC. There is likely a sizeable nonspecific and embedded placebo effect associated with rTMS; by default, patients are behaviorally activated coming into the clinic and there is the close daily interaction with a nurse or technician. This placebo effect should be harnessed in clinical practice, just as it is for other treatments for depression. There is a promising role for the use of rTMS in special populations with depression including, for example, patients with BD, elderly and adolescent populations, and women during pregnancy and postpartum. As the field of rTMS continues to evolve and more research becomes available, novel protocols including TBS and accelerated treatment strategies, as well as alternative stimulation targets beyond the DLFPC, may become more common in clinical practice. Finally, the personalization of rTMS treatments based on underlying neurophysiology or neurocircuitry is on the horizon.

REFERENCES

1. Rush AJ, Trivedi MH, Wisniewski SR, Nierenberg AA, Stewart JW, Warden D, et al. Acute and longer-term outcomes in depressed outpatients requiring one or several treatment steps: A STAR*D report. *Am J Psychiatry.* 2006;163(11):1905–1917.
2. Schatzberg AF, Rush AJ, Arnow BA, Banks PL, Blalock JA, Borian FE, et al. Chronic depression: Medication (nefazodone) or psychotherapy (CBASP) is effective when the other is not. *Arch Gen Psychiatry.* 2005;62(5):513–520.
3. Sackeim HA, Prudic J, Fuller R, Keilp J, Lavori PW, Olfson M. The cognitive effects of electroconvulsive therapy in community settings. *Neuropsychopharmacology.* 2007;32(1):244–254.
4. Ingram A, Saling MM, Schweitzer I. Cognitive side effects of brief pulse electroconvulsive therapy: A review. *J ECT.* 2008;24(1):3–9.
5. Brakemeier EL, Berman R, Prudic J, Zwillenberg K, Sackeim HA. Self-evaluation of the cognitive effects of electroconvulsive therapy. *J ECT.* 2011;27(1):59–66.
6. Bustin J, Rapoport MJ, Krishna M, Matusevich D, Finkelsztein C, Strejilevich S, et al. Are patients' attitudes towards and knowledge of electroconvulsive therapy transcultural? A multi-national pilot study. *Int J Geriatr Psychiatry.* 2008;23(5):497–503.

7. Weir D. The media's damaging impact on public perception of electroconvulsive therapy 2013. http://healthydebate.ca/opinions/the-medias-damaging-impact-on-public-perception-of-electroconvulsive-therapy

8. Pascual-Leone A, Valls-Sole J, Wassermann EM, Hallett M. Responses to rapid-rate transcranial magnetic stimulation of the human motor cortex. *Brain.* 1994;117 (Pt 4):847–858.

9. Kolbinger HM, Höflich G, Hufnagel A, Müller H-J, Kasper S. Transcranial magnetic stimulation (TMS) in the treatment of major depression: A pilot study. *Hum Psychopharmacol Clin Exp.* 1995;10:305–310.

10. George MS, Wassermann EM, Williams WA, Callahan A, Ketter TA, Basser P, et al. Daily repetitive transcranial magnetic stimulation (rTMS) improves mood in depression. *Neuroreport.* 1995;6(14):1853–1856.

11. Pascual-Leone A, Rubio B, Pallardo F, Catala MD. Rapid-rate transcranial magnetic stimulation of left dorsolateral prefrontal cortex in drug-resistant depression. *Lancet.* 1996;348(9022):233–237.

12. Bajbouj M, Lisanby SH, Lang UE, Danker-Hopfe H, Heuser I, Neu P. Evidence for impaired cortical inhibition in patients with unipolar major depression. *Biol Psychiatry.* 2006;59(5):395–400.

13. Salustri C, Tecchio F, Zappasodi F, Bevacqua G, Fontana M, Ercolani M, et al. Cortical excitability and rest activity properties in patients with depression. *J Psychiatry Neurosci.* 2007;32(4):259–266.

14. Fitzgerald PB, Oxley TJ, Laird AR, Kulkarni J, Egan GF, Daskalakis ZJ. An analysis of functional neuroimaging studies of dorsolateral prefrontal cortical activity in depression. *Psychiatry Res.* 2006;148(1):33–45.

15. Fitzgerald PB, Laird AR, Maller J, Daskalakis ZJ. A meta-analytic study of changes in brain activation in depression. *Hum Brain Mapp.* 2008;29(6):683–695.

16. Peng Z, Zhou C, Xue S, Bai J, Yu S, Li X, et al. Mechanism of repetitive transcranial magnetic stimulation for depression. *Shanghai Arch Psychiatry.* 2018;30(2):84–92.

17. Philip NS, Barredo J, Aiken E, Carpenter LL. Neuroimaging mechanisms of therapeutic transcranial magnetic stimulation for major depressive disorder. *Biol Psychiatry Cogn Neurosci Neuroimaging.* 2018;3(3):211–222.

18. Chen R, Gerloff C, Classen J, Wassermann EM, Hallett M, Cohen LG. Safety of different inter-train intervals for repetitive transcranial magnetic stimulation and recommendations for safe ranges of stimulation parameters. *Electroencephalogr Clin Neurophysiol.* 1997;105(6):415–421.

19. Sanacora G, Mason GF, Rothman DL, Behar KL, Hyder F, Petroff OA, et al. REDUCED cortical gamma-aminobutyric acid levels in depressed patients determined by proton magnetic resonance spectroscopy. *Arch Gen Psychiatry.* 1999;56(11):1043–1047.

20. Krystal JH, Sanacora G, Blumberg H, Anand A, Charney DS, Marek G, et al. Glutamate and GABA systems as targets for novel antidepressant and mood-stabilizing treatments. *Mol Psychiatry.* 2002;7 Suppl 1:S71–80.

21. Sanacora G, Mason GF, Rothman DL, Hyder F, Ciarcia JJ, Ostroff RB, et al. Increased cortical GABA concentrations in depressed patients receiving ECT. *Am J psychiatry.* 2003;160(3):577–579.

22. Fitzgerald PB. An update on the clinical use of repetitive transcranial magnetic stimulation in the treatment of depression. *J Affect Dis.* 2020;276:90–103.

23. Fitzgerald PB, Brown TL, Marston NA, Daskalakis ZJ, De Castella A, Kulkarni J. Transcranial magnetic stimulation in the treatment of depression: A double-blind, placebo-controlled trial. *Arch Gen Psychiatry.* 2003;60(10):1002–1008.

24. Avery DH, Holtzheimer PE, 3rd, Fawaz W, Russo J, Neumaier J, Dunner DL, et al. A controlled study of repetitive transcranial magnetic stimulation in medication-resistant major depression. *Biol Psychiatry.* 2006;59(2):187–194.

25. Tarhan N, Sayar FG, Tan O, Kagan G. Efficacy of high-frequency repetitive transcranial magnetic stimulation in treatment-resistant depression. *Clin EEG Neurosci.* 2012;43(4):279–284.

26. O'Reardon JP, Solvason HB, Janicak PG, Sampson S, Isenberg KE, Nahas Z, et al. Efficacy and safety of transcranial magnetic stimulation in the acute treatment of major depression: A multisite randomized controlled trial. *Biol Psychiatry.* 2007;62(11):1208–1216.

27. George MS, Lisanby SH, Avery D, McDonald WM, Durkalski V, Pavlicova M, et al. Daily left prefrontal transcranial magnetic stimulation therapy for major depressive disorder: A sham-controlled randomized trial. *Arch Gen Psychiatry.* 2010;67(5):507–516.

28. Loo C, Mitchell P, Sachdev P, McDarmont B, Parker G, Gandevia S. Double-blind controlled investigation of transcranial magnetic stimulation for the treatment of resistant major depression. *Am J Psychiatry.* 1999;156(6):946–948.

29. Padberg F, Zwanzger P, Thoma H, Kathmann N, Haag C, Greenberg BD, et al. Repetitive transcranial magnetic stimulation (rTMS) in pharmacotherapy-refractory major depression: Comparative study of fast, slow and sham rTMS. *Psychiatry Res.* 1999;88(3):163–171.

30. Yesavage JA, Fairchild JK, Mi Z, Biswas K, Davis-Karim A, Phibbs CS, et al. Effect of repetitive transcranial magnetic stimulation on treatment-resistant major depression in US Veterans: A randomized clinical trial. *JAMA Psychiatry.* 2018;75(9):884–893.

31. Berlim MT, van den Eynde F, Tovar-Perdomo S, Daskalakis ZJ. Response, remission and drop-out rates following high-frequency repetitive transcranial magnetic stimulation (rTMS) for treating major depression: A systematic review and meta-analysis of randomized, double-blind and sham-controlled trials. *Psychol Med.* 2014;44(2):225–239.

32. Lefaucheur JP, Andre-Obadia N, Antal A, Ayache SS, Baeken C, Benninger DH, et al. Evidence-based guidelines on the therapeutic use of repetitive transcranial magnetic stimulation (rTMS). *Clin Neurophysiol.* 2014;125(11):2150–2206.

33. Lefaucheur JP, Aleman A, Baeken C, Benninger DH, Brunelin J, Di Lazzaro V, et al. Evidence-based guidelines on the therapeutic use of repetitive transcranial magnetic stimulation (rTMS): An update (2014–2018). *Clin Neurophysiol.* 2020;131(2):474–528.

34. Couturier JL. Efficacy of rapid-rate repetitive transcranial magnetic stimulation in the treatment of depression: A systematic review and meta-analysis. *J Psychiatry Neurosci.* 2005;30(2):83–90.

35. Klein E, Kreinin I, Chistyakov A, Koren D, Mecz L, Marmur S, et al. Therapeutic efficacy of right prefrontal slow repetitive transcranial magnetic stimulation in major depression: A double-blind controlled study. *Arch Gen Psychiatry.* 1999;56(4):315–320.

36. Feinsod M, Kreinin B, Chistyakov A, Klein E. Preliminary evidence for a beneficial effect of low-frequency, repetitive transcranial magnetic stimulation in patients with major depression and schizophrenia. *Depress Anxiety.* 1998;7(2):65–68.

37. Berlow YA, Zandvakili A, Philip NS. Low frequency right-sided and high frequency left-sided repetitive transcranial magnetic stimulation for depression: The evidence of equivalence. *Brain Stimul.* 2020;13(6):1793–1795.

38. Mutz J, Edgcumbe DR, Brunoni AR, Fu CHY. Efficacy and acceptability of non-invasive brain stimulation for the treatment of adult unipolar and bipolar depression: A systematic review and meta-analysis of randomised sham-controlled trials. *Neurosci Biobehav Rev.* 2018;92:291–303.

39. Schutter DJ. Quantitative review of the efficacy of slow-frequency magnetic brain stimulation in major depressive disorder. *Psychol Med.* 2010;40(11):1789–1795.

40. Chen J, Zhou C, Wu B, Wang Y, Li Q, Wei Y, et al. Left versus right repetitive transcranial magnetic stimulation in treating major depression: A meta-analysis of randomised controlled trials. *Psychiatry Res.* 2013;210(3):1260–1264.

41. Kaur M, Michael JA, Fitzgibbon BM, Hoy KE, Fitzgerald PB. Low-frequency rTMS is better tolerated than high-frequency rTMS in healthy people: Empirical evidence from a single session study. *J Psychiatr Res.* 2019;113:79–82.

42. Kellner CH, Knapp R, Husain MM, Rasmussen K, Sampson S, Cullum M, et al. Bifrontal, bitemporal and right unilateral electrode placement in ECT: Randomised trial. *Br J Psychiatry.* 2010;196(3):226–234.

43. Loo CK, Mitchell PB, Croker VM, Malhi GS, Wen W, Gandevia SC, et al. Double-blind controlled investigation of bilateral prefrontal transcranial magnetic stimulation for the treatment of resistant major depression. *Psychol med.* 2003;33(1):33–40.

44. Fitzgerald PB, Benitez J, de Castella A, Daskalakis ZJ, Brown TL, Kulkarni J. A randomized, controlled trial of sequential bilateral repetitive transcranial magnetic stimulation for treatment-resistant depression. *Am J Psychiatry.* 2006;163(1):88–94.

45. Blumberger DM, Mulsant BH, Fitzgerald PB, Rajji TK, Ravindran AV, Young LT, et al. A randomized double-blind sham-controlled comparison of unilateral and bilateral repetitive transcranial magnetic stimulation for treatment-resistant major depression. *World J Biol Psychiatry.* 2012;13(6):423–435.

46. Pallanti S, Bernardi S, Di Rollo A, Antonini S, Quercioli L. Unilateral low frequency versus sequential bilateral repetitive transcranial magnetic stimulation: Is simpler better for treatment of resistant depression? *Neuroscience.* 2010;167(2):323–328.

47. Fitzgerald PB, Hoy K, Gunewardene R, Slack C, Ibrahim S, Bailey M, et al. A randomized trial of unilateral and bilateral prefrontal cortex transcranial magnetic stimulation in treatment-resistant major depression. *Psychol Med.* 2011;41(6):1187–1196.

48. Fitzgerald PB, Hoy KE, Singh A, Gunewardene R, Slack C, Ibrahim S, et al. Equivalent beneficial effects of unilateral and bilateral prefrontal cortex transcranial magnetic stimulation in a large randomized trial in treatment-resistant major depression. *Int J Neuropsychopharmacol.* 2013;16(9):1975–1984.

49. Chen JJ, Liu Z, Zhu D, Li Q, Zhang H, Huang H, et al. Bilateral vs. unilateral repetitive transcranial magnetic stimulation in treating major depression: A meta-analysis of randomized controlled trials. *Psychiatry Res.* 2014;219(1):51–57.

50. Berlim MT, Van den Eynde F, Daskalakis ZJ. A systematic review and meta-analysis on the efficacy and acceptability of bilateral repetitive transcranial magnetic stimulation (rTMS) for treating major depression. *Psychol Med.* 2013;43(11):2245–2254.

51. Huang YZ, Edwards MJ, Rounis E, Bhatia KP, Rothwell JC. Theta burst stimulation of the human motor cortex. *Neuron.* 2005;45(2):201–206.

52. Trevizol AP, Blumberger DM. An update on repetitive transcranial magnetic stimulation for the treatment of major depressive disorder. *Clin Pharmacol Ther.* 2019;106(4):747–762.

53. Berlim MT, McGirr A, Rodrigues Dos Santos N, Tremblay S, Martins R. Efficacy of theta burst stimulation (TBS) for major depression: An exploratory meta-analysis of randomized and sham-controlled trials. *J Psychiatr Res.* 2017;90:102–109.

54. Blumberger DM, Vila-Rodriguez F, Thorpe KE, Feffer K, Noda Y, Giacobbe P, et al. Effectiveness of theta burst versus high-frequency repetitive transcranial magnetic stimulation in patients with depression (THREE-D): A randomised non-inferiority trial. *Lancet.* 2018;391(10131):1683–1692.

55. Levkovitz Y, Isserles M, Padberg F, Lisanby SH, Bystritsky A, Xia G, et al. Efficacy and safety of deep transcranial magnetic stimulation for major depression: A prospective multicenter randomized controlled trial. *World Psychiatry.* 2015;14(1):64–73.

56. Tavares DF, Myczkowski ML, Alberto RL, Valiengo L, Rios RM, Gordon P, et al. Treatment of bipolar depression with deep TMS: Results from a double-blind, randomized, parallel group, sham-controlled clinical trial. *Neuropsychopharmacology.* 2017;42(13):2593–2601.

57. Kaster TS, Daskalakis ZJ, Noda Y, Knyahnytska Y, Downar J, Rajji TK, et al. Efficacy, tolerability, and cognitive effects of deep transcranial magnetic stimulation for late-life depression: A prospective randomized controlled trial. *Neuropsychopharmacology.* 2018;43(11):2231–2238.

58. Filipcic I, Simunovic Filipcic I, Milovac Z, Sucic S, Gajsak T, Ivezic E, et al. Efficacy of repetitive transcranial magnetic stimulation using a figure-8-coil or an H1-Coil in treatment of major depressive disorder; A randomized clinical trial. *J Psychiatr Res.* 2019;114:113–119.

59. Cullen KR, Jasberg S, Nelson B, Klimes-Dougan B, Lim KO, Croarkin PE. Seizure induced by deep transcranial magnetic stimulation in an adolescent with depression. *J Child Adolesc Psychopharmacol.* 2016;26(7):637–641.

60. Iyer MB, Schleper N, Wassermann EM. Priming stimulation enhances the depressant effect of low-frequency repetitive transcranial magnetic stimulation. *J Neurosci.* 2003;23(34):10867–10872.

61. Fitzgerald PB, Hoy K, McQueen S, Herring S, Segrave R, Been G, et al. Priming stimulation enhances the effectiveness of low-frequency right prefrontal cortex transcranial magnetic stimulation in major depression. *J Clin Psychopharmacol.* 2008;28(1):52–58.

62. Nongpiur A, Sinha VK, Praharaj SK, Goyal N. Theta-patterned, frequency-modulated priming stimulation enhances low-frequency, right prefrontal cortex repetitive transcranial magnetic stimulation (rTMS) in depression: A randomized, sham-controlled study. *J Neuropsychiatry Clin Neurosci.* 2011;23(3):348–357.

63. Koenigs M, Grafman J. The functional neuroanatomy of depression: Distinct roles for ventromedial and dorsolateral prefrontal cortex. *Behav Brain Res.* 2009;201(2):239–243.

64. Bora E, Fornito A, Pantelis C, Yucel M. Gray matter abnormalities in major depressive disorder: A meta-analysis of voxel based morphometry studies. *J Affect Dis.* 2012;138(1–2):9–18.

65. Bakker N, Shahab S, Giacobbe P, Blumberger DM, Daskalakis ZJ, Kennedy SH, et al. rTMS of the dorso-medial prefrontal cortex for major depression: Safety, tolerability, effectiveness, and outcome predictors for 10 Hz versus intermittent theta-burst stimulation. *Brain Stimul.* 2015;8(2):208–215.

66. Schulze L, Wheeler S, McAndrews MP, Solomon CJ, Giacobbe P, Downar J. Cognitive safety of dorsomedial prefrontal repetitive transcranial magnetic stimulation in major depression. *Eur Neuropsychopharmacol.* 2016;26(7):1213–1226.

67. Vanneste S, Ost J, Langguth B, De Ridder D. TMS by double-cone coil prefrontal stimulation for medication resistant chronic depression: A case report. *Neurocase.* 2014;20(1):61–68.

68. Kreuzer PM, Schecklmann M, Lehner A, Wetter TC, Poeppl TB, Rupprecht R, et al. The ACDC pilot trial: Targeting the anterior cingulate by double cone coil rTMS for the treatment of depression. *Brain Stimul.* 2015;8(2):240–246.

69. Feffer K, Fettes P, Giacobbe P, Daskalakis ZJ, Blumberger DM, Downar J. 1Hz rTMS of the right orbito-frontal cortex for major depression: Safety, tolerability and clinical outcomes. *Eur Neuropsychopharmacol.* 2018;28(1):109–117.

70. Loo CK, Mitchell PB, McFarquhar TF, Malhi GS, Sachdev PS. A sham-controlled trial of the efficacy and safety of twice-daily rTMS in major depression. *Psychol Med.* 2007;37(3):341–349.

71. Theleritis C, Sakkas P, Paparrigopoulos T, Vitoratou S, Tzavara C, Bonaccorso S, et al. Two versus one high-frequency repetitive transcranial magnetic stimulation session per day for treatment-resistant depression: A randomized sham-controlled trial. response to Andrade and colleagues. *J ECT.* 2017;33(2):143.

72. Schulze L, Feffer K, Lozano C, Giacobbe P, Daskalakis ZJ, Blumberger DM, et al. Number of pulses or number of sessions? An open-label study of trajectories of improvement for once-vs. twice-daily dorso-medial prefrontal rTMS in major depression. *Brain Stimul.* 2018;11(2):327–336.

73. Modirrousta M, Meek BP, Wikstrom SL. Efficacy of twice-daily vs once-daily sessions of repetitive transcranial magnetic stimulation in the treatment of major depressive disorder: A retrospective study. *Neuropsychiatr Dis Treat.* 2018;14:309–316.

74. Desbeaumes Jodoin V, Miron JP, Lesperance P. Safety and efficacy of accelerated repetitive transcranial magnetic stimulation protocol in elderly depressed unipolar and bipolar patients. *Am J Geriatr Psychiatry.* 2019;27(5):548–558.

75. Fitzgerald PB, Hoy KE, Elliot D, Susan McQueen RN, Wambeek LE, Daskalakis ZJ. Accelerated re-petitive transcranial magnetic stimulation in the treatment of depression. *Neuropsychopharmacol.* 2018;43(7):1565–1572.

76. Baeken C, Vanderhasselt MA, Remue J, Herremans S, Vanderbruggen N, Zeeuws D, et al. Intensive high-frequency-rTMS treatment in refractory medication-resistant unipolar depressed patients. *J Affect Dis.* 2013;151(2):625–631.

77. Holtzheimer PE, 3rd, McDonald WM, Mufti M, Kelley ME, Quinn S, Corso G, et al. Accelerated repetitive transcranial magnetic stimulation for treatment-resistant depression. *Depress Anxiety.* 2010;27(10):960–963.

78. Desmyter S, Duprat R, Baeken C, Van Autreve S, Audenaert K, van Heeringen K. Accelerated intermit-tent theta burst stimulation for suicide risk in therapy-resistant depressed patients: A randomized, sham-controlled trial. *Front Hum Neurosci.* 2016;10:480.

79. Duprat R, Desmyter S, Rudi de R, van Heeringen K, Van den Abbeele D, Tandt H, et al. Accelerated intermittent theta burst stimulation treatment in medication-resistant major depression: A fast road to remission? *J Affect Dis.* 2016;200:6–14.

80. Cole EJ, Stimpson KH, Bentzley BS, Gulser M, Cherian K, Tischler C, et al. Stanford accelerated intelligent neuromodulation therapy for treatment-resistant depression. *Am J Psychiatry.* 2020;177(8):716–726.

81. Senova S, Cotovio G, Pascual-Leone A, Oliveira-Maia AJ. Durability of antidepressant response to repetitive transcranial magnetic stimulation: Systematic review and meta-analysis. *Brain Stimul.* 2019;12(1):119–128.

82. Cohen RB, Boggio PS, Fregni F. Risk factors for relapse after remission with repetitive transcranial mag-netic stimulation for the treatment of depression. *Depress Anxiety.* 2009;26(7):682–688.

83. Mantovani A, Pavlicova M, Avery D, Nahas Z, McDonald WM, Wajdik CD, et al. Long-term efficacy of repeated daily prefrontal transcranial magnetic stimulation (TMS) in treatment-resistant depression. *Depress Anxiety.* 2012;29(10):883–890.

84. Dunner DL, Aaronson ST, Sackeim HA, Janicak PG, Carpenter LL, Boyadjis T, et al. A multisite, naturalistic, observational study of transcranial magnetic stimulation for patients with pharmacoresistant major depressive disorder: Durability of benefit over a 1-year follow-up period. *J Clin Psychiatry.* 2014;75(12):1394–1401.

85. Demirtas-Tatlidede A, Mechanic-Hamilton D, Press DZ, Pearlman C, Stern WM, Thall M, et al. An open-label, prospective study of repetitive transcranial magnetic stimulation (rTMS) in the long-term treatment of refractory depression: Reproducibility and duration of the antidepressant effect in medication-free patients. *J Clin Psychiatry.* 2008;69(6):930–934.

86. Janicak PG, Nahas Z, Lisanby SH, Solvason HB, Sampson SM, McDonald WM, et al. Durability of clinical benefit with transcranial magnetic stimulation (TMS) in the treatment of pharmacoresistant major depression: Assessment of relapse during a 6-month, multisite, open-label study. *Brain Stimul.* 2010;3(4):187–199.

87. Philip NS, Dunner DL, Dowd SM, Aaronson ST, Brock DG, Carpenter LL, et al. Can medication free, treatment-resistant, depressed patients who initially respond to TMS be maintained off medications? a prospective, 12-month multisite randomized pilot study. *Brain Stimul.* 2016;9(2):251–257.

88. Haesebaert F, Moirand R, Schott-Pethelaz AM, Brunelin J, Poulet E. Usefulness of repetitive transcranial magnetic stimulation as a maintenance treatment in patients with major depression. *World J Biol Psychiatry.* 2018;19(1):74–78.

89. Benadhira R, Thomas F, Bouaziz N, Braha S, Andrianisaina PS, Isaac C, et al. A randomized, sham-controlled study of maintenance rTMS for treatment-resistant depression (TRD). *Psychiatry research.* 2017;258:226–233.

90. Fitzgerald PB, Grace N, Hoy KE, Bailey M, Daskalakis ZJ. An open label trial of clustered maintenance rTMS for patients with refractory depression. *Brain Stimul.* 2013;6(3):292–297.

91. Wang HN, Wang XX, Zhang RG, Wang Y, Cai M, Zhang YH, et al. Clustered repetitive transcranial magnetic stimulation for the prevention of depressive relapse/recurrence: A randomized controlled trial. *Transl Psychiatry.* 2017;7(12):1292.

92. McClintock SM, Reti IM, Carpenter LL, McDonald WM, Dubin M, Taylor SF, et al. Consensus recommendations for the clinical application of repetitive transcranial magnetic stimulation (rTMS) in the treatment of depression. *J Clin Psychiatry.* 2018;79(1).

93. Hett D, Marwaha S. Repetitive transcranial magnetic stimulation in the treatment of bipolar disorder. *Ther Adv Psychopharmacol.* 2020;10:2045125320973790.

94. McGirr A, Karmani S, Arsappa R, Berlim MT, Thirthalli J, Muralidharan K, et al. Clinical efficacy and safety of repetitive transcranial magnetic stimulation in acute bipolar depression. *World Psychiatry.* 2016;15(1):85–86.

95. Carnell BL, Clarke P, Gill S, Galletly CA. How effective is repetitive transcranial magnetic stimulation for bipolar depression? *J Affect Dis.* 2017;209:270–272.

96. Fitzgerald PB, Huntsman S, Gunewardene R, Kulkarni J, Daskalakis ZJ. A randomized trial of low-frequency right-prefrontal-cortex transcranial magnetic stimulation as augmentation in treatment-resistant major depression. *Int J Neuropsychopharmacol.* 2006;9(6):655–666.

97. Fitzgerald PB, Hoy KE, Elliot D, McQueen S, Wambeek LE, Daskalakis ZJ. A negative double-blind controlled trial of sequential bilateral rTMS in the treatment of bipolar depression. *J Affect Dis.* 2016;198:158–162.

98. Hu SH, Lai JB, Xu DR, Qi HL, Peterson BS, Bao AM, et al. Efficacy of repetitive transcranial magnetic stimulation with quetiapine in treating bipolar II depression: A randomized, double-blinded, control study. *Sci Rep.* 2016;6:30537.

99. Hausmann A, Kramer-Reinstadler K, Lechner-Schoner T, Walpoth M, Rupp CI, Hinterhuber H, et al. Can bilateral prefrontal repetitive transcranial magnetic stimulation (rTMS) induce mania? A case report. *J Clin Psychiatry.* 2004;65(11):1575–1576.

100. Kaster TS, Knyahnytska Y, Noda Y, Downar J, Daskalakis ZJ, Blumberger DM. Treatment-emergent mania with psychosis in bipolar depression with left intermittent theta-burst rTMS. *Brain Stimul.* 2020;13(3):705–706.

101. Xia G, Gajwani P, Muzina DJ, Kemp DE, Gao K, Ganocy SJ, et al. Treatment-emergent mania in unipolar and bipolar depression: Focus on repetitive transcranial magnetic stimulation. *Int J Neuropsychopharmacol.* 2008;11(1):119–130.

102. McGirr A, Vila-Rodriguez F, Cole J, Torres IJ, Arumugham SS, Keramatian K, et al. Efficacy of active vs sham intermittent theta burst transcranial magnetic stimulation for patients with bipolar depression: A randomized clinical trial. *JAMA Netw Open.* 2021;4(3):e210963.

103. Fregni F, Marcolin MA, Myczkowski M, Amiaz R, Hasey G, Rumi DO, et al. Predictors of antidepressant response in clinical trials of transcranial magnetic stimulation. *Int J Neuropsychopharmacol.* 2006;9(6):641–654.

104. Manes F, Jorge R, Morcuende M, Yamada T, Paradiso S, Robinson RG. A controlled study of repetitive transcranial magnetic stimulation as a treatment of depression in the elderly. *Intl Psychogeriatr IPA.* 2001;13(2):225–231.

105. Kozel FA, Nahas Z, deBrux C, Molloy M, Lorberbaum JP, Bohning D, et al. How coil-cortex distance relates to age, motor threshold, and antidepressant response to repetitive transcranial magnetic stimulation. *J Neuropsychiatry Clin Neurosci.* 2000;12(3):376–384.

106. Figiel GS, Epstein C, McDonald WM, Amazon-Leece J, Figiel L, Saldivia A, et al. The use of rapid-rate transcranial magnetic stimulation (rTMS) in refractory depressed patients. *J Neuropsychiatry Clin Neurosci.* 1998;10(1):20–25.

107. Nahas Z, Li X, Kozel FA, Mirzki D, Memon M, Miller K, et al. Safety and benefits of distance-adjusted prefrontal transcranial magnetic stimulation in depressed patients 55-75 years of age: A pilot study. *Depress Anxiety.* 2004;19(4):249–256.

108. Sabesan P, Lankappa S, Khalifa N, Krishnan V, Gandhi R, Palaniyappan L. Transcranial magnetic stimulation for geriatric depression: Promises and pitfalls. *World J Psychiatry.* 2015;5(2):170–181.

109. Jorge RE, Moser DJ, Acion L, Robinson RG. Treatment of vascular depression using repetitive transcranial magnetic stimulation. *Arch Gen Psychiatry.* 2008;65(3):268–276.

110. Fitzgerald PB, Hoy KE, Anderson RJ, Daskalakis ZJ. A study of the pattern of response to rTMS treatment in depression. *Depress Anxiety.* 2016;33(8):746–753.

111. Conelea CA, Philip NS, Yip AG, Barnes JL, Niedzwiecki MJ, Greenberg BD, et al. Transcranial magnetic stimulation for treatment-resistant depression: Naturalistic treatment outcomes for younger versus older patients. *J Affect Dis.* 2017;217:42–47.

112. Lisanby SH, Husain MM, Rosenquist PB, Maixner D, Gutierrez R, Krystal A, et al. Daily left prefrontal repetitive transcranial magnetic stimulation in the acute treatment of major depression: Clinical predictors of outcome in a multisite, randomized controlled clinical trial. *Neuropsychopharmacology.* 2009;34(2):522–534.

113. Trevizol AP, Goldberger KW, Mulsant BH, Rajji TK, Downar J, Daskalakis ZJ, et al. Unilateral and bilateral repetitive transcranial magnetic stimulation for treatment-resistant late-life depression. *Int J Geriatr Psychiatry.* 2019;34(6):822–827.

114. Croarkin PE, MacMaster FP. Transcranial magnetic stimulation for adolescent depression. *Child Adolesc Psychiatr Clin N Am.* 2019;28(1):33–43.

115. Bloch Y, Grisaru N, Harel EV, Beitler G, Faivel N, Ratzoni G, et al. Repetitive transcranial magnetic stimulation in the treatment of depression in adolescents: An open-label study. *J ECT.* 2008;24(2):156–159.

116. MacMaster FP, Croarkin PE, Wilkes TC, McLellan Q, Langevin LM, Jaworska N, et al. Repetitive transcranial magnetic stimulation in youth with treatment resistant major depression. *Front Psychiatry.* 2019;10:170.

117. Croarkin PE, Nakonezny PA, Deng ZD, Romanowicz M, Voort JLV, Camsari DD, et al. High-frequency repetitive TMS for suicidal ideation in adolescents with depression. *J Affect Dis.* 2018;239:282–290.

118. Zhang T, Zhu J, Xu L, Tang X, Cui H, Wei Y, et al. Add-on rTMS for the acute treatment of depressive symptoms is probably more effective in adolescents than in adults: Evidence from real-world clinical practice. *Brain Stimul.* 2019;12(1):103–109.

119. Croarkin PE, Elmaadawi AZ, Aaronson ST, Schrodt GR, Jr., Holbert RC, Verdoliva S, et al. Left pre-frontal transcranial magnetic stimulation for treatment-resistant depression in adolescents: A double-blind, randomized, sham-controlled trial. *Neuropsychopharmacology.* 2021;46(2):462–469.

120. Rosenich E, Gill S, Clarke P, Paterson T, Hahn L, Galletly C. Does rTMS reduce depressive symptoms in young people who have not responded to antidepressants? *Early Interv Psychiatry.* 2019;13(5):1129–1135.

121. Hall P. Current considerations of the effects of untreated maternal perinatal depression and the National Perinatal Depression Initiative. *J Dev Orig Health Dis.* 2012;3(4):293–295.

122. Vigod SN, Wilson CA, Howard LM. Depression in pregnancy. *Br Med J.* 2016;352:i1547.

123. Ververs T, Kaasenbrood H, Visser G, Schobben F, de Jong-van den Berg L, Egberts T. Prevalence and patterns of antidepressant drug use during pregnancy. *Eur J Clin Pharmacol.* 2006;62(10):863–870.

124. Yanamadala J, Borwankar R, Makarov S, Pascual-Leone A. Estimates of peak electric fields induced by transcranial magnetic stimulation in pregnant women as patients or operators using an FEM full-body model. In Makarov S, Horner M, Noetscher G, eds. *Brain and Human Body Modeling: Computational Human Modeling at EMBC 2018.* Cham (CH): 2019: 49–73.

125. Kim DR, Epperson N, Pare E, Gonzalez JM, Parry S, Thase ME, et al. An open label pilot study of tran-scranial magnetic stimulation for pregnant women with major depressive disorder. *J Womens Health (Larchmt).* 2011;20(2):255–261.

126. Klirova M, Novak T, Kopecek M, Mohr P, Strunzova V. Repetitive transcranial magnetic stimulation (rTMS) in major depressive episode during pregnancy. *Neuro Endocrinol Lett.* 2008;29(1):69–70.

127. Zhang X, Liu K, Sun J, Zheng Z. Safety and feasibility of repetitive transcranial magnetic stimu-lation (rTMS) as a treatment for major depression during pregnancy. *Arch Womens Ment Health.* 2010;13(4):369–370.

128. Trevizol AP, Vigod SN, Daskalakis ZJ, Vila-Rodriguez F, Downar J, Blumberger DM. Intermittent theta burst stimulation for major depression during pregnancy. *Brain Stimul.* 2019;12(3):772–774.

129. Kim DR, Wang E, McGeehan B, Snell J, Ewing G, Iannelli C, et al. Randomized controlled trial of transcranial magnetic stimulation in pregnant women with major depressive disorder. *Brain Stimul.* 2019;12(1):96–102.

130. Hizli Sayar G, Ozten E, Tufan E, Cerit C, Kagan G, Dilbaz N, et al. Transcranial magnetic stimulation during pregnancy. *Arch Womens Ment Health.* 2014;17(4):311–315.

131. Eryilmaz G, Sayar GH, Ozten E, Gul IG, Yorbik O, Isiten N, et al. Follow-up study of children whose mothers were treated with transcranial magnetic stimulation during pregnancy: Preliminary results. *Neuromodulation.* 2015;18(4):255–260.

132. Cole J, Bright K, Gagnon L, McGirr A. A systematic review of the safety and effectiveness of repet-itive transcranial magnetic stimulation in the treatment of peripartum depression. *J Psychiatr Res.* 2019;115:142–150.

133. Myczkowski ML, Dias AM, Luvisotto T, Arnaut D, Bellini BB, Mansur CG, et al. Effects of repetitive transcranial magnetic stimulation on clinical, social, and cognitive performance in postpartum depres-sion. *Neuropsychiatr Dis Treat.* 2012;8:491–500.

134. Garcia KS, Flynn P, Pierce KJ, Caudle M. Repetitive transcranial magnetic stimulation treats post-partum depression. *Brain Stimul.* 2010;3(1):36–41.

135. Kedzior KK, Azorina V, Reitz SK. More female patients and fewer stimuli per session are associated with the short-term antidepressant properties of repetitive transcranial magnetic stimulation (rTMS): A meta-analysis of 54 sham-controlled studies published between 1997-2013. *Neuropsychiatr Dis Treat.* 2014;10:727–756.

136. Yip AG, George MS, Tendler A, Roth Y, Zangen A, Carpenter LL. 61% of unmedicated treatment re-sistant depression patients who did not respond to acute TMS treatment responded after four weeks of twice weekly deep TMS in the Brainsway pivotal trial. *Brain Stimul.* 2017;10(4):847–849.

137. McDonald WM, Durkalski V, Ball ER, Holtzheimer PE, Pavlicova M, Lisanby SH, et al. Improving the antidepressant efficacy of transcranial magnetic stimulation: Maximizing the number of stimulations and treatment location in treatment-resistant depression. *Depress Anxiety.* 2011;28(11):973–980.

138. Avery DH, Isenberg KE, Sampson SM, Janicak PG, Lisanby SH, Maixner DF, et al. Transcranial magnetic stimulation in the acute treatment of major depressive disorder: Clinical response in an open-label extension trial. *J Clin Psychiatry*. 2008;69(3):441–451.

139. Fitzgerald PB, McQueen S, Herring S, Hoy K, Segrave R, Kulkarni J, et al. A study of the effectiveness of high-frequency left prefrontal cortex transcranial magnetic stimulation in major depression in patients who have not responded to right-sided stimulation. *Psychiatry Res*. 2009;169(1):12–15.

140. Cristancho P, Trapp NT, Siddiqi SH, Dixon D, Miller JP, Lenze EJ. Crossover to bilateral repetitive transcranial magnetic stimulation: A potential strategy when patients are not responding to unilateral left-sided high-frequency repetitive transcranial magnetic stimulation. *J ECT*. 2019;35(1):3–5.

141. Rostami R, Kazemi R, Nitsche MA, Gholipour F, Salehinejad MA. Clinical and demographic predictors of response to rTMS treatment in unipolar and bipolar depressive disorders. *Clin Neurophysiol*. 2017;128(10):1961–1970.

142. Kar SK. Predictors of response to repetitive transcranial magnetic stimulation in depression: A review of recent updates. *Clin Psychopharmacol Neurosci*. 2019;17(1):25–33.

143. Nettekoven C, Volz LJ, Leimbach M, Pool EM, Rehme AK, Eickhoff SB, et al. Inter-individual variability in cortical excitability and motor network connectivity following multiple blocks of rTMS. *NeuroImage*. 2015;118:209–218.

144. Berlim MT, Van den Eynde F, Daskalakis ZJ. Efficacy and acceptability of high frequency repetitive transcranial magnetic stimulation (rTMS) versus electroconvulsive therapy (ECT) for major depression: A systematic review and meta-analysis of randomized trials. *Depress Anxiety*. 2013;30(7):614–623.

145. Bailey NW, Hoy KE, Rogasch NC, Thomson RH, McQueen S, Elliot D, et al. Differentiating responders and non-responders to rTMS treatment for depression after one week using resting EEG connectivity measures. *J Affect Dis*. 2019;242:68–79.

146. Corlier J, Wilson A, Hunter AM, Vince-Cruz N, Krantz D, Levitt J, et al. Changes in functional connectivity predict outcome of repetitive transcranial magnetic stimulation treatment of major depressive disorder. *Cerebral Cortex*. 2019;29(12):4958–4967.

147. Siddiqi SH, Weigand A, Pascual-Leone A, Fox MD. Identification of personalized transcranial magnetic stimulation targets based on subgenual cingulate connectivity: An independent replication. *Biol Psychiatry*. 2021.

148. Cash RFH, Weigand A, Zalesky A, Siddiqi SH, Downar J, Fitzgerald PB, et al. Using brain imaging to improve spatial targeting of transcranial magnetic stimulation for depression. *Biol Psychiatry*. 2020.

149. Siddiqi SH, Taylor SF, Cooke D, Pascual-Leone A, George MS, Fox MD. Distinct symptom-specific treatment targets for circuit-based neuromodulation. *Am J Psychiatry*. 2020;177(5):435–446.

rTMS for Other Psychiatric Disorders

14.1 INTRODUCTION

Research since the late 1990s has explored the use of repetitive magnetic stimulation (rTMS) in the treatment of a wide variety of psychiatric disorders. Although many of these studies have been small and not well-replicated, there are a growing number of disorders for which there is accumulating evidence for the potential use of rTMS as a therapeutic intervention; the most significant and advanced of these are reviewed in this chapter. Of note, there is an increasing range of applications for rTMS approved by regulatory authorities. At the time of writing, in addition to the treatment of depression, rTMS had been approved by the US Food and Drug Administration (FDA) for the treatment of obsessive-compulsive disorder (OCD) and smoking cessation.

14.2 SCHIZOPHRENIA

Schizophrenia is typically a difficult disorder to treat.[1] At least 30% of patients continue to have substantial positive symptoms despite adequate treatment with antipsychotic medications. These so-called positive symptoms include disordered thoughts, delusions, and auditory hallucinations. Patients with schizophrenia also commonly experience negative symptoms. These seem to be mediated by abnormalities in prefrontal function and include an inability to experience pleasure and a lack of motivation drive and energy. Negative symptoms tend to respond very poorly to any form of treatment and have a major impact on long-term prognosis. Prefrontal dysfunction also appears to underline aspects of the cognitive impairment seen in patients with schizophrenia. These are also poorly responsive to standard antipsychotic medication treatments and appear to be a major contributor to long-term disability. Due to the frequently refractory nature of the symptoms of schizophrenia, there has been persistent interest in the potential use of brain stimulation, especially rTMS in the treatment of this condition.

Although early approaches to the use of TMS in the treatment of schizophrenia were nonspecific, there generally has been an attempt to develop interventional approaches in which specific symptom domains are targeted with appropriately oriented rTMS stimulation and an acceptance that a single brain stimulation approach is unlikely to ameliorate the totality of the symptoms seen in this disorder. Two main brain regions have been the focus for treatment approaches adopted to date. First, the dorsolateral prefrontal cortex (DLPFC) has been the main site for treatment approaches aimed at ameliorating negative or cognitive symptoms.[2] It has been hypothesized that high-frequency rTMS applied to the DLPFC may improve these by increasing cortical excitability or activity in prefrontal regions or potentially ameliorate deficits in prefrontal cortical–subcortical connectivity.[3] The other main cortical region targeted in rTMS studies has been the temporoparietal cortex (TPC). Although there are some contradictory findings and a variety of hypotheses about the pathogenesis of hallucinations, a number of studies have suggested that the pathophysiology of auditory hallucinations is related to hyperactivity in the left TPC.[4,5] Based on this notion, Hoffman et al. developed a low-frequency rTMS protocol applied to the left TPC to modulate the potentially "overactive state" underpinning auditory hallucinations.[6,7]

14.2.1 Prefrontal Stimulation: Negative and Cognitive Symptoms

Some of the earliest rTMS studies conducted in patients with schizophrenia essentially adopted therapeutic models developed for the treatment of depression, applying either high- or low-frequency rTMS to the DLPFC without really establishing substantial therapeutic effects.[8–10] One early study specifically targeted positive symptoms with high-frequency DLPFC stimulation in a crossover design.[11] A significant reduction in Brief Psychiatric Rating Scale (BPRS) scores was seen with active but not sham stimulation. However, three other studies of high-frequency stimulation of the left DLPFC have failed to demonstrate an improvement in positive symptoms,[12–14] and a lack of an effect of high-frequency stimulation of prefrontal regions on positive symptoms was indicated in a meta-analysis of a number of studies conducted of this approach.[15]

A more consistent body of research has attempted to ameliorate negative symptoms with prefrontal rTMS. This body of literature predominately contains a series of small parallel design trials, although the sample sizes of more recent trials has grown somewhat. Considering the enduring nature of negative symptoms, these studies have also been quite short term and, by modern standards, have used relatively low doses of rTMS. They have also been predominantly unilateral, with the focus on left-sided stimulation. Given the short-term nature and small scale of these clinical trials, it is not at all surprising that there have been a number of negative studies.[12,16,17] In fact, given the limitations of this research, it is somewhat surprising that as many studies have reported positive effects as have done so.[14,18–20] Three of these studies[14,18,19] used higher stimulation intensity (>100% of the standard resting motor threshold), and one of the studies used a longer treatment duration (15 days) than most of negative studies (10 days).[18] Some of these studies have failed to adequately control for potential improvements in depressed mood although this was the case in one of the more carefully conducted trials. This study carefully controlled for the possible confound of improved depressive symptoms using scores on the Calgary Depression Scale for Schizophrenia. Depression scores were included as a covariate: improved depression did not account for the observed improvement in negative symptoms.[14]

There have been a number of other less standard approaches. For example, a three-arm parallel study compared 20 Hz stimulation to stimulation provided at the patient's individual alpha frequency and to a sham condition.[21] Alpha frequency stimulation was provided at the patient's peak alpha frequency assessed from five frontal electroencephalogram (EEG) leads. The rationale for enhancing activation by using the patient's own alpha frequency was based on the hypothesis that a deficiency in oscillations at this frequency was potentially related to the underlying pathophysiology of negative symptoms. Stimulation at the patient's α-frequency resulted in a significantly greater reduction in negative symptoms than the other conditions. More recently, studies have also provided stimulation in a bilateral manner, based on the observation that patients with negative symptoms demonstrate bilateral underactivity in prefrontal brain regions. Despite this, both studies reported no improvement in negative symptoms.[22,23] Finally, one small trial showed some benefits of deep TMS with an H coil on negative symptoms over a 20-day treatment period.[24]

Several more recent attempts have been made to conduct more substantive evaluations of rTMS treatment for negative symptoms. In the largest study to date, 175 patients across multiple sites were randomized to receive either active (10 Hz rTMS applied to the left DLPC) or sham stimulation for 3 weeks.[25] No statistically significant differences were seen between active or sham treatment at the end of treatment or during subsequent follow-up. In contrast to this report, Quan et al. randomized 117 patients to a longer 20-day course of left prefrontal 10 Hz stimulation (this actually consisted of two 10-day periods of treatment separated by a break of 2 weeks).[26] The overall dose of stimulation was quite low (800 pulses per day applied at only 80% of the motor threshold), and stimulation was applied with a circular coil. It is not clear from the report how the coil was orientated and whether this would have resulted in any bilateral stimulation. A significant benefit of active over sham treatment was seen at 2 and 6 weeks for negative but not positive symptoms. A third smaller multicenter trial randomized 32 patients to active or sham treatment, provided again at 10 Hz, but this time bilaterally over 3 weeks[27] A significant difference between active and sham treatment was found for negative but not positive symptoms which persisted at 3-month follow-up.

Finally, a study was recently reported that compared the application of three forms of rTMS applied to the left DLPFC (10Hz, 20Hz, and intermittent theta burst stimulation [iTBS]) to a sham group.[28] All three active groups produced better outcomes in regards to negative symptoms than the control group. The TBS condition produced greater effects than the 10 and 20 Hz rTMS approaches.

The results of these studies have been summarized in several meta-analyses. These have generally shown moderate positive and statistically significant treatment effects (for example [29,30]). Of note, there is some limited emerging evidence that similar benefits may be found with an "activating" form of transcranial direct current stimulation (tDCS) applied to the left DLPFC,[29,30] providing additional support for this brain region as a stimulation target in the treatment of negative symptoms.

Many fewer studies have explicitly targeted the treatment of cognitive symptoms. Impaired cognition has been increasingly recognized as a primary deficit in schizophrenia.[31] Recent data suggest that high-frequency rTMS applied to DLPFC can improve performance on higher order cognitive functions and selectively modulate gamma oscillations, which have been shown to be abnormal in schizophrenia, in frontal regions.[32] In one study, bilateral rTMS applied at 20 Hz and targeted to the DLPFC was shown to improve working memory deficits in patients with schizophrenia in a study including 27 patients.[33] Working memory was assessed using the N-back task. rTMS significantly improved 3-back accuracy to targets compared to sham. There was also a trend toward significance on the effects of rTMS on the 1- versus 3-back, suggesting that rTMS was more effective on working memory performance as difficulty increased. However, this finding was not replicated in a larger, more recent study of 4 weeks of double-blind 20 Hz treatment in 83 patients[34] or in a third study of 25 patients who received 3 weeks of 10 Hz stimulation, with cognitive outcomes and working memory–related functional magnetic resonance imaging (fMRI) activation unchanged after treatment.[35] No benefits were seen in a second study of 10 Hz stimulation, this time applied over 20 days in a sham controlled design,[36] and no benefits on cognitive performance were seen in a trial of 20 Hz stimulation targeting negative symptoms and cognition.[37] A recent study exploring the use of rTMS, predominantly in the treatment of negative symptoms, found that both 10 and 20 Hz rTMS appeared to produce some improvements in cognition that persisted for 6 months following an 8-week period of treatment.[28]

A meta-analysis in 2018 identified nine studies including 351 patients and found that rTMS treatment was associated with an improvement in working memory but no improvements in other cognitive domains.[38]

In summary, there is certainly a strong suggestion from the studies conducted to date that prefrontal rTMS may produce therapeutic benefits for patients with enduring negative symptoms. The effects seem to be greater in clinical trials conducted for longer periods of time, although there does not appear to be a strong relationship between stimulation dose and response to treatment or laterality. TBS also appears a promising approach that warrants further investigation. Limited data to date have addressed the question of whether rTMS has the capacity to improve cognitive function, with the most promising findings to date being in the modulation of working memory.

14.2.2 Temporoparietal Cortex Stimulation: Auditory Hallucinations

Research for 20 years has investigated the use of rTMS in the treatment of persistent auditory hallucinations in patients with schizophrenia. This application of rTMS was initially proposed based on the observation in early neuroimaging studies that patients with auditory hallucinations appeared to have overactivity in auditory processing regions in the area of the temporoparietal junction.

Based on this observation, Ralph Hoffman initiated an important series of studies progressively evaluating the application of low-frequency stimulation (1 Hz) to this site.[6,7] These studies began by exploring the duration of stimulation required to produce transient benefits with single stimulation trains, with the greatest reduction in hallucination produced with 16 min of stimulation. The effectiveness of rTMS was then tested in a number of parallel controlled studies. Therapeutic benefits were seen that were noted to persist in the months after treatment ceased.[39] Treatment in larger samples was also found to be safe and well-tolerated, something that has been a consistent finding in many subsequent studies.[40]

A relatively extensive series of randomized sham-controlled trials have explored this type of treatment although these have been mostly of limited sample size.[41–52] Interestingly, two of the randomized controlled studies have found significant reduction in frequency and intensity of auditory hallucinations with less than 10 days of treatment.[41,42] Not all studies have produced positive results, but several meta-analyses have suggested that rTMS does have beneficial effects.[53–57] For example, one analysis found that left temporoparietal stimulation was effective, with an effect size of 0.63,[53] but stimulation on the right was not found to be effective. Heterogeneity issues were raised as a concern in earlier analyses but several issues, for example in relationship to sample size, have not shown to be significantly influencing the result in sensitivity analyses.[54]

Along with left-sided stimulation, studies have attempted to explore the possibility of bilateral and right-sided temporoparietal cortex rTMS. As suggested earlier, meta-analyses have not yet supported the efficacy of these approaches, although there are little data collected to date. Although early, some studies are also starting to test whether high-frequency stimulation applied to the left temporoparietal cortex might have therapeutic benefits[58] and the potential value of theta burst stimulation.[59] Researchers are also investigating the use of neuronavigational targeting to improve clinical outcomes. One study of this type found no specific benefit of rTMS or of MRI-based localization,[60] and a second found an overall benefit with rTMS but, again, no improvement with functional MRI-based localization.[61]

In summary, a substantial number of studies have explored the possibility of treating persistent auditory hallucinations with temporoparietal cortex stimulation, predominantly on the left and at low frequency. There appears to be relatively consistent evidence for a therapy benefit of this type of stimulation although this has not been replicated in large multisite trials, and the optimal stimulation parameters have not been well-defined.

14.3 MANIA

Mania is a disorder for which there was early interest in the potential use of rTMS treatment, but it is also a disorder for which there has been little progression of this therapeutic approach. Early models of the use of rTMS in depression suggested that its efficacy was potentially mediated through increasing reduced levels of activity in the left prefrontal cortex in patients with depression. Alternatively, rTMS could be applied at low frequency to reduce an overactive right prefrontal cortex. It was proposed that mania may involve a reversed pattern of brain dysfunction: in particular, that mania may be related to an underactivity of the right prefrontal cortex. Partly on this basis, an initial study was conducted randomizing patients to either right- or left-sided treatment with high-frequency stimulation. In this study involving 16 patients, greater therapeutic benefits were reported with right-sided compared to left-sided treatment.[62] Further support for this approach came from two case series.[63,64]

However, few more substantive sham-controlled trials have been conducted, probably reflecting the difficulty of conducting trials in patients with mania. The first involved 25 patients and found no difference between active and sham stimulation.[65] A more recent study of 41 patients using 20 Hz rTMS found a significant benefit of active over sham stimulation over a 10-day period.[66]

In summary, a limited body of research has systematically evaluated the use of high-frequency stimulation applied to the right DLPFC in patients with mania. The research conducted to date suggests that this might have some effects, but the body of evidence must be considered preliminary.

14.4 OBSESSIVE COMPULSIVE DISORDER

There has been considerable interest in the use of rTMS to treat OCD due to the often refractory nature of this disorder and the limited range of currently available and effective treatments. The neural pathways and networks involved in OCD have been relatively well-defined through neuroimaging studies, and, given that these pathways involve prefrontal brain regions, these may well be amenable to targeted brain stimulation techniques.

The first study exploring rTMS for OCD involved 20 patients who received high-frequency stimulation to the left or right prefrontal cortex or a control site.[67] Stimulation was provided at a relatively low intensity, but right prefrontal stimulation was found to decrease compulsions and improve mood. This was seen to a greater degree than in left-sided stimulation or control site stimulation. Following on from this study, several groups have explored high-frequency stimulation to prefrontal areas, although, somewhat oddly, most of these have focused on the left prefrontal region rather than the right. These did not produce promising results.[68,69] A more recent high-frequency approach applied stimulation based on the individual alpha frequency recorded with EEG to bilateral prefrontal cortex. This approach appeared to produce a reduction in OCD symptoms acutely, with a later reduction in depression.[70]

Studies have also utilized low-frequency stimulation applied to the DLPFC with fairly unimpressive outcomes. For example, 1 Hz rTMS applied to the right DLPFC over eighteen 20 min daily sessions[71] produced no significant effects on obsessions or compulsions. 1 Hz stimulation applied to the left DLPFC[72] also failed to find therapeutic effects.

There seems to be more promise in approaches that target brain regions away from the DLPFC. One of the first alternative brain regions to gain attention was the supplementary motor area. A number of modestly sized studies have evaluated low-frequency stimulation applied bilaterally to the supplementary motor area in the midline,[70,73,74] generally with positive results. The rationale for this approach is based on the observation that the supplementary motor area is strongly connected to the anterior cingulate and areas of the striatum, brain regions known to be abnormally active in patients with OCD[74] (see Figure 14.1). A second novel approach has been to provide stimulation to the orbitofrontal cortex, either on the left or right, with the stimulation coil placed just above the eyebrow; these studies have had promising early reports of success.[75,76]

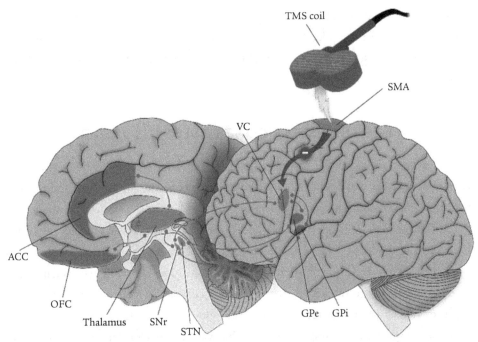

FIGURE 14.1 *The proposed mechanism of action of supplementary motor cortex (SMA) low-frequency repetitive transcranial magnetic stimulation (rTMS) in the treatment of obsessive-compulsive disorder. Stimulation of the SMA reduces local activity and activity in the connected ventral caudate (VC), part of the circuit of overactive regions in OCD. ACC, anterior cingulate cortex; OFC, orbitofrontal cortex, SNr, substantia nigra; STN, subthalamic nucleus; GPe, globus pallidus externa; GPi, globus pallidus interna.*

The approach that has had the most impact on clinical practice, however, has been the development of deep TMS stimulation, coupled with symptom provocation for the treatment of OCD. This was evaluated in a multicenter trial of 99 patients with OCD who received either high-frequency (20 Hz) or sham deep TMS targeting the medial prefrontal cortex/anterior cingulate cortex.[77] Immediately prior to each stimulation session patients underwent a brief provocation procedure designed to induce significant OCD-related anxiety. Deep TMS resulted in a 38% response rate with active treatment compared to 11% in the sham group, with persistent benefit at 1-month follow-up. The results of this trial resulted in FDA approval of deep TMS using the Brainsway TMS system in the United States, and, more recently, a second TMS coil/system has also been approved for clinical use in OCD.

In summary, the application of deep TMS to the medial prefrontal cortex appears to have efficacy in the treatment of OCD and has been sufficient for clinical approval, the second established psychiatric indication for rTMS therapy. There is also more limited evidence for the potential use of low-frequency stimulation applied to the supplementary motor and orbitofrontal cortical regions.

14.5 POSTTRAUMATIC STRESS DISORDER

A growing body of research has explored the use of rTMS in posttraumatic stress disorder (PTSD). The first uncontrolled study explored the application of very low-frequency stimulation (0.3 Hz) applied to both the left and right motor cortex, producing a reduction in PTSD symptoms.[78] Subsequently, studies have investigated a variety of stimulation paradigms including low- and high-frequency stimulation applied to the left DLPFC and low- and high-frequency stimulation applied to the right DLPFC.[79-82]

Although an increasing number of studies are exploring the use of TMS in PTSD, these have been generally modest in size. A recent meta-analysis of 11 randomized controlled trials found that rTMS produced a significant reduction in core PTSD symptoms, with a large effect size, and that significant effects were seen with both high- and low-frequency stimulation of the right DLPFC.[83] These effects were seen to be durable at 2 and 4 weeks after the cessation of treatment. Studies are also now emerging on the effects of iTBS in PTSD. For example, Philip et al. found therapeutic benefits of a relatively short course of right DLPFC iTBS on a variety of symptom dimensions.[84]

Several studies have explored the potential integration of rTMS stimulation with some form of psychological treatment or symptom provocation. Using deep TMS to stimulate medial prefrontal cortex, one study found a significant benefit of active treatment when combined with pretreatment symptom provocation.[85] The therapeutic benefit was seen when rTMS was applied immediately after exposure to a trauma-related events script. However, this effect was not replicated in a subsequent multisite trial.[86] A third study combined a weekly session of TMS provided in conjunction with 12–15 weeks of cognitive processing therapy[87]: combining TMS and therapy produced greater benefits than sham stimulation and therapy, with benefit sustained for 6 months after the end of treatment.

In summary, more research is required to evaluate the use of rTMS in PTSD but there appears to be significant potential for the use of stimulation, especially when applied to the right DLPFC.

14.6 OTHER ANXIETY DISORDERS

Although there is a high degree of comorbidity between depression and anxiety disorders, a surprising paucity of research has explored the specific treatment of these conditions with rTMS. In regards to panic disorder, the research literature includes a number of case reports and several small randomized controlled trials. Two studies have utilized low-frequency stimulation applied to the right DLPFC. One small study was negative,[88] and a slightly larger study demonstrated a positive therapeutic benefit on panic disorder symptoms in patients with comorbid panic disorder and depression.[89]

Very limited research has also explored rTMS in generalized anxiety disorder (GAD). In an initial open-label study, 1 Hz stimulation was applied to the right DLPFC with the site determined by an fMRI activation scan.[90] Six out of ten patients met remission criteria for reduction in anxiety symptoms within this study. A significant benefit of active over sham stimulation was seen in a small randomized controlled trial of 1 Hz stimulation applied to the right DLPFC.[91] Of note, improvements in anxiety symptoms are commonly seen when depression is treated in patients with anxiety comorbidity, and these improvements in anxiety have been noted with both right, left, and bilateral forms of rTMS.[92] No studies other than case reports have explored the use of rTMS in social anxiety disorder other than case reports.[93,94]

In summary, insufficient evidence has explored the use of rTMS in anxiety disorders other than PTSD to make meaningful clinical recommendations.

14.7 DISORDERS OF ADDICTION

Disorders of addiction comprise a therapeutic area where, as with chronic pain, there has been a reasonably considerable body of research, but this is relatively shallow with a few studies in multiple addictive conditions and a relative absence of substantial large or definitive clinical trials. The main approach to treating disorders of addiction with TMS has been to apply high-frequency stimulation to the DLPFC to reduce craving, but it is also possible that stimulation of this area may enhance inhibitory control.[95] The literature includes multiple studies exploring the effects of single stimulation sessions on craving, but an increasing number of studies explore the repeated application of stimulation, most commonly exploring the potential use of TMS to decrease smoking or alcohol consumption. There is a considerably smaller number of trials investigating addiction to substances such as opiates, cocaine, and cannabis.[95]

In regards to smoking, this has been explored in at least 10 clinical trials to date, although most of these have been quite small. In the largest study, bilateral stimulation of the bilateral prefrontal cortices and insula resulted in a significant reduction in smoking-related variables when applied at high but not low frequency.[96] In a recent follow-up to this, the manufacturer of deep TMS coils, Brainsway, has completed a pivotal study of deep TMS in smoking cessation that has been used in a successful FDA application for licensing in the United States, although the clinical data supporting this application have not yet been published.

A growing number of studies explore the use of TMS in the treatment of alcohol dependence, although these have had somewhat mixed results. These have mostly targeted the right DLPFC, but studies have also delivered stimulation to the left DLPFC and the

TABLE 14.1 Status of applications of repetitive transcranial magnetic stimulation (rTMS) treatment

In widespread use	Increasing clinical use	Emerging clinical trial data	Pilot studies
Depression	Obsessive compulsive disorder	Posttraumatic stress disorder	Autism
	Smoking cessation	Schizophrenia: Negative symptoms	Mania
	Schizophrenia: Auditory hallucinations	Dementia/Alzheimer's disease	Other anxiety disorders

medial prefrontal cortex. High-frequency stimulation has been the most commonly utilized approach.[95]

In summary, across multiple approaches, emerging evidence suggests that prefrontal applications of rTMS may well be effective in modulating meaningful therapeutic outcomes in disorders of addiction. The recent demonstration of significant benefits of rTMS in smoking cessation resulting in FDA approval is likely to result in a significant escalation of interest in establishing more formally the role of rTMS in other addictive conditions.

14.8 CONCLUSION

Although depression is clearly the most well-established and intensively explored mental health condition for which rTMS may be useful, this chapter has explored a wide range of studies that have been conducted investigating its application in other conditions (see Table 14.1). Recent clinical approvals for the use of rTMS in the treatment of OCD and smoking cessation are likely to be followed by increasingly intense interest in the potential use of rTMS in other addictive disorders, especially chronic pain and PTSD.

REFERENCES

1. Lieberman JA, Stroup TS, McEvoy JP, Swartz MS, Rosenheck RA, Perkins DO, et al. Effectiveness of antipsychotic drugs in patients with chronic schizophrenia. *N Engl J Med*. 2005;353:1209–1223.
2. Andreasen NC, O'Leary DS, Flaum M, Nopoulos P, Watkins GL, Boles Ponto LL, et al. Hypofrontality in schizophrenia: Distributed dysfunctional circuits in neuroleptic-naive patients. *Lancet*. 1997;349:1730–1734.
3. Cohen E, Bernardo M, Masana J, Arrufat FJ, Navarro V, Valls S, et al. Repetitive transcranial magnetic stimulation in the treatment of chronic negative schizophrenia: A pilot study. *J Neurol Neurosurg Psychiatry*. 1999;67:129–130.
4. Shergill SS, Brammer MJ, Williams SC, Murray RM, McGuire PK. Mapping auditory hallucinations in schizophrenia using functional magnetic resonance imaging. *Arch Gen Psychiatry*. 2000;57:1033–1038.

5. Silbersweig DA, Stern E, Frith C, Cahill C, Holmes A, Grootoonk S, et al. A functional neuroanatomy of hallucinations in schizophrenia. *Nature.* 1995;378:176–179.

6. Hoffman RE, Boutros NN, Berman RM, Roessler E, Belger A, Krystal JH, et al. Transcranial magnetic stimulation of left temporoparietal cortex in three patients reporting hallucinated "voices." *Biol Psychiatry.* 1999;46:130–132.

7. Hoffman RE, Boutros NN, Hu S, Berman RM, Krystal JH, Charney DS. Transcranial magnetic stimulation and auditory hallucinations in schizophrenia. *Lancet.* 2000;355:1073–1075.

8. Geller V, Grisaru N, Abarbanel JM, Lemberg T, Belmaker RH. Slow magnetic stimulation of prefrontal cortex in depression and schizophrenia. *Prog Neuropsychopharmacol Biol Psychiatry.* 1997;21:105–110.

9. Feinsod M, Kreinin B, Chistyakov A, Klein E. Preliminary evidence for a beneficial effect of low-frequency, repetitive transcranial magnetic stimulation in patients with major depression and schizophrenia. *Depress Anxiety.* 1998;7:65–68.

10. Klein E, Kolsky Y, Puyerovsky M, Koren D, Chistyakov A, Feinsod M. Right prefrontal slow repetitive transcranial magnetic stimulation in schizophrenia: A double-blind sham-controlled pilot study. *Biol Psychiatry.* 1999;46:1451–1454.

11. Rollnik JD, Huber TJ, Mogk H, Siggelkow S, Kropp S, Dengler R, et al. High frequency repetitive transcranial magnetic stimulation (rTMS) of the dorsolateral prefrontal cortex in schizophrenic patients. *Neuroreport.* 2000;11:4013–4015.

12. Holi MM, Eronen M, Toivonen K, Toivonen P, Marttunen M, Naukkarinen H. Left prefrontal repetitive transcranial magnetic stimulation in schizophrenia. *Schizophr Bull.* 2004;30:429–434.

13. Sachdev P, Loo C, Mitchell P, Malhi G. Transcranial magnetic stimulation for the deficit syndrome of schizophrenia: A pilot investigation. *Psychiatry Clin Neurosci.* 2005;59:354–357.

14. Hajak G, Marienhagen J, Langguth B, Werner S, Binder H, Eichhammer P. High-frequency repetitive transcranial magnetic stimulation in schizophrenia: A combined treatment and neuroimaging study. *Psychol Med.* 2004;34:1157–1163.

15. Freitas C, Fregni F, Pascual-Leone A. Meta-analysis of the effects of repetitive transcranial magnetic stimulation (rTMS) on negative and positive symptoms in schizophrenia. *Schizophr Res.* 2009;108:11–24.

16. Mogg A, Purvis R, Eranti S, Contell F, Taylor JP, Nicholson T, et al. Repetitive transcranial magnetic stimulation for negative symptoms of schizophrenia: A randomized controlled pilot study. *Schizophr Res.* 2007;93:221–228.

17. Novak T, Horacek J, Mohr P, Kopecek M, Skrdlantova L, Klirova M, et al. The double-blind sham-controlled study of high-frequency rTMS (20 Hz) for negative symptoms in schizophrenia: Negative results. *Neuro Endocrinol Lett.* 2006;27:209–213.

18. Prikryl R, Kasparek T, Skotakova S, Ustohal L, Kucerova H, Ceskova E. Treatment of negative symptoms of schizophrenia using repetitive transcranial magnetic stimulation in a double-blind, randomized controlled study. *Schizophr Res.* 2007;95:151–157.

19. Jandl M, Bittner R, Sack A, Weber B, Gunther T, Pieschl D, et al. Changes in negative symptoms and EEG in schizophrenic patients after repetitive transcranial magnetic stimulation (rTMS): An open-label pilot study. *J Neural Transm.* 2005;112:955–967.

20. Goyal N, Nizamie SH, Desarkar P. Efficacy of adjuvant high frequency repetitive transcranial magnetic stimulation on negative and positive symptoms of schizophrenia: Preliminary results of a double-blind sham-controlled study. *J Neuropsychiatry Clin Neurosci.* 2007;19:464–467.

21. Jin Y, Potkin SG, Kemp AS, Huerta ST, Alva G, Thai TM, et al. Therapeutic effects of individualized alpha frequency transcranial magnetic stimulation (alphaTMS) on the negative symptoms of schizophrenia. *Schizophr Bull.* 2006;32:556–561.

22. Barr MS, Farzan F, Tran LC, Fitzgerald PB, Daskalakis ZJ. A randomized controlled trial of sequentially bilateral prefrontal cortex repetitive transcranial magnetic stimulation in the treatment of negative symptoms in schizophrenia. *Brain Stimul.* 2012;5:337–346.

23. Fitzgerald PB, Herring S, Hoy K, McQueen S, Segrave R, Kulkarni J, et al. A study of the effectiveness of bilateral transcranial magnetic stimulation in the treatment of the negative symptoms of schizophrenia. *Brain Stimul.* 2008;1:27–32.

24. Rabany L, Deutsch L, Levkovitz Y. Double-blind, randomized sham controlled study of deep-TMS add-on treatment for negative symptoms and cognitive deficits in schizophrenia. *J Psychopharmacol.* 2014;28:686–690.

25. Wobrock T, Guse B, Cordes J, Wolwer W, Winterer G, Gaebel W, et al. Left prefrontal high-frequency repetitive transcranial magnetic stimulation for the treatment of schizophrenia with predominant negative symptoms: A sham-controlled, randomized multicenter trial. *Biol Psychiatry.* 2015;77:979–988.

26. Quan WX, Zhu XL, Qiao H, Zhang WF, Tan SP, Zhou DF, et al. The effects of high-frequency repetitive transcranial magnetic stimulation (rTMS) on negative symptoms of schizophrenia and the follow-up study. *Neurosci Lett.* 2015;584:197–201.

27. Dlabac-de Lange JJ, Bais L, van Es FD, Visser BG, Reinink E, Bakker B, et al. Efficacy of bilateral repetitive transcranial magnetic stimulation for negative symptoms of schizophrenia: Results of a multicenter double-blind randomized controlled trial. *Psychol Med.* 2015;45:1263–1275.

28. Zhao S, Kong J, Li S, Tong Z, Yang C, Zhong H. Randomized controlled trial of four protocols of repetitive transcranial magnetic stimulation for treating the negative symptoms of schizophrenia. *Shanghai Arch Psychiatry.* 2014;26:15–21.

29. Aleman A, Enriquez-Geppert S, Knegtering H, Dlabac-de Lange JJ. Moderate effects of noninvasive brain stimulation of the frontal cortex for improving negative symptoms in schizophrenia: Meta-analysis of controlled trials. *Neurosci Biobehav Rev.* 2018;89:111–118.

30. Osoegawa C, Gomes JS, Grigolon RB, Brietzke E, Gadelha A, Lacerda ALT, et al. Non-invasive brain stimulation for negative symptoms in schizophrenia: An updated systematic review and meta-analysis. *Schizophr Res.* 2018;197:34–44.

31. Heinrichs RW. The primacy of cognition in schizophrenia. *Am Psychol.* 2005;60:229–242.

32. Barr MS, Farzan F, Rusjan PM, Chen R, Fitzgerald PB, Daskalakis ZJ. Potentiation of gamma oscillatory activity through repetitive transcranial magnetic stimulation of the dorsolateral prefrontal cortex. *Neuropsychopharmacology.* 2009;34:2359–2367.

33. Barr MS, Farzan F, Arenovich T, Chen R, Fitzgerald PB, Daskalakis ZJ. The effect of repetitive transcranial magnetic stimulation on gamma oscillatory activity in schizophrenia. *PLoS One.* 2011;6:e22627.

34. Voineskos AN, Blumberger DM, Schifani C, Hawco C, Dickie EW, Rajji TK, et al. Effects of repetitive transcranial magnetic stimulation on working memory performance and brain structure in people with schizophrenia spectrum disorders: A double-blind, randomized, sham-controlled trial. *Biol Psychiatry Cogn Neurosci Neuroimaging.* 2021;6:449–458.

35. Guse B, Falkai P, Gruber O, Whalley H, Gibson L, Hasan A, et al. The effect of long-term high frequency repetitive transcranial magnetic stimulation on working memory in schizophrenia and healthy controls: A randomized placebo-controlled, double-blind fMRI study. *Behav Brain Res.* 2013;237:300–307.

36. Mittrach M, Thunker J, Winterer G, Agelink MW, Regenbrecht G, Arends M, et al. The tolerability of rTMS treatment in schizophrenia with respect to cognitive function. *Pharmacopsychiatry.* 2010;43:110–117.

37. Zhuo K, Tang Y, Song Z, Wang Y, Wang J, Qian Z, et al. Repetitive transcranial magnetic stimulation as an adjunctive treatment for negative symptoms and cognitive impairment in patients with schizophrenia: A randomized, double-blind, sham-controlled trial. *Neuropsychiatr Dis Treat.* 2019;15:1141–1150.

38. Jiang Y, Guo Z, Xing G, He L, Peng H, Du F, et al. Effects of high-frequency transcranial magnetic stimulation for cognitive deficit in schizophrenia: A meta-analysis. *Front Psychiatry.* 2019;10:135.

39. Hoffman RE, Hawkins KA, Gueorguieva R, Boutros NN, Rachid F, Carroll K, et al. Transcranial magnetic stimulation of left temporoparietal cortex and medication-resistant auditory hallucinations. *Arch Gen Psychiatry.* 2003;60:49–56.

40. Hoffman RE, Gueorguieva R, Hawkins KA, Varanko M, Boutros NN, Wu YT, et al. Temporoparietal transcranial magnetic stimulation for auditory hallucinations: Safety, efficacy and moderators in a fifty patient sample. *Biol Psychiatry.* 2005;58:97–104.

41. Brunelin J, Poulet E, Bediou B, Kallel L, Dalery J, D'Amato T, et al. Low frequency repetitive transcranial magnetic stimulation improves source monitoring deficit in hallucinating patients with schizophrenia. *Schizophr Res.* 2006;81:41–45.

42. Chibbaro G, Daniele M, Alagona G, Di Pasquale C, Cannavo M, Rapisarda V, et al. Repetitive transcranial magnetic stimulation in schizophrenic patients reporting auditory hallucinations. *Neurosci Lett.* 2005;383:54–57.

43. d'Alfonso AA, Aleman A, Kessels RP, Schouten EA, Postma A, van Der Linden JA, et al. Transcranial magnetic stimulation of left auditory cortex in patients with schizophrenia: Effects on hallucinations and neurocognition. *J Neuropsychiatry Clin Neurosci.* 2002;14:77–79.

44. Fitzgerald PB, Benitez J, Daskalakis JZ, Brown TL, Marston NA, de Castella A, et al. A double-blind sham-controlled trial of repetitive transcranial magnetic stimulation in the treatment of refractory auditory hallucinations. *J Clin Psychopharmacol.* 2005;25:358–362.

45. Jandl M, Steyer J, Weber M, Linden DE, Rothmeier J, Maurer K, et al. Treating auditory hallucinations by transcranial magnetic stimulation: A randomized controlled cross-over trial. *Neuropsychobiology.* 2006;53:63–69.

46. McIntosh AM, Semple D, Tasker K, Harrison LK, Owens DG, Johnstone EC, et al. Transcranial magnetic stimulation for auditory hallucinations in schizophrenia. *Psychiatry Res.* 2004;127:9–17.

47. Poulet E, Brunelin J, Bediou B, Bation R, Forgeard L, Dalery J, et al. Slow transcranial magnetic stimulation can rapidly reduce resistant auditory hallucinations in schizophrenia. *Biol Psychiatry.* 2005;57:188–191.

48. Saba G, Schurhoff F, Leboyer M. Therapeutic and neurophysiologic aspects of transcranial magnetic stimulation in schizophrenia. *Neurophysiol Clin.* 2006;36:185–194.

49. Horacek J, Brunovsky M, Novak T, Skrdlantova L, Klirova M, Bubenikova-Valesova V, et al. Effect of low-frequency rTMS on electromagnetic tomography (LORETA) and regional brain metabolism (PET) in schizophrenia patients with auditory hallucinations. *Neuropsychobiology.* 2007;55:132–142.

50. Bagati D, Nizamie SH, Prakash R. Effect of augmentatory repetitive transcranial magnetic stimulation on auditory hallucinations in schizophrenia: Randomized controlled study. *Aust N Z J Psychiatry.* 2009;43:386–392.

51. Vercammen A, Knegtering H, Bruggeman R, Westenbroek HM, Jenner JA, Slooff CJ, et al. Effects of bilateral repetitive transcranial magnetic stimulation on treatment resistant auditory-verbal hallucinations in schizophrenia: A randomized controlled trial. *Schizophr Res.* 2009;114:172–179.

52. Rosa MO, Gattaz WF, Rosa MA, Rumi DO, Tavares H, Myczkowski M, et al. Effects of repetitive transcranial magnetic stimulation on auditory hallucinations refractory to clozapine. *J Clin Psychiatry.* 2007;68:1528–1532.

53. Slotema CW, Blom JD, van Lutterveld R, Hoek HW, Sommer IE. Review of the efficacy of transcranial magnetic stimulation for auditory verbal hallucinations. *Biol Psychiatry.* 2014;76:101–110.

54. Otani VH, Shiozawa P, Cordeiro Q, Uchida RR. A systematic review and meta-analysis of the use of repetitive transcranial magnetic stimulation for auditory hallucinations treatment in refractory schizophrenic patients. *Int J Psychiatry Clin Pract.* 2014:1–6.

55. Slotema CW, Blom JD, Hoek HW, Sommer IE. Should we expand the toolbox of psychiatric treatment methods to include repetitive transcranial magnetic stimulation (rTMS)? A meta-analysis of the efficacy of rTMS in psychiatric disorders. *J Clin Psychiatry.* 2010;71:873–884.

56. He H, Lu J, Yang L, Zheng J, Gao F, Zhai Y, et al. Repetitive transcranial magnetic stimulation for treating the symptoms of schizophrenia: A PRISMA compliant meta-analysis. *Clin Neurophysiol.* 2017;128:716–724.

57. Kennedy NI, Lee WH, Frangou S. Efficacy of non-invasive brain stimulation on the symptom dimensions of schizophrenia: A meta-analysis of randomized controlled trials. *Eur Psychiatry.* 2018;49:69–77.

58. de Weijer AD, Sommer IE, Lotte Meijering A, Bloemendaal M, Neggers SF, Daalman K, et al. High frequency rTMS: A more effective treatment for auditory verbal hallucinations? *Psychiatry Res.* 2014;224:204–210.

59. Kindler J, Homan P, Flury R, Strik W, Dierks T, Hubl D. Theta burst transcranial magnetic stimulation for the treatment of auditory verbal hallucinations: Results of a randomized controlled study. *Psychiatry Res.* 2013;209:114–117.

60. Schonfeldt-Lecuona C, Gron G, Walter H, Buchler N, Wunderlich A, Spitzer M, et al. Stereotaxic rTMS for the treatment of auditory hallucinations in schizophrenia. *Neuroreport.* 2004;15:1669–1673.

61. Sommer IE, de Weijer AD, Daalman K, Neggers SF, Somers M, Kahn RS, et al. Can fMRI-guidance improve the efficacy of rTMS treatment for auditory verbal hallucinations? *Schizophr Res.* 2007;93:406–408.

62. Grisaru N, Chudakov B, Yaroslavsky Y, Belmaker RH. Transcranial magnetic stimulation in mania: A controlled study. *Am J Psychiatry.* 1998;155:1608–1610.

63. Michael N, Erfurth A. Treatment of bipolar mania with right prefrontal rapid transcranial magnetic stimulation. *J Affect Disord.* 2004;78:253–257.

64. Saba G, Rocamora JF, Kalalou K, Benadhira R, Plaze M, Lipski H, et al. Repetitive transcranial magnetic stimulation as an add-on therapy in the treatment of mania: A case series of eight patients. *Psychiatry Res.* 2004;128:199–202.

65. Kaptsan A, Yaroslavsky Y, Applebaum J, Belmaker RH, Grisaru N. Right prefrontal TMS versus sham treatment of mania: A controlled study. *Bipolar Disord.* 2003;5:36–39.

66. Praharaj SK, Ram D, Arora M. Efficacy of high frequency (rapid) suprathreshold repetitive transcranial magnetic stimulation of right prefrontal cortex in bipolar mania: A randomized sham controlled study. *J Affect Disord.* 2009;117:146–150.

67. Greenberg BD, Martin JD, Cora-Locatelli G, Wassermann EM, Benjamin J, Grafman J, et al. Effects of single treatment with rTMS at different brain sites in depression. *Electroencephalogr Clin Neurophysiol.* 1997;103:A77.

68. Sachdev PS, Loo CK, Mitchell PB, McFarquhar TF, Malhi GS. Repetitive transcranial magnetic stimulation for the treatment of obsessive compulsive disorder: A double-blind controlled investigation. *Psychol Med.* 2007;37:1645–1649.

69. Sarkhel S, Sinha VK, Praharaj SK. Adjunctive high-frequency right prefrontal repetitive transcranial magnetic stimulation (rTMS) was not effective in obsessive-compulsive disorder but improved secondary depression. *J Anxiety Disord.* 2010;24:535–539.

70. Ma X, Huang Y, Liao L, Jin Y. A randomized double-blinded sham-controlled trial of alpha electroencephalogram-guided transcranial magnetic stimulation for obsessive-compulsive disorder. *Chin Med J (Engl).* 2014;127:601–606.

71. Alonso P, Pujol J, Cardoner N, Benlloch L, Deus J, Menchon JM, et al. Right prefrontal repetitive transcranial magnetic stimulation in obsessive-compulsive disorder: A double-blind, placebo-controlled study. *Am J Psychiatry.* 2001;158:1143–1145.

72. Prasko J, Paskova B, Zalesky R, Novak T, Kopecek M, Bares M, et al. The effect of repetitive transcranial magnetic stimulation (rTMS) on symptoms in obsessive compulsive disorder. A randomized, double blind, sham controlled study. *Neuro Endocrinol Lett.* 2006;27:327–332.

73. Mantovani A, Lisanby SH, Pieraccini F, Ulivelli M, Castrogiovanni P, Rossi S. Repetitive transcranial magnetic stimulation (rTMS) in the treatment of obsessive-compulsive disorder (OCD) and Tourette's syndrome (TS). *Int J Neuropsychopharmacol.* 2006;9:95–100.

74. Mantovani A, Simpson HB, Fallon BA, Rossi S, Lisanby SH. Randomized sham-controlled trial of repetitive transcranial magnetic stimulation in treatment-resistant obsessive-compulsive disorder. *Int J Neuropsychopharmacol.* 2010;13:217–227.

75. Ruffini C, Locatelli M, Lucca A, Benedetti F, Insacco C, Smeraldi E. Augmentation effect of repetitive transcranial magnetic stimulation over the orbitofrontal cortex in drug-resistant obsessive-compulsive disorder patients: A controlled investigation. *Prim Care Companion J Clin Psychiatry.* 2009;11:226–230.

76. Nauczyciel C, Le Jeune F, Naudet F, Douabin S, Esquevin A, Verin M, et al. Repetitive transcranial magnetic stimulation over the orbitofrontal cortex for obsessive-compulsive disorder: A double-blind, cross-over study. *Transl Psychiatry.* 2014;4:e436.

77. Carmi L, Tendler A, Bystritsky A, Hollander E, Blumberger DM, Daskalakis J, et al. Efficacy and safety of deep transcranial magnetic stimulation for obsessive-compulsive disorder: A prospective multicenter randomized double-blind placebo-controlled trial. *Am J Psychiatry.* 2019;176:931–938.

78. Grisaru N, Amir M, Cohen H, Kaplan Z. Effect of transcranial magnetic stimulation in posttraumatic stress disorder: A preliminary study. *Biol Psychiatry.* 1998;44:52–55.

79. Rosenberg PB, Mehndiratta RB, Mehndiratta YP, Wamer A, Rosse RB, Balish M. Repetitive transcranial magnetic stimulation treatment of comorbid posttraumatic stress disorder and major depression. *J Neuropsychiatry Clin Neurosci.* 2002;14:270–276.

80. Cohen H, Kaplan Z, Kotler M, Kouperman I, Moisa R, Grisaru N. Repetitive transcranial magnetic stimulation of the right dorsolateral prefrontal cortex in posttraumatic stress disorder: A double-blind, placebo-controlled study. *Am J Psychiatry.* 2004;161:515–524.

81. Boggio PS, Rocha M, Oliveira MO, Fecteau S, Cohen RB, Campanha C, et al. Noninvasive brain stimulation with high-frequency and low-intensity repetitive transcranial magnetic stimulation treatment for posttraumatic stress disorder. *J Clin Psychiatry*. 2010;71:992–999.

82. Watts BV, Landon B, Groft A, Young-Xu Y. A sham controlled study of repetitive transcranial magnetic stimulation for posttraumatic stress disorder. *Brain Stimul*. 2012;5:38–43.

83. Kan RLD, Zhang BBB, Zhang JJQ, Kranz GS. Non-invasive brain stimulation for posttraumatic stress disorder: A systematic review and meta-analysis. *Transl Psychiatry*. 2020;10:168.

84. Philip NS, Barredo J, Aiken E, Larson V, Jones RN, Shea MT, et al. Theta-burst transcranial magnetic stimulation for posttraumatic stress disorder. *Am J Psychiatry*. 2019;176:939–948.

85. Isserles M, Shalev AY, Roth Y, Peri T, Kutz I, Zlotnick E, et al. Effectiveness of deep transcranial magnetic stimulation combined with a brief exposure procedure in post-traumatic stress disorder--a pilot study. *Brain Stimul*. 2013;6:377–383.

86. Isserles M, Tendler A, Roth Y, Bystritsky A, Blumberger DM, Ward H, et al. Deep transcranial magnetic stimulation combined with brief exposure for posttraumatic stress disorder: A prospective multisite randomized trial. *Biol Psychiatry*. 2021;90(10):721–728.

87. Kozel FA, Motes MA, Didehbani N, DeLaRosa B, Bass C, Schraufnagel CD, et al. Repetitive TMS to augment cognitive processing therapy in combat veterans of recent conflicts with PTSD: A randomized clinical trial. *J Affect Disord*. 2018;229:506–514.

88. Prasko J, Zalesky R, Bares M, Horacek J, Kopecek M, Novak T, et al. The effect of repetitive transcranial magnetic stimulation (rTMS) add on serotonin reuptake inhibitors in patients with panic disorder: A randomized, double blind sham controlled study. *Neuro Endocrinol Lett*. 2007;28:33–38.

89. Mantovani A, Aly M, Dagan Y, Allart A, Lisanby SH. Randomized sham controlled trial of repetitive transcranial magnetic stimulation to the dorsolateral prefrontal cortex for the treatment of panic disorder with comorbid major depression. *J Affect Disord*. 2013;144:153–159.

90. Bystritsky A, Kaplan JT, Feusner JD, Kerwin LE, Wadekar M, Burock M, et al. A preliminary study of fMRI-guided rTMS in the treatment of generalized anxiety disorder. *J Clin Psychiatry*. 2008;69:1092–1098.

91. Diefenbach GJ, Bragdon LB, Zertuche L, Hyatt CJ, Hallion LS, Tolin DF, et al. Repetitive transcranial magnetic stimulation for generalised anxiety disorder: A pilot randomised, double-blind, sham-controlled trial. *Br J Psychiatry*. 2016;209:222–228.

92. Chen L, Hudaib AR, Hoy KE, Fitzgerald PB. Is rTMS effective for anxiety symptoms in major depressive disorder? An efficacy analysis comparing left-sided high-frequency, right-sided low-frequency, and sequential bilateral rTMS protocols. *Depress Anxiety*. 2019;36:723–731.

93. Paes F, Machado S, Arias-Carrion O, Silva AC, Nardi AE. rTMS to treat social anxiety disorder: A case report. *Rev Bras Psiquiatr*. 2013;35:99–100.

94. Paes F, Baczynski T, Novaes F, Marinho T, Arias-Carrion O, Budde H, et al. Repetitive transcranial magnetic stimulation (rTMS) to treat social anxiety disorder: Case reports and a review of the literature. *Clin Pract Epidemiol Ment Health*. 2013;9:180–188.

95. Hanlon CA, Dowdle LT, Henderson JS. Modulating neural circuits with transcranial magnetic stimulation: Implications for addiction treatment development. *Pharmacol Rev*. 2018;70:661–683.

96. Dinur-Klein L, Dannon P, Hadar A, Rosenberg O, Roth Y, Kotler M, et al. Smoking cessation induced by deep repetitive transcranial magnetic stimulation of the prefrontal and insular cortices: A prospective, randomized controlled trial. *Biol Psychiatry*. 2014;76:742–749.

Safety Considerations and Management of TMS Side Effects

15.1 INTRODUCTION

Following the pioneering research and early proof-of-principle studies uncovering the therapeutic potential of transcranial magnetic stimulation (TMS), researchers and clinicians were faced with numerous ethical and safety considerations. The transition from using TMS as an investigational device to implementing lengthy and repetitive protocols (i.e., rTMS) led to a growing concern regarding the long-term effects of this intervention. While several studies investigated the safety of rTMS,[1,2] the field remained apprehensive, with one letter published in *the Lancet* entitled "Shocking Safety Concerns."[3] In 1996, several leaders in the field met to detail the potential risks and establish procedural standards and guidelines for the safe use of TMS.[4]

The decades following this early consensus conference saw a growth in the interest and widespread implementation of TMS in research and rTMS clinical settings, leading to the approval by regulatory agencies in several countries. Continued research during this time also led to numerous methodological advancements, from modified device features to novel stimulation paradigms, all of which were known to impact the safety profile of TMS. As such, the safety guidelines developed in 1998 were reviewed in a consensus conference 10 years later. While many of the initial guidelines remained, the updated guidelines focused on reducing potential risks by limiting the train durations, combination of frequencies, and intensities of current rTMS protocols.[5] Once again, a decade following this publication, key researchers and clinicians in the field met to review and update the 2009 guidelines. This new guideline aimed to focus on novel issues associated with the expansion of the clinical application of TMS, technological advancements, and the implementation of cross-modality research.[6] Drawing primarily from these three key guidelines, this chapter focuses on the safety concerns and potential side effects of TMS, as well as on strategies to mitigate and manage risks.

15.2 SAFETY CONSIDERATIONS

15.2.1 Implanted Devices and Nonremovable Metal

15.2.1.1 Implanted Electrodes

Additional safety precautions must be taken for individuals who have electrodes implanted within the central or peripheral nervous system. Implanted electrodes can include deep brain electrodes, epidural or subdural electrodes, peripheral or cranial nerve stimulating electrodes, and cardiac pacemakers. Numerous studies have investigated the effects of single, paired, and repetitive TMS in those with implanted devises, assessing the effects on the TMS evoked responses and electroencephalogram (EEG) activity.[5]

In general, studies conducted both ex vivo and in vivo have found that TMS can be safely administered using the figure-of-eight coil in individuals with implanted electrodes or devices, provided the coil is not located in close proximity (i.e., <10 cm) to an internal pulse generator (IPG) system or other electronic components (i.e., leads and loops) in the neck or chest.[6] While studies have not reported adverse effects specifically in these individuals, TMS administered close to the implanted wires connecting the electrodes with the IPG have been shown to induce currents between the device components, leading to unintended motor responses.[7,8] Therefore, if possible, it is recommended to turn off the IPG system during TMS and avoid lead loops in implanted devices to reduce the potential of electromagnetic induction. Furthermore, TMS should initially be administered at a low intensity with gradual increases in intensity as a precaution in these cases.

15.2.1.2 Heating

While heating produced in the brain by TMS is considered to be negligible (>0.1°C),[9] TMS may heat implanted electrodes and devices via induced currents.[10] The potential for such heating depends on a number of factors, including the TMS parameters (i.e., coil, configuration, and protocol) and the conductivity of the device and surrounding tissue, as well as the shape, size, and placement of the implant. The material is another important factor; for example, electrodes composed of gold or silver are highly conductive and therefore are at an increased risk of heating, leading to potential skin burns.[11] In contrast, low-conductivity plastic electrodes, electrodes or plates with radial slits, and implanted titanium plates or rods are less likely to heat up.[10,12] Ex vivo studies have shown that rTMS administered over implantable electrodes[13,14] and vascular stents[15] does not significantly heat these objects and is therefore considered safe. In spite of these findings, extra caution should be taken when TMS is administered to those with implanted devices or nonremovable metal.

15.2.1.3 Forces and Magnetization

The magnetic field generated by TMS can exert forces on ferromagnetic and conductive materials, thus posing a risk for the displacement of implanted electrodes. However, studies have shown that implanted objects made from titanium, including rods, clips, and plates, are not significantly impacted by TMS forces.[10,12,16] Similarly, ex vivo[13,14] and modeling studies[17] suggest that the risk of movement of implanted electrodes caused by TMS is minimal. Implants that contain magnets (e.g., cochlear implants) are at an increased risk of movement or demagnetization with TMS, and TMS has traditionally been considered unsafe in these cases.[5] However, a recent study found that a new generation of cochlear implants remained intact and fully functional during focal TMS stimulation when the intensity was equal or below 2.2 Tesla (T). The induced forces exerted on the implant were negligible, even when stimulation parameters exceeded current safety guidelines.[18] Thus, those with new-generation cochlear implants may be permitted to receive TMS treatment under certain parameters; however, continued research is needed. Additional research is also needed regarding the use of TMS in individuals with permanent makeup and scalp tattoos, which may contain ferromagnetic particles. It is recommended that, when possible, objects worn on the head that could contain ferromagnetic and conductive materials, including jewelry, glasses, hearing aids, and some forms of make-up, be removed prior to stimulation.

15.2.1.4 Induced Electrical Current

As mentioned, the TMS coil can induce high voltages and currents in devices and wires when in close proximity to one another, leading to unintended stimulation and outcomes.[7,8] This can occur even when the device is turned off. Studies investigating deep brain and cortical implants have demonstrated relatively high voltages of currents induced between the electrode or lead and IPG of these devices, thus posing a safety risk.[13,14,19] The current induction depends on a number of factors including the proximity of stimulation and lead. The largest current induction occurs when the center of the coil is placed directly over the lead and the current orientation of the coil is aligned with the lead or when the coil loops and the loops of the electrode lead are centered over one another.[14,19] This may result in exceeding the maximum charge density stipulated by the device manufacturer,[13,14] and additional care must be taken. One approach to minimize the potential for inductive loops is to group and twist external leads together and orient them as far from the coil as possible. Additionally, when possible, electronically isolate the amplifier input or external stimulator output from the ground.[6]

This section highlights the risks and safety considerations associated with implanted devices and nonremovable metal implants. To ensure the safety of the patient, risk analyses should be conducted on a case-by-case basis.

15.2.2 Combining TMS with Other Devices

TMS combined with other neurophysiological and neuroimaging modalities is known to improve targeting accuracy and clinical efficacy.[20–22] However, combining different modalities and devices poses a unique set of safety concerns. TMS with magnetic resonance imaging (MRI), for example, is most often assessed "offline," whereby TMS is delivered before and after the MRI, outside of the scanner room. This approach does not result in any additional safety concerns beyond those of any standard TMS protocol. However, recent technological advances have allowed for the interleaved combination of TMS and MRI, which requires MR-approved TMS coils. These coils and any other TMS equipment cannot contain ferromagnetic material and must be able to withstand the mechanic stress associated with the static magnetic field of the MR scanner.[5] To ensure the integrity of the coil over time, as a precaution, MR-approved TMS coils are only able to deliver a certain number of pulses.

TMS is also commonly combined with transcranial electric stimulation (TES; e.g., transcranial direct current stimulation [tDCS]/transcranial alternating current stimulation [tACS]) as a means to prime and enhance the neurophysiological effects of either protocol.[23] Similar to TMS-MRI, these protocols can be applied simultaneously or consecutively. To date studies have assessed TMS-TES, including single-pulse TMS and theta burst stimulation (TBS) in healthy individuals,[24–27] as well as a few studies in clinical populations.[28,29] While current studies are limited both in number and sample size and were not designed primarily to assess safety, no serious adverse effects have been reported, and only one study reported an adverse effect of scalp pain.[29] While there is a proposed risk of heating or magnetically induced currents associated with the TES electrodes, current evidence suggests that combined TMS-TES is safe.[6]

15.3 POTENTIAL ADVERSE EFFECTS

15.3.1 Seizures

While rare, TMS-induced seizures have been reported, with the majority occurring prior to the development of the safety guidelines. Seizures result from an inhibitory/excitatory imbalance leading to hypersynchronized discharges of large groups of neurons. Seizures can present as a loss of consciousness, unresponsiveness, tonus (muscle stiffness), clonus (repetitive involuntary movement), loss of bowel or bladder control, and postictal disorientation.

In an attempt to characterize the incidence of seizures among TMS protocols, Lerner et al. gathered data from more than 100 TMS researchers and clinicians and 300,000 TMS sessions. Overall, 24 seizures were reported (standardized risk: 7/100,000 sessions), 19 of which occurred in individuals with a heightened risk of seizures due to medical or other reasons. Furthermore, 16 TMS-related seizures occurring in more than 200,000 sessions (standardized risk of 8/100,000 sessions) in high- and low-risk individuals were observed during single, paired (13), and low-frequency stimulation (3) (≤1 Hz). Regarding rTMS at frequencies higher than 1 Hz, eight seizures have been reported, including one associated with intermittent TBS (iTBS) (standardized risk: 7/100,000 sessions). Of note, one of the risks identified in this report was a lack of previous TMS exposure, as more than 75% occurred within the first three sessions. For more details regarding the specific risks of TMS protocols see Lerner et al.[30]

In addition to lack of exposure, a number of factors are known to lower the seizure threshold and therefore increase the risk of inducing a seizure during TMS. For example, an elevated risk of seizure has been reported in a number of disorders in addition to epilepsy, including patients with neurodegenerative diseases and acquired brain injury.[6] Furthermore, few studies report an elevated risk in several psychiatric disorders, including depression and bipolar disorder,[31,32] autism,[33] and substance abuse.[34] Beyond these disorders, a number of known medical conditions and medications (reviewed in Section 15.5.1.3) may increase the risk of TMS-induced seizures.[6] Finally, several general factors which have been suggested to trigger seizures in those with epilepsy and that may therefore be applicable in TMS include but are not limited to sleep deprivation, anxiety and stress, and increased alcohol use.[35–37] As such, additional precautions must be considered when administering TMS to individuals who present with these risk factors.

15.3.2 Syncope

Vasodepressor syncope can often be misinterpreted as a seizure in those who present with certain features, including myoclonic jerks, tonic stiffening, and oral and motor automatisms, among others. One key distinguishing feature of syncope versus seizures is rapid recovery (i.e., within seconds) of consciousness in the absence of confusion or disorientation and without loss of pulse or breathing.[38] Additionally, tongue-biting, incontinence, and oral frothing are more common in seizures than syncope. Regardless of the presence of a seizures or syncope, TMS should be terminated and medical attention should be summoned.[5]

15.3.3 Hearing

Although reports vary, the estimated acoustic artifact generated from the TMS pulse is reported to be around 140 dB sound pressure level (SPL),[39] a volume that surpasses recommended safety levels (US Occupational Safety and Health Administration-OSHA). The sound level experienced by the study participant depends on a number of factors including the number of frequency of pulses, the stimulus intensity, the coil type and site of stimulation, and, importantly, the use of hearing protection.[6,40] A few studies have shown that a small subset of adults experienced transient modification in hearing sensitivity,[41] which may be minimized with the use of hearing protection.[42,43] Additionally, there is a reportedly low risk of aggravating preexisting auditory symptoms.[44]

As such, the TMS safety guidelines[6] have outlined a number of recommendations and considerations including that (1) participants and TMS operators should use well-fitted and approved hearing protection; (2) any individuals experiencing hearing loss, tinnitus, or aural fullness following TMS should be referred for an auditory assessment; (3) TMS should only be administered to those with preexisting noise-induced hearing loss or concurrent treatment with ototoxic medications (aminoglycosides, cisplatin) if the risk-benefit ratio is favorable; (4) caution should be taken when administering TMS to the affected auditory cortex in patients treated for tinnitus (or even auditory hallucinations) with hyperacusis; (5) although limited data currently exist, single-pulse and paired-pulse TMS appear to be safe in children 2 years and older with appropriate hearing protection; (6) TMS should not be given to those with cochlear implants (though a recent cochlear implant may be safe, see Section 15.2.1); and (7) it is important to consider the sound levels of TMS to be potentially hazardous to hearing without the use of hearing protection.

15.3.4 Local Pain and Headaches

The most common side effect to TMS is pain, and, as such, individuals should be advised that stimulation may be uncomfortable. It is reported that in active rTMS, around 28% of patients with depression experienced headaches and 39% experienced pain or discomfort, while sham stimulation was associated with rates of 16% and 15%, respectively.[45] Neck pain is also commonly experienced, due in large part to the posture and head immobilization required during rTMS.[46] While discomfort may occur, very few individuals (i.e., 2%) discontinue treatment because of it, and pain usually subsides quickly.[5] If headaches persist following treatment, acetaminophen, ibuprofen, or other nonsteroidal anti-inflammatory agents may be recommended. Of note, rTMS was not shown to induce migraines in healthy controls or in those who sought treatment for chronic migraines.[47]

In an attempt to minimize pain experienced during TMS, researchers have investigated the use of topical anesthetics, injection of 1% lidocaine, and the use of air-filled foam pads. Results showed that lidocaine was the most successful in reducing pain intensity (50%), followed by the foam pad (7%).[48] A more practical approach to reducing pain includes applying a ramping-up algorithm, whereby the intensity of stimulation is started below target dose and gradually increased over the first few treatments.

15.3.5 Cognitive Changes

With respect to cognition, TMS has been shown to both impair or enhance functioning, as indexed by reaction times and error rates or signal detection measures. For example, rTMS administered over the Wernicke's or Broca's area elicits inhibition and facilitation of language, respectively.[49] Similarly, rTMS applied to the parietal[50] and prefrontal regions improved reaction time and action naming,[51] respectively. The effects are generally modest and temporary and, as such, do not pose as a significant safety concern.

When TMS is applied in clinical settings, especially in targeting the dorsolateral prefrontal cortex (DLPFC), the potential cognitive effects are often difficult to differentiate from the clinical improvements. While recent reviews highlight the potential of rTMS in depression and other neuropsychiatric disorders to improve cognitive functioning, the presence of numerous negative findings suggest that the pro-cognitive effects of TMS are not robust.[52–54] While there is significant heterogeneity within studies, a lack of long-term follow-up, and a paucity of research specifically focusing on cognitive safety, it appears that TMS is not associated with any significant, lasting cognitive adverse outcomes in healthy individuals.[5]

15.3.6 Acute Psychiatric Changes

There are a few reported cases of treatment-emergent mania in patients with uni- and bipolar depression following left prefrontal low- or high-frequency rTMS. With 13 cases reported across 53 randomized control studies, the rate TMS-emergent mania was found to be 0.84% for the active rTMS group and 0.73% for the sham group; thus, results did not significantly differ between groups. Of note, most of the rTMS protocols were within the safety guidelines and the majority of these cases were bipolar patients taking medication during the course of rTMS.[55] With the advent of iTBS for depression, there have been several reports of mania induced in bipolar depressed patients treated with iTBS of the left DLPFC.[56,57]

In addition to mania, transient psychotic symptoms, anxiety, agitation, suicidal ideation, and insomnia have been reported during rTMS treatments[42,58]; however, the causal relationship is not known and the rate at which these symptoms occurred may be comparable to that of the natural course of the disease.[5] Importantly, significant changes in mood are not reported in healthy individuals undergoing rTMS.[59] It is recommended that patients receiving rTMS should be aware of the potential yet unlikely outcome of developing such acute psychiatric side effects.[5]

15.4 SAFETY GUIDELINES

The safety guidelines first outlined in 1998 and more recently updated following the 2009 and 2019 consensus conferences stipulate that the use of TMS for research or clinical applications must follow three key ethical principles: (1) informed consent, (2) expected benefits must outweigh the risks, and (3) there must be an equal distribution of the expected burdens and potential benefits of the research.[5] Building on these basic requirements and the available research at the time, Wassermann et al. developed a safety table with respect to specific frequencies and intensities for the appropriate use of rTMS.[4] While these guidelines drew from limited research conducted in healthy participants, employing only a figure-of-eight coil and conventional rTMS protocols, they have been fairly successful in preventing seizures and ensuring the safe use of TMS over the years. Importantly, despite the development and implementation of numerous novel TMS protocols and parameters, the rate of adverse events remains low and thus TMS appears to be relatively safe regardless of the protocol.

15.4.1 Conventional rTMS

The 2009 guidelines, following early research by Chen at el., built on the original safety tables to include not only safe parameters for motor rTMS at each frequency and stimulus intensity, but also included guidelines for safe intertrain intervals and the maximum duration of pulses per rTMS trains at each intensity. The guidelines were also modified to reduce the maximum stimulus intensity from 220% to 130%, given available research. Consensus was also reached regarding situations in which motor threshold cannot be determined, whereby the intensity used should be that of the lower 95% confidence interval of the average threshold associated with the specific population, coil, and device. Finally, it was recommended that investigators follow the safety guidelines conservatively, especially in the case of Class 2 (indirect benefit, moderate risk) and Class 3 (indirect benefit, low risk) studies. Class 1 studies associated with a direct benefit but higher degree of risk may consider employing parameters that exceed these recommendations if the anticipated clinical benefits outweigh the expected risks.[5]

Conventional rTMS protocols applied outside of the motor cortex are generally considered safe. This may be due in part to the fact that the motor cortex is considered the most epileptogenic cortical brain region,[60] and the original safety guidelines were based on motor cortical evidence. While more research specifically investigating the safety of nonmotor rTMS is needed, several reviews have investigated various nonmotor rTMS parameters in the absence of serious adverse events.[45,46]

While no recent study has directly examined the safety profiles of different combinations of TMS parameters, the development of novel protocols employing new stimulation parameters and locations, treatment schedules, equipment, etc. continues to grow. Importantly, the reported occurrence of seizures and other serious adverse effects remain consistently low, suggesting that, regardless of the chosen protocol, rTMS can be considered fairly safe.[6] Thus, the original safety guidelines outlined in 2009 appear to remain effective in preventing seizures. The most recent 2021 guidelines have instead included operational guidelines and suggest that the potential combination of intensity, frequency, and duration of conventional rTMS remains below the current stimulation parameters used for magnetic seizure therapy (MST) (i.e., 100% of maximal stimulator output, frequency of 25 Hz, delivered in a single train lasting up to 10 seconds).[6] Additionally, several recommendations are outlined for clinical trials in which the combination of stimulation parameters exceeds the 2009 guidelines. In summary, these include balancing the risk-benefit ratio, employing neurophysiological monitoring, reconsidering the study protocol if a seizure occurs, and reporting safety findings to the scientific community.[6]

15.4.2 Patterned rTMS

The use of alternative rTMS protocols including quadripulse (QPS) and TBS have become increasingly popular over the past several years. Quadripulse stimulation uses monophasic magnetic/electric pulses to induce long-term potentiation/depression in the brain.[61,62] Since its development, QPS has been studied in both healthy and clinical populations. In these studies, including those that used stimulation parameters that were outside the originally reported protocol,[62] no adverse effects were reported.[63] As such, the most recent TMS safety guidelines reported that QPS using a figure-of-eight coil in normal participants is considered safe and outlined guidelines for this protocol.[6]

Similarly, studies employing TBS have used fairly consistent parameters first described in Huang et al. (i.e., 50 Hz bursts of 3 pulses repeated at 5 Hz; 80% active motor threshold).[64] However, intensities have ranged from 80% to 100% of the motor threshold, with the exception of studies using 110% intensity in alcohol and cocaine users[65] and using 120% in patients with depression.[66] Of note, a few studies have reported the induction of seizures in healthy individuals, one of which occurred following standard conventional TBS parameters.[67-69] Despite these incidences, recent studies on the use of TBS in clinical populations and in adolescents did not report any seizures.[70,71] Given these findings, the most recent safety guidelines concluded that TBS using standard parameters is safe.[6] Beyond this, future research should continue to investigate the safety of novel patterned TMS protocols, including safe guidelines regarding the intervals between TBS sessions and the cumulative use of TBS with respect to accelerated protocols.

15.5 MITIGATING AND MANAGING RISKS

15.5.1 Important Patient Considerations

15.5.1.1 Contraindications and Patient Screening

A number of known factors are contraindications for TMS/rTMS or may enhance the risk of adverse effects. Therefore, clinicians and investigators should consider using a screening questionnaire (e.g., TMS Adult Safety Screen [TASS]) when informed consent is obtained. In addition to screening questionnaires, a more extensive pre-TMS evaluation may be warranted, including a medical examination, an evaluation of current medications to rule out the presence of seizure threshold-lowering medications (see Section 14.5.1.3), screening for substance use disorders, and pregnancy testing.

The only absolute contraindication to TMS/rTMS is presence of a metallic hardware component in close contact to the TMS coil (such as cochlear implants, an internal pulse generator, or medication pumps). In such instances there is a risk of inducing malfunctions in these implanted devices.[6] Caution is advised when using paradigms and parameters that have not been studied extensively, as well as with protocols that go beyond the safety tables listed in the current guidelines.[6] In general, a history of seizure disorder is a relative contraindication.

15.5.1.2 Treatment and Testing in Special Populations

Pediatrics. Certain technical challenges and added ethical issues[72] must be considered when administering TMS in children. Additionally, numerous neurological changes underlying the development process likely impact the risk and potential long-term effects of TMS-related adverse events. For example, enhanced cortical excitability, higher resting thresholds and therefore stimulation intensities, and the ongoing maturation of the external auditory canal in children, especially neonates, represent some of the factors that may impact TMS safety. Thus, nontherapeutic research in children should only be conducted using a protocol that has been deemed safe in adults.[5]

In spite of these potential concerns and challenges, there are a growing number of physiological and clinical studies conducted in healthy children and those with neurodevelopmental and motor disorders.[73,74] The majority of these studies employed single- or paired-pulse paradigms although some studies have used rTMS and TBS.[71,75] Importantly, these studies reported minimal to no side effects. Thus, single- and paired-pulse paradigms appear to be relatively safe in children 2 years and older with appropriate hearing protection[6]; however, continued research is needed.

Pregnancy. Due in part to the potential risk to the fetus associated with the use of pharmacological interventions in pregnancy, noninvasive brain stimulation may be considered an alternative intervention. Drawing from computerized modeling research, studies suggest that the E-field generated from standard rTMS (i.e., figure-of-eight coil to the DLPFC, ≥60 cm from the uterus)[76] and single-pulse TMS applied to the occiput in pregnant patients with migraines[77] are well below the safety threshold.[78]

The risk of seizure in the mother represents an important potential complication. Current research, including high-frequency, low-frequency, and bilateral DLPFC stimulation for depression and other conditions during pregnancy, reports fairly high rates of clinical improvement (around 58% taken together) and mild, transient adverse effects.[79-82] Of note, there was one report of supine hypotension syndrome, as well as concentration difficulty and anxiety. Taken together, the rate of adverse effects among the 12 available studies in pregnancy for left, right, and bilateral rTMS were 11% (4/36), 50% (6/12), and 0% (0/2), respectively. There has also been a case report of iTBS in a depressed pregnant woman.[83] Therefore, it appears that single-, paired-pulse TMS, and rTMS likely pose minimal risk for the mother and fetus.[6] However, continued investigation on the long-term effects on the child, as well as the use of alternative protocols and coils, is needed.

Therapeutic and Nontherapeutic Research. Conducting research in vulnerable populations, including children, pregnant women, prisoners, and those who are unable to give informed consent, presents a unique set of safety, ethical, and legal considerations. As one important ethical implication of including populations who are unable to give consent, additional effort must be made to ensure that the participant understands the risks and benefits, if possible, including the use of consent partners. Regarding potential safety issues in vulnerable populations, the risk of seizure may be enhanced in certain groups (i.e., those with substance or medication use or traumatic brain injury). Therefore, investigators must consider the risks associated with continuing, modifying, or discontinuing certain medications for research purposes. It should be noted that, in general, these individuals should not be excluded from research on this basis alone, but that certain legal or medical regulations may be in place and must be consulted prior to participation. As with any safety consideration, the potential benefits of including vulnerable populations in research must outweigh the risks of not treating or using an alternative treatment.[6]

15.5.1.3 Concurrent Medication Use

Given that some of the rTMS-induced seizures observed in early research occurred in individuals who were on medications known to lower the seizure threshold, it was assumed that those receiving rTMS who also were taking certain drugs would be at heightened risk for seizure induction. As such, a list of potentially hazardous medications was reported in Rossi et al.[5] This list included imipramine, chlorpromazine, clozapine, amphetamines, cocaine, phencyclidine, ketamine, gamma-hydroxybutyrate, alcohol, and theophylline. The potential hazards of withdrawal of several drugs was also noted, including alcohol, barbiturates, benzodiazepines, meprobamate, and chloral hydrate. For a more complete list of strong or relatively hazardous drugs, see Rossi et al.[5]

However, since the publication of the 2009 guidelines and the administration of TMS in thousands of patients likely taking one of more of these medications, there does not appear to be evidence for a significantly enhanced risk of seizure induction in patients taking the listed medications.[6] While this does not completely rule out the potential for a seizure in those taking these medications, it is more likely that this risk may be related to additional factors including the drug dose and speed of increase or withdrawal, sleep deprivation, and alcohol and cannabis use.[5] Therefore, the recommendations set out by the updated guidelines suggest that while empirical evidence may not provide support for an enhanced risk due to certain medications, rTMS providers should continue to report the presence of any factors, including medications, which may lower seizure threshold.[6] Continued investigation is required as novel TMS protocols and equipment becomes available.

15.5.2 Additional Testing and Treatment Considerations

15.5.2.1 Monitoring During Testing

Physiological Monitoring. Physiological monitoring, via EEG or electromyogram (EMG) measures, is recommended especially when the rTMS protocol exceeds the recommended safety guidelines.[4] Early signs of seizure activity may be observed as a spread of activation across neighboring cortical regions and the presence of EEG discharges after stimulation has ceased. While EEG monitoring may provide a reliable and logical measure of rTMS effects, the rare occurrence of TMS-induced epileptiform activity and lack of predictive value of epileptiform activity with regards to seizure induction suggest that routine EEG monitoring may not significantly enhance rTMS safety.[5] EMG monitoring may also provide a measure of rTMS effects whereby the presence of motor-evoked potentials (MEPs) when they are not expected to be elicited by rTMS or MEPs elicited in neighboring muscles may indicate the spread of cortical excitation beyond the motor cortex. Finally, visual monitoring of the participant or patient during stimulation is always necessary.

Neuropsychological Monitoring. Self-reports and objective neurophysiological measures detect subtle changes in cognitive functioning although rTMS does not appear to cause any significant long-term cognitive effects (refer to Chapter 6). Like physiological monitoring, this is especially important when novel parameters or protocols for which cognitive safety profiles are not well known are employed. The appropriate cognitive battery should be selected based on the potential effects and site of stimulation.[5]

15.5.2.2 TMS Settings

The setting in which TMS is being administered, whether for research or clinical purposes, represents an important safety consideration. Setting requirements are based on the application and class of study as well as the specific rules set out by institutional review boards (IRB). According to current guidelines,[6,84] for research applications (i.e., Class 3 studies of indirect benefit, low risk and Class 2 studies of indirect benefit, moderate risk, in healthy individuals), single-, paired-, and repetitive TMS may not need to be conducted in a medical setting unless the rTMS parameters exceed current safety limits. All relevant information regarding the potential risks, risk-benefit ratio, and the roles of the study personnel responsible for the delivery of TMS, as well as the level of medical supervision required, should be outlined in the study protocol.[6] Given the potential for adverse effects, the principal investigator should receive input and ongoing support from a medically responsible physician who is familiar with the protocol if they are not a licensed physician. Whether the physician is required to be on site during the administration of TMS/rTMS depends on the anticipated risks associated with the protocol of interest and is to be determined by the investigators and IRB.[5]

With respect to clinical applications (i.e., Class 1 studies of direct benefit, potential high risk and Class 2 studies in patients for diagnostic and therapeutic purposes), single-, paired-, and repetitive TMS are required to be administered in a medical setting. Decisions regarding prescribing TMS for therapeutic use in clinical and psychiatric disorders and obtaining informed consent are the responsibility of an adequately trained physician. TMS may be administered by the physician or by an adequately trained technician under a physician's supervision.[6] Medical settings include hospitals and outpatient clinics equipped with the necessary life-support equipment, emergency medical protocols, and facilities.[5]

15.5.2.3 Training for TMS Providers

Training among TMS providers, either in a research or clinical setting, is an important step toward minimizing the risks associated with unsafe practices and potentially less effective clinical outcomes. Additionally, training ensures a measure of quality control, reliability, and validity of TMS practices. As such, the International Federation of Clinical Neurophysiology (IFNC) committee came together to outline a consensus training guideline.[84] This guideline provides specific definitions and core competencies required for (1) technicians (i.e., those who administer TMS, monitor the participant/patient during stimulation, and may collect outcome assessments), (2) clinicians (i.e., those who determine the indication, prescription, and protocol and who supervise the technician), and (3) scientists (i.e., those investigators responsible for the overall study protocol and who may administer TMS or supervise the technician). For a detailed description of the roles and responsibilities of each group see Fried et al.[84]

While the training protocol across different labs, clinics, or institutions should be individualized to suit their needs, all training programs should combine didactic learning, hands-on training, and supervised practice. Furthermore, training should cover topics including basic knowledge and theoretical aspects of brain stimulation, key safety and ethical concepts, and skills competencies including device operations, coil handling, and motor threshold assessments.[84] Finally, training protocols should consider implementing a structured final evaluation to formally assess and document that the training requirements have been met by each trainee.

15.6 MANAGING EMERGENCIES

While each TMS lab or clinic may have its own safety and emergency medical protocols, there are a number of universally accepted steps for managing adverse events. All TMS providers should be familiar with the institution's protocols and be aware of how and when to activate emergency medical services. While a detailed description of medical procedures is beyond the scope of this chapter, important steps taken to manage syncope and seizures are briefly reviewed. TMS should be stopped immediately if syncope or seizure is suspected and emergency medical support activated. In the case of syncope, the individual may be placed in a supine position on the floor with their legs elevated. Regarding suspected seizures, following emergency medical activation, the medical team should take steps to protect the individual's airway and prevent potential injury due to motor convulsions or falls. If tonic-clonic seizure activity does not occur, the individual may be turned onto their side to avoid aspiration. The medical team is responsible for performing the appropriate assessments to determine the differential diagnosis (i.e., syncope vs. seizure vs. other), potential etiology, and care plan. In a research setting, the participant should be withdrawn from the study unless medically cleared, and the event should be reported to the IRB and sponsors, if applicable. Finally, medical and psychological support should be provided to those who experience a TMS-induced seizure or serious adverse event.

15.7 CONCLUSION

Taken together, the evidence presented in this chapter and gathered over the past several decades has demonstrated that, in general, TMS is safe and the risk of seizures is relatively low. However, one can expect an enhanced level of risk if TMS parameters exceed the values outlined in current safety guidelines.[6] Given the rapid growth in the field of TMS and continual development of novel protocols, devices, and applications, the ethical and safety regulations must continue to evolve. As such, clinicians and researchers using TMS have a duty to understand current risks, be prepared for potential unknown risks, and document and report to the scientific community any findings relating to safety. Furthermore, future research should prioritize investigating the safety of TMS, with a focus on larger and more diverse samples and long-term follow-ups.

REFERENCES

1. Pascual-Leone A, Houser CM, Reese K, Shotland LI, Grafman J, Sato S, et al. Safety of rapid-rate transcranial magnetic stimulation in normal volunteers. *Electroencephalogr Clin Neurophysiol.* 1993;89(2):120–130.
2. Hufnagel A, Claus D, Brunhoelzl C, Sudhop T. Short-term memory: No evidence of effect of rapid-repetitive transcranial magnetic stimulation in healthy individuals. *J Neurol.* 1993;240(6):373–376.
3. Brown P. Shocking safety concerns. *Lancet.* 1996;348(9032):959.
4. Wassermann EM. Risk and safety of repetitive transcranial magnetic stimulation: Report and suggested guidelines from the International Workshop on the Safety of Repetitive Transcranial Magnetic Stimulation, June 5–7, 1996. *Electroencephalogr Clin Neurophysiol.* 1998;108(1):1–16.
5. Rossi S, Hallett M, Rossini PM, Pascual-Leone A. Safety of TMSCG. Safety, ethical considerations, and application guidelines for the use of transcranial magnetic stimulation in clinical practice and research. *Clin Neurophysiol.* 2009;120(12):2008–2039.
6. Rossi S, Antal A, Bestmann S, Bikson M, Brewer C, Brockmoller J, et al. Safety and recommendations for TMS use in healthy subjects and patient populations, with updates on training, ethical and regulatory issues: Expert Guidelines. *Clin Neurophysiol.* 2021;132(1):269–306.
7. Hidding U, Baumer T, Siebner HR, Demiralay C, Buhmann C, Weyh T, et al. MEP latency shift after implantation of deep brain stimulation systems in the subthalamic nucleus in patients with advanced Parkinson's disease. *Movem Dis.* 2006;21(9):1471–1476.
8. Kuhn AA, Trottenberg T, Kupsch A, Meyer BU. Pseudo-bilateral hand motor responses evoked by transcranial magnetic stimulation in patients with deep brain stimulators. *Clin Neurophysiol.* 2002;113(3):341–345.
9. Brix G, Seebass M, Hellwig G, Griebel J. Estimation of heat transfer and temperature rise in partial-body regions during MR procedures: An analytical approach with respect to safety considerations. *Magn Reson Imaging.* 2002;20(1):65–76.
10. Rotenberg A, Harrington MG, Birnbaum DS, Madsen JR, Glass IE, Jensen FE, et al. Minimal heating of titanium skull plates during 1Hz repetitive transcranial magnetic stimulation. *Clin Neurophysiol.* 2007;118(11):2536–2538.

11. Roth BJ, Pascual-Leone A, Cohen LG, Hallett M. The heating of metal electrodes during rapid-rate magnetic stimulation: A possible safety hazard. *Electroencephalogr Clin Neurophysiol.* 1992;85(2):116–123.

12. Petrosyan HA, Alessi V, Sniffen J, Sisto SA, Fiore S, Davis R, et al. Safety of titanium rods used for spinal stabilization during repetitive magnetic stimulation. *Clin Neurophysiol.* 2015;126(12):2405–2406.

13. Phielipp NM, Saha U, Sankar T, Yugeta A, Chen R. Safety of repetitive transcranial magnetic stimulation in patients with implanted cortical electrodes. An ex-vivo study and report of a case. *Clin Neurophysiol.* 2017;128(6):1109–1115.

14. Shimojima Y, Morita H, Nishikawa N, Kodaira M, Hashimoto T, Ikeda S. The safety of transcranial magnetic stimulation with deep brain stimulation instruments. *Parkinsonism Relat Disord.* 2010;16(2):127–131.

15. Varnerin N, Mirando D, Potter-Baker KA, Cardenas J, Cunningham DA, Sankarasubramanian V, et al. Assessment of Vascular Stent Heating with Repetitive Transcranial Magnetic Stimulation. *J Stroke Cerebrovasc Dis.* 2017;26(5):1121–1127.

16. Pridmore S, Lawson F. Transcranial magnetic stimulation and movement of aneurysm clips. *Brain Stimul.* 2017;10(6):1139–1140.

17. Golestanirad L, Rouhani H, Elahi B, Shahim K, Chen R, Mosig JR, et al. Combined use of transcranial magnetic stimulation and metal electrode implants: A theoretical assessment of safety considerations. *Phys Med Biol.* 2012;57(23):7813–7827.

18. Mandala M, Baldi TL, Neri F, Mencarelli L, Romanella S, Ulivelli M, et al. Feasibility of TMS in patients with new generation cochlear implants. *Clin Neurophysiol.* 2021;132(3):723–729.

19. Deng ZD, Lisanby SH, Peterchev AV. Transcranial magnetic stimulation in the presence of deep brain stimulation implants: Induced electrode currents. *Annu Int Conf IEEE Eng Med Biol Soc.* 2010;2010:6821–6824.

20. Fitzgerald PB, Hoy K, McQueen S, Maller JJ, Herring S, Segrave R, et al. A randomized trial of rTMS targeted with MRI based neuro-navigation in treatment-resistant depression. *Neuropsychopharmacology.* 2009;34(5):1255–1262.

21. Fox MD, Liu H, Pascual-Leone A. Identification of reproducible individualized targets for treatment of depression with TMS based on intrinsic connectivity. *NeuroImage.* 2013;66:151–160.

22. Sack AT, Cohen Kadosh R, Schuhmann T, Moerel M, Walsh V, Goebel R. Optimizing functional accuracy of TMS in cognitive studies: A comparison of methods. *J Cogn Neurosci.* 2009;21(2):207–221.

23. Karabanov A, Ziemann U, Hamada M, George MS, Quartarone A, Classen J, et al. Consensus paper: Probing homeostatic plasticity of human cortex with non-invasive transcranial brain stimulation. *Brain Stimul.* 2015;8(3):442–454.

24. Bocci T, Vannini B, Torzini A, Mazzatenta A, Vergari M, Cogiamanian F, et al. Cathodal transcutaneous spinal direct current stimulation (tsDCS) improves motor unit recruitment in healthy subjects. *Neurosci Lett.* 2014;578:75–79.

25. Cosentino G, Fierro B, Paladino P, Talamanca S, Vigneri S, Palermo A, et al. Transcranial direct current stimulation preconditioning modulates the effect of high-frequency repetitive transcranial magnetic stimulation in the human motor cortex. *Eur J Neurosci.* 2012;35(1):119–124.

26. Doeltgen SH, McAllister SM, Ridding MC. Simultaneous application of slow-oscillation transcranial direct current stimulation and theta burst stimulation prolongs continuous theta burst stimulation-induced suppression of corticomotor excitability in humans. *Euro J Neurosc.* 2012;36(5):2661–2668.

27. Guerra A, Suppa A, Bologna M, D'Onofrio V, Bianchini E, Brown P, et al. Boosting the LTP-like plasticity effect of intermittent theta-burst stimulation using gamma transcranial alternating current stimulation. *Brain Stimul.* 2018;11(4):734–842.

28. Antal A, Lang N, Boros K, Nitsche M, Siebner HR, Paulus W. Homeostatic metaplasticity of the motor cortex is altered during headache-free intervals in migraine with aura. *Cerebral Cortex.* 2008;18(11):2701–2705.

29. Loo C, Martin D, Pigot M, Arul-Anandam P, Mitchell P, Sachdev P. Transcranial direct current stimulation priming of therapeutic repetitive transcranial magnetic stimulation: A pilot study. *J ECT.* 2009;25(4):256–260.

30. Lerner AJ, Wassermann EM, Tamir DI. Seizures from transcranial magnetic stimulation 2012-2016: Results of a survey of active laboratories and clinics. *Clin Neurophysiol.* 2019;130(8):1409–1416.

31. Hesdorffer DC, Ishihara L, Mynepalli L, Webb DJ, Weil J, Hauser WA. Epilepsy, suicidality, and psychiatric disorders: A bidirectional association. *Ann Neurol.* 2012;72(2):184–191.

32. Sucksdorff D, Brown AS, Chudal R, Jokiranta-Olkoniemi E, Leivonen S, Suominen A, et al. Parental and comorbid epilepsy in persons with bipolar disorder. *J Affect Dis.* 2015;188:107–111.

33. Bolton PF, Carcani-Rathwell I, Hutton J, Goode S, Howlin P, Rutter M. Epilepsy in autism: Features and correlates. *Br J Psychiatry.* 2011;198(4):289–294.

34. Samokhvalov AV, Irving H, Mohapatra S, Rehm J. Alcohol consumption, unprovoked seizures, and epilepsy: A systematic review and meta-analysis. *Epilepsia.* 2010;51(7):1177–1184.

35. Balamurugan E, Aggarwal M, Lamba A, Dang N, Tripathi M. Perceived trigger factors of seizures in persons with epilepsy. *Seizure.* 2013;22(9):743–747.

36. Haut SR, Hall CB, Masur J, Lipton RB. Seizure occurrence: Precipitants and prediction. *Neurology.* 2007;69(20):1905–1910.

37. Wassenaar M, Kasteleijn-Nolst Trenite DG, de Haan GJ, Carpay JA, Leijten FS. Seizure precipitants in a community-based epilepsy cohort. *J Neurol.* 2014;261(4):717–724.

38. McKeon A, Vaughan C, Delanty N. Seizure versus syncope. *Lancet Neurol.* 2006;5(2):171–180.

39. Counter SA, Borg E. Analysis of the coil generated impulse noise in extracranial magnetic stimulation. *Electroencephalogr Clin Neurophysiol.* 1992;85(4):280–288.

40. Dhamne SC, Kothare RS, Yu C, Hsieh TH, Anastasio EM, Oberman L, et al. A measure of acoustic noise generated from transcranial magnetic stimulation coils. *Brain Stimul.* 2014;7(3):432–434.

41. Loo C, Sachdev P, Elsayed H, McDarmont B, Mitchell P, Wilkinson M, et al. Effects of a 2- to 4-week course of repetitive transcranial magnetic stimulation (rTMS) on neuropsychologic functioning, electroencephalogram, and auditory threshold in depressed patients. *Biol Psychiatry.* 2001;49(7):615–623.

42. Janicak PG, O'Reardon JP, Sampson SM, Husain MM, Lisanby SH, Rado JT, et al. Transcranial magnetic stimulation in the treatment of major depressive disorder: A comprehensive summary of safety experience from acute exposure, extended exposure, and during reintroduction treatment. *J Clin Psychiatry.* 2008;69(2):222–232.

43. O'Reardon JP, Solvason HB, Janicak PG, Sampson S, Isenberg KE, Nahas Z, et al. Efficacy and safety of transcranial magnetic stimulation in the acute treatment of major depression: A multisite randomized controlled trial. *Biol Psychiatry.* 2007;62(11):1208–1216.

44. Muller PA, Pascual-Leone A, Rotenberg A. Safety and tolerability of repetitive transcranial magnetic stimulation in patients with pathologic positive sensory phenomena: A review of literature. *Brain Stimul.* 2012;5(3):320–329 e27.

45. Loo CK, McFarquhar TF, Mitchell PB. A review of the safety of repetitive transcranial magnetic stimulation as a clinical treatment for depression. *Int J Neuropsychopharmacol.* 2008;11(1):131–147.

46. Machii K, Cohen D, Ramos-Estebanez C, Pascual-Leone A. Safety of rTMS to non-motor cortical areas in healthy participants and patients. *Clin Neurophysiol.* 2006;117(2):455–471.

47. Brighina F, Piazza A, Vitello G, Aloisio A, Palermo A, Daniele O, et al. rTMS of the prefrontal cortex in the treatment of chronic migraine: A pilot study. *J Neurol Sci.* 2004;227(1):67–71.

48. Borckardt JJ, Smith AR, Hutcheson K, Johnson K, Nahas Z, Anderson B, et al. Reducing pain and unpleasantness during repetitive transcranial magnetic stimulation. *J ECT.* 2006;22(4):259–264.

49. Drager B, Breitenstein C, Helmke U, Kamping S, Knecht S. Specific and nonspecific effects of transcranial magnetic stimulation on picture-word verification. *Eur J Neurosci.* 2004;20(6):1681–1687.

50. Luber B, Kinnunen LH, Rakitin BC, Ellsasser R, Stern Y, Lisanby SH. Facilitation of performance in a working memory task with rTMS stimulation of the precuneus: Frequency- and time-dependent effects. *Brain Res.* 2007;1128(1):120–129.

51. Cappa SF, Sandrini M, Rossini PM, Sosta K, Miniussi C. The role of the left frontal lobe in action naming: RTMS evidence. *Neurology.* 2002;59(5):720–723.

52. Iimori T, Nakajima S, Miyazaki T, Tarumi R, Ogyu K, Wada M, et al. Effectiveness of the prefrontal repetitive transcranial magnetic stimulation on cognitive profiles in depression, schizophrenia, and Alzheimer's disease: A systematic review. *Prog Neuro-Psychopharmacol Biol Psychiatry.* 2019;88:31–40.

53. McClintock SM, Kallioniemi E, Martin DM, Kim JU, Weisenbach SL, Abbott CC. A Critical review and synthesis of clinical and neurocognitive effects of noninvasive neuromodulation antidepressant therapies. *Focus (Am Psychiatr Publ)*. 2019;17(1):18–29.

54. Serafini G, Pompili M, Belvederi Murri M, Respino M, Ghio L, Girardi P, et al. The effects of repetitive transcranial magnetic stimulation on cognitive performance in treatment-resistant depression: A systematic review. *Neuropsychobiology*. 2015;71(3):125–139.

55. Xia G, Gajwani P, Muzina DJ, Kemp DE, Gao K, Ganocy SJ, et al. Treatment-emergent mania in unipolar and bipolar depression: Focus on repetitive transcranial magnetic stimulation. *Int J Neuropsychopharmacol*. 2008;11(1):119–130.

56. McGirr A, Vila-Rodriguez F, Cole J, Torres IJ, Arumugham SS, Keramatian K, et al. Efficacy of active vs sham intermittent theta burst transcranial magnetic stimulation for patients with bipolar depression: A randomized clinical trial. *JAMA Netw Open*. 2021;4(3):e210963.

57. Kaster TS, Knyahnytska Y, Noda Y, Downar J, Daskalakis ZJ, Blumberger DM. Treatment-emergent mania with psychosis in bipolar depression with left intermittent theta-burst rTMS. *Brain Stimul*. 2020;13(3):705–706.

58. Zwanzger P, Ella R, Keck ME, Rupprecht R, Padberg F. Occurrence of delusions during repetitive transcranial magnetic stimulation (rTMS) in major depression. *Biol Psychiatry*. 2002;51(7):602–603.

59. Grossheinrich N, Rau A, Pogarell O, Hennig-Fast K, Reinl M, Karch S, et al. Theta burst stimulation of the prefrontal cortex: Safety and impact on cognition, mood, and resting electroencephalogram. *Biol Psychiatry*. 2009;65(9):778–784.

60. Penfield W, Jasper H. *Epilepsy and the Functional Anatomy of the Human Brain*. Boston, MA: Little, Brown; 1954.

61. Hamada M, Ugawa Y. Quadripulse stimulation: A new patterned rTMS. *Restor Neurol Neurosci*. 2010;28(4):419–424.

62. Hamada M, Terao Y, Hanajima R, Shirota Y, Nakatani-Enomoto S, Furubayashi T, et al. Bidirectional long-term motor cortical plasticity and metaplasticity induced by quadripulse transcranial magnetic stimulation. *J Physiol*. 2008;586(16):3927–3947.

63. Matsumoto H, Ugawa Y. Quadripulse stimulation (QPS). *Exp Brain Res*. 2020;238(7–8):1619–1625.

64. Huang YZ, Edwards MJ, Rounis E, Bhatia KP, Rothwell JC. Theta burst stimulation of the human motor cortex. *Neuron*. 2005;45(2):201–206.

65. Hanlon CA, Dowdle LT, Correia B, Mithoefer O, Kearney-Ramos T, Lench D, et al. Left frontal pole theta burst stimulation decreases orbitofrontal and insula activity in cocaine users and alcohol users. *Drug Alcohol Depend*. 2017;178:310–317.

66. Blumberger DM, Vila-Rodriguez F, Thorpe KE, Feffer K, Noda Y, Giacobbe P, et al. Effectiveness of theta burst versus high-frequency repetitive transcranial magnetic stimulation in patients with depression (THREE-D): A randomised non-inferiority trial. *Lancet*. 2018;391(10131):1683–1692.

67. Lenoir C, Algoet M, Mouraux A. Deep continuous theta burst stimulation of the operculo-insular cortex selectively affects A delta-fibre heat pain. *J Physiology*. 2018;596(19):4767–4787.

68. Lenoir C, Algoet M, Vanderclausen C, Peeters A, Santos SF, Mouraux A. Report of one confirmed generalized seizure and one suspected partial seizure induced by deep continuous theta burst stimulation of the right operculo-insular cortex. *Brain Stimul*. 2018;11(5):1187–1188.

69. Oberman LM, Pascual-Leone A. Report of seizure induced by continuous theta burst stimulation. *Brain Stimul*. 2009;2(4):246–247.

70. Rachid F. Safety and efficacy of theta-burst stimulation in the treatment of psychiatric disorders: A review of the literature. *J Nerv Ment Dis*. 2017;205(11):823–839.

71. Hong YH, Wu SW, Pedapati EV, Horn PS, Huddleston DA, Laue CS, et al. Safety and tolerability of theta burst stimulation vs. single and paired pulse transcranial magnetic stimulation: A comparative study of 165 pediatric subjects. *Front Hum Neurosci*. 2015;9:29.

72. Hameed MQ, Dhamne SC, Gersner R, Kaye HL, Oberman LM, Pascual-Leone A, et al. Transcranial magnetic and direct current stimulation in children. *Curr Neurol Neurosci Rep*. 2017;17(2):11.

73. Gilbert DL, Huddleston DA, Wu SW, Pedapati EV, Horn PS, Hirabayashi K, et al. Motor cortex inhibition and modulation in children with ADHD. *Neurology*. 2019;93(6):e599–e610.

74. Oberman LM, Pascual-Leone A, Rotenberg A. Modulation of corticospinal excitability by transcranial magnetic stimulation in children and adolescents with autism spectrum disorder. *Front Hum Neurosci.* 2014;8:627.

75. Zewdie E, Ciechanski P, Kuo HC, Giuffre A, Kahl C, King R, et al. Safety and tolerability of transcranial magnetic and direct current stimulation in children: Prospective single center evidence from 3.5 million stimulations. *Brain Stimul.* 2020;13(3):565–575.

76. Yanamadala J, Borwankar R, Makarov S, Pascual-Leone A. Estimates of Peak electric fields induced by transcranial magnetic stimulation in pregnant women as patients or operators using an FEM full-body model. In Makarov S, Horner M, Noetscher G, eds. *Brain and Human Body Modeling: Computational Human Modeling at EMBC* 2018. Cham (CH); 2019: 49–73.

77. Dodick DW, Schembri CT, Helmuth M, Aurora SK. Transcranial magnetic stimulation for migraine: A safety review. *Headache.* 2010;50(7):1153–1163.

78. McRobbie D. Concerning guidelines for limiting exposure to time-varying electric, magnetic, and electromagnetic fields (1 Hz-100 kHz). *Health Phys.* 2011;100(4):442; author reply

79. Burton C, Gill S, Clarke P, Galletly C. Maintaining remission of depression with repetitive transcranial magnetic stimulation during pregnancy: A case report. *Arch Womens Ment Health.* 2014;17(3):247–250.

80. Ferrao YA, da Silva RMF. Repetitive transcranial magnetic stimulation for the treatment of major depression during pregnancy. *Braz J Psychiatry.* 2018;40(2):227–228.

81. Gahr M, Blacha C, Connemann BJ, Freudenmann RW, Schonfeldt-Lecuona C. Successful treatment of major depression with electroconvulsive therapy in a pregnant patient with previous non-response to prefrontal rTMS. *Pharmacopsychiatry.* 2012;45(2):79–80.

82. Hizli Sayar G, Ozten E, Tufan E, Cerit C, Kagan G, Dilbaz N, et al. Transcranial magnetic stimulation during pregnancy. *Arch Womens Ment Health.* 2014;17(4):311–315.

83. Trevizol AP, Vigod SN, Daskalakis ZJ, Vila-Rodriguez F, Downar J, Blumberger DM. Intermittent theta burst stimulation for major depression during pregnancy. *Brain Stimul.* 2019;12(3):772–774.

84. Fried PJ, Santarnecchi E, Antal A, Bartres-Faz D, Bestmann S, Carpenter LL, et al. Training in the practice of noninvasive brain stimulation: Recommendations from an IFCN committee. *Clin Neurophysiol.* 2021;132(3):819–837.

Index

Figures and tables are indicated by *f* and *t* following the page number.